M. Joyce. 215 Cleveland
Tower, Holloway Head
Biham.

Immediate and
Replacement Dentures

To Mary and Mary

Immediate and Replacement Dentures

JOHN N. ANDERSON

M.D.S., L.D.S. (Sheffield)

Professor of Dental Prosthetics, University of Dundee. Consultant in Dental Prosthetics, Eastern Regional Hospital Board, Scotland. External Examiner in Dental Prosthetics, Universities of Bristol and Liverpool. Formerly External Examiner in the University of Birmingham and The Royal College of Surgeons in Ireland. Author of Applied Dental Materials

AND

ROY STORER

M.Sc., F.D.S.R.C.S.

Professor of Prosthodontics, University of Newcastle upon Tyne. Consultant Dental Surgeon, Newcastle Regional Hospital Board. External Examiner in Dental Prosthetics, University of Birmingham and The Royal College of Surgeons of England. Formerly Visiting Associate Professor, Northwestern University Dental School, Chicago. Formerly External Examiner in Dental Subjects, Universities of Newcastle upon Tyne, Dundee and Bristol, Queen's University, Belfast and Trinity College, Dublin.

SECOND EDITION

BLACKWELL SCIENTIFIC PUBLICATIONS

OXFORD LONDON EDINBURGH MELBOURNE

© 1966, 1973 Blackwell Scientific Publications
Osney Mead, Oxford,
3 Nottingham Street, London W1,
9 Forrest Road, Edinburgh,
P.O. Box 9, North Balwyn, Victoria, Australia.

ISBN 0 632 09560 1

First published 1966
Second edition 1973

Printed and bound in Great Britain by
W & J Mackay Limited, Chatham.

Contents

Foreword to First Edition

During the last decade or two the pattern of prosthetic treatment has changed. From the days when it was normal procedure to extract all the remaining teeth and leave the patient 'sans teeth, sans everything' for many months, we have progressed to a more logical sequence of transition from natural to artificial occlusion. When a patient is destined to become edentulous, progression from partial dentures to immediate complete dentures is now considered normal practice. The first part of this book clarifies many of the problems that may be encountered in the provision of immediate complete dentures.

Many textbooks on complete denture prosthetics take, as their starting point, the hypothetical patient who arrives at the dentist edentulous, never apparently, having had any dentures previously, and with the alveolar ridges well-formed, smooth and healthy. In reality, most edentulous patents arrive with immediate dentures requiring modification, or with old dentures in need of replacement. More often than not, the mucosal supporting tissues have been abused by the dentures and their condition is far from the textbook ideal.

In this book, the authors have faced these problems realistically and have dealt with the complete denture problem as one of denture replacement. There is no doubt that a need exists for more knowledge to be disseminated about such denture service. Any prosthetic consultant will confirm that a high percentage of his patients are referred with problems that have arisen following the provision of new dentures after the patient had been a successful denture wearer for many years.

This book fills a gap in prosthetic literature—and does it well.

1966   JOHN OSBORNE *Birmingham*

Preface to Second Edition

This is a textbook for undergraduates and practitioners on the complete denture phase of dental treatment. Unlike all other textbooks on the subject it deals with the transition from the partially edentulous to the edentulous state, via the immediate denture; then follows the maintenance and replacement of these dentures when this becomes necessary. This is the normal linear progression of treatment in modern dental practice.

In a practical subject such as dental prosthetics, knowledge cannot be gained from theory alone and it is assumed that practical tuition and experience will accompany the reading of this text. Therefore, precise details of technique have generally been omitted and their place taken by reasoned comparisons of ideas and techniques. As in many disciplines, the important thing is not the method but the knowledge which lies behind it.

In recent years the emphasis in dentistry has moved from a concentration on technical procedures to one of appreciation of the part that a dentist plays in providing a health service for the patient. Dentures must be designed so as to maintain the residual tissues in the best possible state of health.

On looking retrospectively at the first edition, we are aware (as we were at the time of writing) of the difficulties imposed in writing a book which followed the normal treatment pattern of immediate dentures followed by replacement dentures. There was inevitably some duplication of content and subdivision of some arguments. In this second edition, the general principles applicable both to immediate and replacement dentures have been dealt with separately.

JOHN N ANDERSON, Dundee
ROY STORER, Newcastle upon Tyne

1973

Acknowledgements

Interest, advice and encouragement are invaluable during the preparation of any book and the authors are most grateful to their many professional colleagues who have helped in any way.

To Mr P. R. H. Brown, Mr M. R. Y. Dyer, Mr J. A. Hobkirk, Mr F. F. Lyon, Dr J. W. McCrorie, Mr D. R. McMillan, Dr T. H. Melville, Mr J. Murgatroyd, Mr H. E. Simpson, Mr D. C. Williamson and Mr A. W. Wolland, we express our thanks for their specialist advice. We are particularly indebted to Professor Niels Brill for his comments on Chapter 7 and to Mr W. M. Oliver for help with Chapter 3. Several other colleagues have read the manuscript and have offered comments on various chapters.

The photographs in the book are the work of Mr David Chalmers, Mr Brian Hill and Mr Melford Paisley.

The typing of the manuscript has been in the capable hands of Mrs M. High and Mrs O. McKevitt. Our thanks are also due to our wives for assistance in typing, proof reading and indexing.

To all our friends and colleagues we are grateful for their competent and willing help.

We wish to thank Professor A. O. Mack for the loan of the photographs used for Fig. 20.12, Blackwell Scientific Publications for permission to use the block for Fig. 22.11, an illustration from the late Dr U. Posselt's book The Physiology of Occlusion and Rehabilitation, and the Editor of the British Dental Journal for permission to use the blocks for Figs 3.1, 17.7, 18.1 and 21.10.

Section One
General Principles

Chapter 1

Limitations of Complete Dentures

As dental health education and dental care improve throughout the world, more people wish to save their teeth and only part with them in small numbers when disease processes have gone too far despite regular dental care. Many consider that the loss of the natural dentition carries with it a social stigma, and every effort is made to repair and maintain the natural teeth. But there are still some patients who look forward to the removal of all their natural teeth as the end to their dental troubles.

WHY NOT COMPLETE DENTURES?

It has often been suggested that dentistry could consist of two procedures: the extraction of natural teeth and their replacement by complete dentures. Why not remove everyone's natural teeth and provide them with complete dentures since these can be acceptable for appearance and also be made to a high degree of technical perfection? It may be argued by some that their natural teeth are ugly and could well be improved by replacing them with artificial substitutes. At times, this is undoubtedly true. But dental beauty is difficult to define; what is acceptable to one person may offend the aesthetic sense of another.

Other people would like to lose their teeth because they have had frequent pain, and because of the discomfort and inconvenience of prolonged dental treatment which they feel can only be relieved permanently by multiple extractions. Whilst this may have been true some years ago, modern methods of cavity preparation and techniques of anaesthesia make this a much less powerful argument today. Tooth substance is cut rapidly and efficiently by the use of high rotational speeds, thus reducing the treatment time necessary. Improvements in local anaesthetics ensure adequate blockage of any painful stimuli during cavity preparation. For the very nervous or handicapped patient, a general anaesthetic may be used for restorative procedures. Thus there is less discomfort in dental treatment today and it is not necessarily as prolonged as it used to be.

A strong argument against the removal of the natural teeth can be put when treating patients up to the age of 21. Teeth, and tooth function, contribute to the growth of the face and jaws and therefore must be retained until this growth is completed. But why not remove all teeth at this age and replace them with complete dentures? First because of appearance, and secondly because dentures do not necessarily restore good oral function for the remainder of the patient's life.

APPEARANCE

The natural teeth and their supporting bone make an important contribution to the contours of the face. Without them, there is a typical appearance of premature senility which is seen often in edentulous patients. Whilst dentures may restore some of the support there are limitations to what can be achieved. Some change in facial appearance is inevitable after the extraction of teeth, as bone is lost from areas where the facial contour cannot be restored by a denture. For example, loss of bone at the base of the nose cannot be restored adequately by a prosthesis. In addition, there is often a loss of tonus of the facial musculature due to the limitation on muscle movements imposed by a denture. This loss of tone is followed by increased skin wrinkling and folding.

The aesthetic qualities of modern denture base materials are good; the appearance of acrylic and porcelain teeth is satisfactory in the cheaper ranges and good in the more expensive. Thus a very realistic effect can be achieved initially in the anterior segment of the mouth.

Acrylic teeth, however, deteriorate fairly rapidly and the initial good appearance is lost as attrition and abrasion cause loss of surface detail. The smoothing of the labial surface gives a flat and lifeless appearance to the teeth. Porcelain anterior teeth retain their aesthetic qualities far longer, but they may chip and do tend to darken towards a grey colour after some years.

Artificial teeth on an immediate denture can resemble the natural dentition closely, provided that the position of the natural teeth is compatible with tooth arrangement in a denture. In later years, however, restoration of appearance may not be possible. Changes in the supporting structures may necessitate a change in anterior tooth position in order to give greater denture stability and better function.

ORAL FUNCTION

Oral function involves mastication, deglutition and speech. The mouth also plays an important part in facial expression. During the movements associated with these functions various forces are applied to the natural or artificial teeth.

In mastication, the major force is directed vertically towards the alveolar bone with smaller forces acting laterally and anteroposteriorly. In moments of stress, the patient may clench the teeth and apply a very large vertical force to the alveolar ridges. On deglutition, there is only a light passing tooth contact. When the patient is speaking and during the soft tissue movements involved in facial expression, the teeth do not meet. Therefore, during oral functions other than mastication, there is little or no vertical force, but the lips, cheeks and tongue press horizontally against the teeth and dentures.

WITH NATURAL TEETH

In the natural dentition, the periodontal membrane resembles a sling which is designed principally to resist forces applied vertically towards the apex of the tooth. Horizontal forces are also resisted but to a lesser extent. However, these horizontal forces are usually weaker than those applied vertically and the design of the periodontal membrane is such that it can usually accept them without damage. Anteroposterior forces are also absorbed by contacts between adjacent teeth in the intact dental arch, so that such forces are spread over many teeth.

Thus, the method of suspension of the natural dentition is well designed and forces within the normal range applied to healthy natural teeth cause no damage or discomfort. Incision of hard or fibrous foodstuffs is efficient and provided that a limited amount of smooth gliding of the teeth over each other can take place, mastication of tough foods causes no difficulty or pain.

The actual loads applied to the teeth can be divided into: (i) static loads—occurring when the teeth are clenched, and (ii) dynamic loads—produced during mastication. The load during clenching is the greatest that can be delivered to the teeth in a vertical direction by the musculature. In one study the maximum static force recorded on the first molar was 90 kg. The loads applied to the teeth during mastication, however, vary with the type of food and the occlusal form and surface area of the teeth. As one is not conscious of a great effort in mastication, it is not surprising that chewing loads between molar teeth can be as low as 15 kg.

The load during tooth clenching is limited by the proprioceptive nerve endings in the periodontal membrane, which reflexly inhibit further contraction of the elevator muscles when the load reaches a certain level. Normally, the masticatory loads borne by the teeth do not reach this level. However, if something hard, such as a piece of shot or bone, is encountered within the bolus of food, a large load is applied and the masticatory cycle is temporarily halted to avoid pain or possible damage to the teeth. A similar situation occurs with a high restoration, where the load developed on the single tooth may be significantly greater than when there is whole arch contact and even distribution of the load. In both instances pain from the tooth will result in modification of the masticatory effort.

WITH DENTURES

The nature of the support for the complete denture is quite different from that of the natural teeth. Static and dynamic loads are applied via the denture to the mucoperiosteum covering the alveolar ridge. On application of chewing forces, this soft tissue is squeezed between the hard denture base and the underlying bone. Under these conditions a much smaller load elicits a painful response from the nerve endings within the mucoperiosteum, with a consequent reduction in the load that can be tolerated. In the premolar region of a complete denture, the maximum static load is of the order of 12 kg whilst the average is only about 7 kg. However, during chewing, the average load used for most foods is only 1·6 kg. The greatest load is tolerated when the denture covers the maximum area of tissue. Therefore in function, there is usually less discomfort with an upper denture than with a lower. However, a denture which has moved slightly away from the tissues during function, may, on being pressed quickly back into place, apply to a small area a very high pressure and thus cause considerable pain. Thus the patient learns painfully to limit the force and type of chewing movement which may be used with dentures.

Hence, fear of pain causes the patient to be less vigorous with chewing movements. As a result, the efficiency of chewing with dentures is only a quarter to a third of that of the natural dentition. Consequently, foods which require chewing to reveal their full flavour and which give enjoyment in the act of chewing can no longer be included in the patient's diet. The complete denture wearer may complain of a diminished sense of taste. This is due partly to the elimination from the diet of this type of food and also because those foods that are included, are not chewed long enough to reveal their full flavour. Appreciation of 'taste' is also due to the sensation of texture of the foodstuffs against the hard palate. A denture blankets this sensation.

Due to the relative inefficiency of complete dentures for mastication, the patient may tend to swallow large particles of food which have not been chewed. Mastication is thought to be necessary to break up the food for easier attack by the gastric juices and it is recognized that many patients suffer from indigestion if they are rendered edentulous and are not provided with dentures for several months. Thus, although it has been shown that digestion and absorption of unmasticated food undoubtedly occurs, such food probably remains longer in the stomach before being passed to the small intestine. It may therefore throw a greater strain on gastric digestion. In the healthy stomach and intestine there is a large spare capacity for adaptation and this extra load is accepted without producing any symptoms. But where the digestive process is impaired, chewing may well be necessary. The act of chewing stimulates the secretion of gastric juices, so preparing the stomach to accept food. On mixing food with saliva during chewing, digestion of carbohydrate commences. Whilst the acidity of the stomach stops this digestion, about half of the carbohydrate is digested by this means, thus reducing the amount of digestion necessary in the small intestine.

Of course, if all food is reduced to a state which does not require mastication, this loss of masticatory efficiency is probably not of great importance. Some patients are quite happy to select foods which require little or no chewing. However, patients who take a more natural diet with a large fibrous content, e.g. vegetarians, find difficulty in swallowing their food without adequate mastication. Consequently, they find dentures to be unsatisfactory because of their masticatory inefficiency and because of their instability during any vigorous chewing movements. The most difficult foods to chew are meat, and fibrous foods such as fresh fruit and vegetables. A patient seeking easily chewed foods avoids these and selects a diet consisting mainly of carbohydrate.

The older person in particular must maintain an interest in food and so ensure a suitable diet. Both economic and masticatory limitations may force an elderly patient to exist on a diet of carbohydrate consisting mainly of white bread and jam, buns and tea. The number of old people is increasing as the years go by and if they are rendered edentulous early in life they may suffer from lack of masticatory power in old age. If their dental inefficiency causes them to select an unsuitable carbohydrate diet, the concomitant lack of protein and the resultant obesity produce a variety of problems in ageing persons.

Some relationship may exist between unsatisfactory denture experience and the level of various constituents of the body fluid. A relationship between carbohydrate, vitamin, mineral and electrolyte metabolism and an unsatisfactory denture tolerance begins to appear. This is one of those frequent occasions when it is difficult to decide which comes first. Inadequate metabolism results in tissues which cannot tolerate the trauma from the denture, but does denture discomfort contribute to inadequate metabolism, by limiting the diet to that which does not cause discomfort on chewing?

Studies in nutrition in recent years indicate that refined sugars and milled cereals form too great a proportion of the diet of highly developed communities. Two hundred years ago this type of carbohydrate provided only 2 per cent of the calories of our diet; one hundred years ago this was 5 per cent and today it is nearly 20 per cent. The total weight of carbohydrate eaten in poor and in more prosperous countries, does not vary widely, but in the poorer countries only 5 per cent of this is in the form of refined sugar as against 33 per cent in the more prosperous areas. Refined sugar is the most important commercial product for giving palatability to manufactured foods. Evidence is accumulating that besides causing dental decay, if eaten in the form of sweets all day long, certain types of carbohydrate may have an influence on the aetiology of heart disease, diabetes, and peptic ulcer. Thus if masticatory efficiency is at a low level, patients may well select palatable manufactured foods requiring little chewing, instead of the more nutritious natural foods which require adequate chewing to bring out their taste.

OTHER ORAL FUNCTIONS

Dentures are frequently dislodged by the horizontal forces exerted by the cheeks, lips and tongue during speech and on swallowing food. To prevent movement of the dentures the patient reduces the amount of movement during speech and facial expression. In many cases, the dentures must be designed to avoid these dislodging forces. Usually, such dentures do not give adequate support to the facial tissues nor is the appearance of the teeth at all similar to that of the natural dentition. As a result, there is an appearance of premature ageing as folds occur in the facial tissues, and also, the general facial appearance of the patient undergoes a marked change.

Resorption of alveolar bone continues for an indefinite period after the loss of the natural teeth. Whilst the patient may have comfortable, functional dentures for some years after extraction of the teeth, in later years the continuing bone resorption frequently creates denture difficulties. In this situation, appearance must give way at least partly to function.

UPPER AND LOWER DENTURES

It would be more precise to differentiate to some degree between replacement of teeth in the upper and lower jaws. Dentists and their patients enjoy some success when replacing the upper teeth by a denture, but the complete lower denture is frequently the 'Sisyphean stone' of a large number of patients. (Sisyphus was condemned to roll a huge stone ceaselessly uphill.) The attempts of these patients to levitate their lower dentures and to prevent them rolling down and damaging the tissues beneath are seldom successful. The necessity of a denture for appearance and mastication conflicts with the ever present discomfort and these poor patients wander from dentist to dentist with a bag full of dentures seeking the impossible.

The necessity of wearing dentures varies with differences in social level. Therefore the proportion of dentures which are not worn, i.e. where the discomforts outweigh the advantages to the patient, varies also between different social groups. However, difficulties have been found to exist for between 10 and 15 per cent of complete denture wearers. The incidence of difficulty is greater in relation to the lower denture.

SOCIAL DISADVANTAGES OF DENTURES

On removal of complete dentures for cleaning, the facial appearance is completely changed. At this time the patient wishes privacy until appearance is restored. Many wives will not be seen without their dentures because of the drastic change in appearance. In family life, or when travelling, such privacy is not always available and the dentures become a social embarrassment.

Unless great care is taken to keep the dentures clean, they stain, particularly in the case of smokers. This staining is typical of dentures and occurs on the gingival portion of the denture base between the teeth as well as on the teeth themselves. In the natural dentition, only the teeth are stained. In addition, a certain degree of denture odour accompanies lack of perfect oral hygiene in the denture wearer.

DISADVANTAGES OF DENTURES IN PARTICULAR WALKS OF LIFE

For persons who can adapt their oral movements to the limitations of dentures, the loss of teeth is not serious. There are others, however, whose livelihood depends upon free movement of lips, cheeks and tongue supported by the teeth. Vocalists and wind-instrument players frequently experience difficulties with complete dentures. During the act of singing the wide-open mouth and tension of the lips may loosen the dentures. Brass wind instrumentalists press the mouthpiece against the lips, whilst woodwind players apply loads directly to the teeth in addition to pressure via the lips. The stability and retention of complete dentures is frequently inadequate to resist these horizontal forces. Consequently, some alteration in playing technique or the provision of a special prosthesis for playing may become necessary. The loss of facility in playing or singing is not limited to the professional performer and many amateurs who derive considerable pleasure from making music, experience a waning of interest after the loss of natural teeth. Not only is the production of the correct sound made more difficult but the quality of the sound made may also be affected.

Public speakers, teachers and lecturers require confidence in their ability to wear complete dentures. They may have a fear of sudden loss of retention, particularly of an upper denture, which would cause considerable embarrassment when speaking in public. In addition, during the weeks immediately after the provision of dentures, lack of confidence in their control is a frequent occurrence.

Thus, whilst extraction of all their natural teeth may for some patients give relief from continuous toothache and protracted dental care, in the majority some loss of efficiency accompanies the change to complete dentures. This change affects people in different ways; some adapt readily and accept the differences between natural teeth and dentures, whereas others regret the irrevocable nature of tooth extraction and realize too late the limitations of complete dentures.

THE INCIDENCE OF EDENTULOUSNESS

Despite dental care and dental health education, a relatively large proportion of people become edentulous. Estimates range from 10 to 50 per cent of the

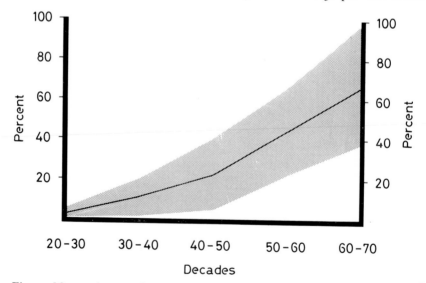

Fig. 1.1 Mean and range of percentages of persons edentulous at various decades of life.

adult population in different countries of the world. The incidence appears to be higher for women than men. Naturally, the risk of edentulousness increases with age. Figure 1.1 shows the percentage of persons edentulous at different decades of life. The wide variations are thought to be due to social class and attitude differences, and to the dentist:patient ratio which varies widely between countries.

Chapter 2

The Patient as a Person

It is of prime importance that we understand something of the person whom we are treating and do not limit our outlook to the dental condition presented. Patients cannot readily be classified into types but broad subdivisions form a useful basis for comparison and treatment.

THE QUIET MIND

The normal patient is one in whom the loss of teeth follows previous satisfactory dental treatment and whose approach is intelligent, understanding and cooperative towards professional opinion and advice for treatment. When given guidance and education this type of patient is a joy to treat. Similarly, the patient who has had satisfactory dentures but who is returning for further service, already has the correct approach to any denture problems.

Some patients in this group may have been dissatisfied with their present dentures over a short period of time. After the completion of satisfactory treatment this episode will soon be forgotten. A small amount of discussion and examination soon reveals the errors which were previously made and as the new patient–dentist relationship is established, treatment proceeds harmoniously to a satisfactory conclusion.

This type of patient sits quietly in the chair showing an interest in treatment but no more than a normal reaction to any stimulus. Fortunately, a great number of dental patients fall into this category.

THE MORE DIFFICULT PATIENT

Whilst it is not intended to deal with the subject of mental health to any great degree, certain patients require more than treatment as a prosthetic case, if they are to be satisfied.

As people grow up they adapt to the responsibilities and difficulties of adult life. Their childhood fears, dependence and lack of restraint are kept under control to an extent which varies between individuals. Under normal circumstances the patient will react normally. In conditions of stress, however, the patient may regress psychologically and some of the veneer of control is lost. Stress may arise from working conditions, home relationships, financial difficulties or various other factors in adult life. The patient may then be classified as mildly neurotic. Such a patient reacts abnormally to normal surroundings and normal life.

Patients who prove difficult to treat are not all of the same type. A further subdivision of the difficult patient group into anxious, suspicious (doubting), aggressive and indifferent groups is therefore suggested.

THE ANXIOUS PATIENT

Whilst prosthetic treatment is generally more unpleasant than painful, the prospect of any dental treatment may produce excitement in the patient. If the patient is simply nervous, then a calm, confident approach will soon bring reassurance and any temporary anxiety will rapidly be overcome. When the confidence of children is gained they are relatively easy to treat provided that unduly painful or unpleasant stimuli are not applied. In adult life, however, the anxious patient under stress from daily life is not changed so readily to a normally reacting patient. The patient is constantly over-stimulated by adrenal secretion with a consequent increase in response to normal treatment stimuli.

This type of neurotic patient may not be able to define with accuracy the precise factors which are causing difficulty. Few people suffer from anxiety neurosis due to such tangible factors as overwork; but more from confusion. In fact, rather than recognize consciously the deeper emotional roots of his other anxiety, such a patient will readily 'explain' anxiety in terms of current bodily disturbance. Thus he may displace his anxiety to the mouth and will then be worried about oral cancer. The patient requests frequent examination of normal oral structures and is often unconvinced by one opinion.

The changes that occur during the climacteric—that period of transition in life between maturity and senility—are in themselves emotionally disturbing to the female patient in the 45 to 60 age group. If to this is added the loss of natural teeth, the patient may become anxious at the thought of becoming 'old' and losing attraction and appearance. Also, at this age there is often loss of family interests such as children getting married and moving away from home. Retirement from active work outside the home at a slightly later age causes difficulties of adjustment. All these factors contribute to the difficult female patient. Men present difficulties related more to their mental type than to their age, though similar emotional disturbances can occur in the male of 50 to 60 years.

THE SUSPICIOUS PATIENT

The very tidy, meticulously dressed lady, fussy about her appearance and about 'appearances' in general requires thoughtful handling. She is often materialistic in outlook and very house-proud. This type of patient may be reluctant to accept advice and may not have confidence in the competence of the dentist to give satisfactory treatment. Provided that this lack of confidence can be overcome, these patients can be treated satisfactorily but more time is required than normal to achieve the high standard demanded by the patient.

THE AGGRESSIVE PATIENT

The dentist will find that some patients appear uncooperative, antagonistic and cynical at the first meeting. They may appear irritated and impatient, particularly during the discussion necessary before treatment is commenced. This type of patient is usually male, and whilst he may be relying considerably upon the dentist he may be over-compensating for his dependent feelings. Such a patient is usually very demanding and returns at frequent intervals to the dentist. He may make impossible demands and react unfavourably, for example by threatening legal action, when these are not met.

THE INDIFFERENT PATIENT

Depression with lack of interest may follow a major personal disappointment or a bereavement. Some patients are not interested in their appearance and also select a diet requiring little mastication. They are passively cooperative, are non-persevering and it is extremely difficult to stimulate their interest in treatment. Their apparently ready acceptance of prognosis and treatment plan should not be assumed to be a tacit agreement. Often these patients are impelled towards treatment by their wife or husband rather than by themselves. This last category is often the most difficult one to treat satisfactorily.

RAPPORT

The dentist–patient relationship is an important one. The phrase 'I like you, if you like me' sums up the rapport between patient and operator. We all respond to those whom we like and give of our best. Some patients, however, are antagonized by us and we by them. In these circumstances, the effect of lack of mutual confidence and respect may be sufficient to reduce markedly the possibility of success.

Everybody likes to have an interest taken in them and most patients wish to be somebody, not just a case for dental treatment. The simple recording by the dentist of the patient's interests in the community, his or her family life or work will give a starting point for a short conversation. This helps, particularly at the early stages of treatment, to bridge the gap of apprehension between dentist and patient.

One's personal appearance, the arrangement, decoration and cleanliness of the surgery and the appearance of the staff of the practice can all affect a patient's confidence. A suitably trained dental nurse or receptionist can do much to calm the nervous patient.

Until an attempt has been made to establish rapport between patient and dentist, no hurried classification of the patient as a person should be made. Just because difficulties exist, the patient should not be immediately classified as neurotic. Whilst with many patients a good atmosphere can be created within minutes, with others more time is necessary in order to gain some understanding of the patient as a person and of his or her problems.

All patients who may be thought of as mildly neurotic should be treated gently. Their story should be listened to with some sympathy, but not at too great a length. The bluff, rough approach will not produce a satisfactory end result to the treatment given. However, once confidence in the dentist is achieved by discussion of the denture problem, the patient usually will accept the prognosis.

There is a great deal of difference between an explanation given to the patient before treatment starts and one given after difficulties have arisen. Whereas the former improves the dentist–patient relationship, the latter appears to many patients to be an excuse for failure. When there are few difficulties, little time need be spent in prior discussion with the patient. As treatment proceeds suitable explanation can accompany it. When it is anticipated that patient reaction will not be good and dental difficulties exist, then prior discussion is essential.

Chapter 3

The Decision to Render the Patient Edentulous

There are many factors which influence the fate of the natural teeth and the speed with which they are lost. Perhaps the main ones are:—

1 The quality of the patient's tissues and their resistance to dental diseases

2 The importance which the patient attaches to tooth retention, which will largely influence——

3 The regularity and quality of the care of the mouth by the patient and will also influence——

4 The quality and regularity of dental care by the patient's practitioner.

When most of these conditions are favourable, then the natural dentition is often retained for life either completely or with the loss of only a few teeth. Other situations arise where the effects of previous neglect and breakdown can be arrested, and from thenceforward, the patient's dentition can be maintained. For many patients, the above factors may be less favourable but the rate of tooth loss is still slow and single teeth are extracted at infrequent intervals when disease processes have proceeded beyond the possibility of dental repair. Even in these circumstances, the necessity of removing all the teeth occurs infrequently. For other patients, however, even with regular dental care, the dentist is fighting a losing battle. Then when only a few teeth remain, the decision arises as to whether or not they should now all be extracted.

But all patients do not enjoy regular dental care. Where disease has produced a condition which is reparable only with considerable effort, and especially if the patient is poorly motivated, then many teeth have to be extracted at one time and the patient proceeds rapidly from the natural to the artificial dentition.

Apart from trauma, the main reasons for extracting several teeth are advanced caries and periodontal disease. On occasion, teeth may also be extracted because of poor appearance, or where there is severe malocclusion.

EXTRACTION BECAUSE OF DENTAL CARIES

Dental caries is a disease that mainly affects the young with the rate of attack usually diminishing as the patient gets older. Patients in whom caries cannot be controlled, may lose teeth in rapid succession in their teens and early twenties. The dentist is often fighting a losing battle, with recurrent caries developing around recently placed restorations. The provision of partial dentures in these cases may accelerate the carious process due to increased stagnation, and ultimately it may be necessary to render the patient edentulous at an early age. In cases of less severe attack, the gradual loss of tooth substance by recurrent caries may leave insufficient tooth remaining for further simple conservative procedures. In such cases endodontic therapy, full coronal restorations and the replacement of missing units by fixed or removable prostheses, is undoubtedly the ideal treatment. Economic factors, time and the skill necessary to carry out this work, together with the degree of patient cooperation, all limit the application of this type of treatment. In some cases, therefore, extraction and provision of one or both complete dentures, may be the most satisfactory means of oral rehabilitation.

It must be remembered, however, that the alveolar processes exist to support the natural teeth. Where there is no periodontal disease, the alveolar bone remains for as long as the teeth are retained, no matter how carious they may be. After teeth are extracted, resorption of this bone takes place at a rate which varies widely between patients and which cannot easily be forecast before extractions. The earlier the age at which teeth are lost, the longer is the time available for resorption to take place. Many edentulous patients in the 45 to 55 age group who present with denture problems, had their teeth removed either through lack of dental care, or from the wrong type of dental treatment in their early twenties. Undoubtedly, at that age, the removal of teeth and their replacement by dentures is not a difficult procedure. The patient adapts well to the dentures and indeed often welcomes them as indicating the end of all dental troubles. Although this type of treatment may be considered to be economically sound when one takes a short-term or short-sighted view, the patient is frequently not a regular attender and after the provision of dentures may not return for many years. A difficult denture problem then exists, since the dentures are likely to have become ill-fitting as a result of bone resorption. With the development of malocclusion and continuous abuse of the tissues of the denture-bearing areas, gross resorption frequently removes one or both ridges.

Therefore, in cases of carious attack, loss of teeth should be delayed until there is no other means of providing oral function and restoring aesthetics within the limitations presented by the patient.

EXTRACTION BECAUSE OF PERIODONTAL DISEASE

Much discussion centres round the advisability of retaining the teeth despite the loss of bone caused by periodontal disease. This is because there are so many factors to be considered and so little factual evidence of their influence is available.

From the point of view of providing prostheses, the philosophy of delaying extraction can lead to many problems and difficulties. A well-formed alveolar ridge is of considerable importance to the retention and stability of complete dentures as it provides resistance to the displacing forces that are applied to dentures during function.

Natural teeth are supported in bone which for convenience, may be divided into alveolar process and basal or body bone. There is, however, no histological evidence to support this subdivision. The alveolar process round the walls of the socket is relatively thin at the neck of the tooth in relation to that at the apex. The bone then thickens further to form the body of the mandible or the maxilla. During active periodontal disease, the alveolar process supporting the tooth is lost. Once the framework of bone has gone, it does not regenerate.

The bone destruction associated with periodontal inflammation, also changes the architecture of the remaining tooth supporting tissues. If the teeth are to be retained, this architecture must be restored to one in which periodontal inflammation will find difficulty in becoming active in the future. In addition, the periodontal 'climate' or 'environment' in the mouth, which was a contributing factor to the disease, must also be altered so that the possibility of future inflammation is greatly reduced. On arrest of the disease and eradication of its effects, the rate of bone loss reduces to a negligible level. Where periodontal treatment achieves the elimination of periodontal inflammation and creates a readily maintained periodontal architecture, then this treatment is preferable to tooth extraction.

Problems may arise, however, due to lapses either in treatment or in home care. Then further bone is lost. If the eventual prognosis is to be one of complete extractions, then this pattern of recurrent bone destruction should not be allowed to continue, otherwise the prognosis for complete dentures deteriorates rapidly with time. The dentition may deteriorate to a state which is not amenable to periodontal therapy nor, after extractions, will the resultant ridges provide favourable bases for complete dentures.

Periodontal treatment which, for whatever cause, does not arrest the loss of supporting bone, is against the best interests of the patient. The continuing ineffectual treatment of the patient whose periodontal disease persists may well be called 'supervised neglect'. All that is happening is that valuable bone is being lost. Eventually when the teeth have to be extracted, the bone remaining will be less than that which was present at the start of such 'periodontal treatment'. The level at which healing of the socket takes place is determined largely by the height of the remaining alveolar bone. It can be no higher than this. Where more alveolar bone is present before extraction, a larger ridge may remain after healing.

Various writers have suggested that extractions should be considered after a certain amount of the root has been denuded of its bony support. Suggestions have been made that a tooth should be extracted when only a half or a third of the root remains supported. Teeth can be maintained, however, even when a large proportion of their support has been lost. Provided that the periodontal tissues are healthy and the bone and soft tissues have a contour which permits them to be maintained in this condition, the teeth need not necessarily be extracted although their proportion of root support is small.

The retention of natural teeth after loss of much of their bony support carries with it some disadvantages. The appearance of such teeth may be unsatisfactory to the patient and also, in some cases, a periodontal splint may mar the patient's appearance or interfere with oral hygiene maintenance. In addition, the teeth may, due to their position, traumatize an already edentulous opposing ridge, causing resorption. Such reasons influence both patient and dentist in deciding whether or not to retain these teeth.

The eradication of periodontal inflammation is not only important during the life of the tooth, but is also important at the time of extraction. Clinically, there is a more rapid change in the shape of the alveolar process in the first few weeks after the extraction of teeth which are affected by periodontal disease than there is following extractions due to caries. This is primarily due to soft tissue collapse and shrinkage since the relation between alveolar bone and gingival tissues is not as close in teeth affected by chronic periodontitis as it is in the unaffected mouth. The alveolar bone crest–gingival margin distance may then be 6 to 7 mm compared with the normal 2 to 3 mm. The change in shape during healing is also influenced by the areas of existing inflammation and the irregular bony contour which the periodontal disease has left behind. Intrabony pockets filled with inflamed tissue may persist after tooth extraction and cause further bone resorption or delay the rate of healing.

Not only must the size of the alveolar ridge be adequate, but the quality of its bone also must be suitable to bear the loads applied by a prosthesis. After the removal of teeth, the persistence of the bony defects characteristic of advanced chronic periodontitis results in a ragged and irregular ridge crest which is sharp to the touch. Removal of the bony defects at extraction by curettage of granulation tissue and bone trimming (alveoloplasty) improves the ridge contour, but may reduce its height. However, if this is not done, the bone defects persist and healing does not appear to be completed by the formation of a smooth cortical layer of bone. This is seen particularly in the lower anterior region and is the cause of much discomfort under a complete lower denture. In marked contrast are the good denture foundations seen in young patients who have had all their natural teeth extracted in their early twenties because of gross caries. In such cases it is more common to find well-rounded alveolar ridges with a good covering of cortical bone.

The rate of bone destruction must be considered as well as the extent. For example, a moderate rate of bone loss in a young patient suggests a more rapid rate of destruction than the same loss in an older patient.

Probably the most important factor in keeping natural teeth is the patient's cooperation. The patient and the dentist working together can often avoid the edentulous state.

As the expectation of life increases, however, the retention of the natural dentition throughout life becomes increasingly difficult. It must be remembered, though, that with advancing age, aesthetics become less important, at least for the male patient. In addition, much oral function can be achieved from a few molar teeth in contact and therefore a mutilated and reduced dentition unacceptable to a younger patient may be adequate for an older patient.

MAKING A DECISION

The decision on whether or not teeth should be extracted because of periodontal involvement may be very easy. In many cases where minimal bone resorption has occurred, it is obvious that sufficient support remains for the retention of the teeth. In other cases where only the apices of several teeth remain in bone, it is equally obvious that they are unsavable.

The borderline cases, where considerable amounts of support have been lost, are the ones in which a decision is difficult to reach. Assuming that the tooth crowns are sound in other respects and are useful for prosthetic purposes, the decision should be guided in general by three main considerations:—

1 The height of the remaining bone support
2 The presence of other pathological changes related to the root
3 The pattern of bone destruction.

As a general rule, when up to two-thirds of the support has been destroyed, teeth can still be quite functional without artificial support provided that they are not subject to excessive loading in either a vertical or a horizontal direction. The prognosis for teeth with more than this amount of loss of support must be considered poor. Periapical infection of pulpal origin or resorption of the apex of the tooth effectively reduces the amount of tooth support.

Where bone has been lost in a fairly even pattern over the whole area of the jaw, the prognosis is relatively good even when a large proportion of the root is unsupported. In this circumstance, there are no discrete areas in which inflammation has spread more rapidly to cause local destruction. When intra-bony pockets are present, especially if they are multiple or root bifurcations are involved, bone destruction has proceeded more rapidly. The elimination of these bone defects may jeopardise the support of the adjacent teeth. The prognosis is then poorer.

Information with which to assess these factors can be obtained readily from:—

1 Measurement of the pocket depth on all four vertical surfaces of each tooth
2 A careful appraisal of radiographs.

Tooth mobility is a poor criterion for assessing the amount of bone loss as frequently teeth become firmer once the inflammation of the periodontal tissues has been successfully treated.

Thus if periodontal treatment and continual care by both patient and dentist can maintain healthy, well contoured periodontal tissues, retention of the existing teeth is advised. If treatment cannot achieve this end, then early, rather than late extraction is preferred.

AGE OF THE PATIENT

The decision to keep or extract teeth must also be related to the patient's age, bearing in mind the possible difference between the chronological and biological age of the patient. In some patients, the ageing processes occur prematurely, whilst in others they are long delayed (Fig. 3.1).

The effects of ageing are seen not only in the tissues of the face and of the denture bearing areas, but also in the central nervous system. Progressive atrophy destroys functional elements of the cerebral cortex and subcortical structures which are involved in the learning processes. Initial signs of cerebral involution may occur in patients in their forties and sometimes earlier with disease, nutritional deficiencies and stress. Thus, young persons usually have a high capacity for learning but this capacity diminishes with age. The initial period of adaptation to complete dentures involves the musculature in a

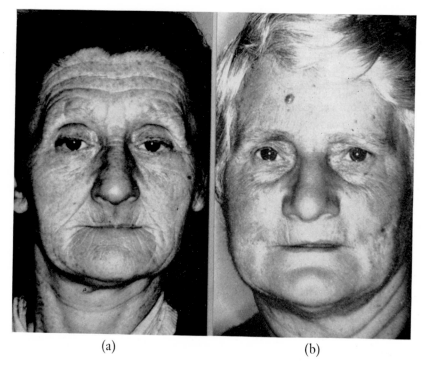

(a)   (b)

Fig. 3.1 Biological and chronological age discrepancies:
(a) patient is aged 45 and is biologically old;
(b) patient is aged 75 and is biologically young.

sometimes lengthy process of learning, in order to control and manipulate the new prosthesis. Thus, the older the patient, the longer the period necessary for adaptation to dentures.

Modern dentistry is combating caries and periodontal disease more effectively than ever before. The result is that total extraction is being delayed, and more and more patients are finally rendered edentulous in the age groups when adaptation to complete dentures occurs more slowly. Some patients may even be beyond the point where new muscular activity can readily be learned. Thus, if we delay extraction in this way until the patient cannot adapt to complete dentures, we are not taking a sufficiently forward view of the patient's dental treatment. All patients beyond the age of 55 should be carefully assessed for prognosis of tooth retention and for signs of premature ageing. If we can keep the teeth for life, no problem arises. But where the eventual loss of all the natural teeth is inevitable, a decision to extract must be made at an age when the patient can still adapt. The actual time of extraction depends upon how much comfort and efficiency the patient is enjoying with the natural dentition. Some patients prefer to continue with their natural teeth for a longer period and are ready to accept the lesser dental efficiency which may ultimately result. Of course, the longer the period during which the natural dentition is retained, the shorter is the period of denture wearing. Other patients prefer to play safe and hope for slightly better denture comfort by accepting the edentulous state at an earlier date.

SPECIAL CONSIDERATIONS

In nervous disorders such as Parkinson's disease, epilepsy, and in the feeble-minded, prosthetic treatment is often difficult and complete denture tolerance also poor. The natural teeth should therefore be retained where possible. This may be difficult, however, due to the inability on the part of the patient to cooperate in home care. Likewise, in cleft palate patients, the natural teeth should be preserved for as long as possible to provide retention for the necessary prosthesis.

EXTRACTION TO IMPROVE AESTHETICS

Gross irregularity or protrusion of the anterior teeth may have an unfortunate psychological effect particularly on the young female patient. Orthodontic treatment or natural development may bring about an improvement in appearance and often an irregularity which at first is displeasing to the patient becomes accepted in later life. On occasion, however, gross irregularity of the anterior teeth continues into early adult life and the patient's mind becomes obsessed with the ugliness of the natural dentition. Whilst adult orthodontic treatment is possible and should always be considered, in some cases removal of the offending teeth is to be preferred. This is particularly so when proclination of the anteriors is associated with loss of bone (Fig. 3.2). When some posterior teeth are also missing, extraction of all the remaining teeth and the provision of a complete denture must be thought of as possibly the best treatment plan.

It must always be remembered, however, that natural teeth function better than dentures and unless appearance causes great displeasure, then preservation of the natural teeth is the treatment of choice.

Of course, what may be aesthetically satisfactory to one patient or to one dentist, may arouse critical comment from another. Discussion between dentist and patient is therefore essential in order to resolve any aesthetic differences which exist.

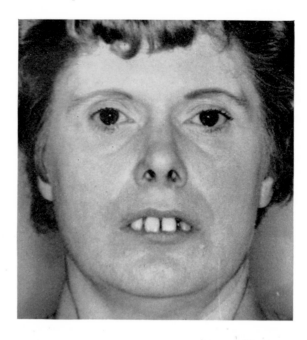

Fig. 3.2 Proclination and spacing of the upper anterior teeth associated with loss of supporting bone.

EXTRACTIONS IN CASES OF MALOCCLUSION

Most malocclusions of young patients can be treated satisfactorily by orthodontic therapy. In the adult dentition where malocclusion is minimal it may
be corrected by selective grinding and the replacement of unsuitably shaped
restorations, by the use of partial dentures with onlays, or by extraction of
malpositioned teeth. A marked malocclusion, however, is likely to be an aesthetic and functional handicap to the patient (Fig. 3.3). When caries or periodontal disease is also present or when a number of teeth have already been
lost, extraction of the remaining teeth and the insertion of complete dentures
must be considered. This argument may be applied unwisely to those patients
with a marked inferior protrusion, often associated with a space between the
anterior teeth. To obtain sufficient room between upper and lower ridges
posteriorly to accommodate two denture bases and the attached teeth, alveolectomy is often necessary. Despite careful prosthetic treatment, many of
these cases are functionally unsuccessful. The overall ridge relation may not be
conducive to the retention and stability of the dentures, and also the environ-

mental musculature may be unable to adapt to the considerable differences in tooth position that have occurred in the change from natural to artificial dentition. This is particularly so when an attempt is made to change an abnormal incisor relation in the natural dentition to a normal incisor relation in the complete dentures. Therefore, in cases of severe malocclusion where total extraction is indicated because of caries or periodontal disease in addition to the defects in occlusion, consideration should be given to surgery to improve the basal jaw relation as well as the appearance. For example, a case of inferior protrusion may be treated by section of either the horizontal or vertical ramus of the mandible. In a case of inferior retrusion, grafting into the body of the mandible may be used to improve the jaw relation and the appearance.

In many centres in this country such treatment is now in the hands of specialist plastic and oral surgeons working in close collaboration. A careful study is made of casts of the jaw relations prior to operation, using an adjustable articulator or special analyser, and with the aid of cephalometric radiographs, the precise change in jaw relation is carefully planned.

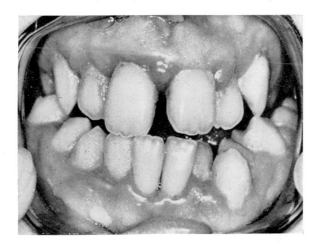

Fig. 3.3 Marked malocclusion—a possible case for total extractions to improve appearance and function.

EXTRACTION TO AVOID
THE SINGLE COMPLETE DENTURE

The construction of a single complete denture in occlusion with natural teeth in the opposing jaw is often difficult. The natural teeth may be so badly positioned that the elimination of displacing contacts between the natural and artificial teeth during function may be impossible. The prognosis is more favourable with a complete upper denture opposing natural lower teeth than with a complete lower denture against natural upper teeth. The small denture-bearing area in the lower jaw gives less retention and there is a great danger of trauma to the remaining lower alveolar ridge. The need for coordination of the occlusal surfaces of the denture and the natural teeth is vital if stability is to be achieved. Modification of the natural occlusal table is often necessary.

When a complete denture opposes natural teeth complemented by a partial denture, similar considerations must be borne in mind. The presence of natural or artificial molar teeth spreads the occlusal load more evenly over the denture area.

Where an unbalanced functional occlusal relationship has been in use against a single complete denture for some time and has caused rapid loss of alveolar bone, extraction of all the remaining teeth should be considered. Rapid resorption of bone frequently follows the continued use of a complete upper denture opposed only by the lower anterior teeth. The rate of resorption depends upon the quality and quantity of the alveolar bone under the complete denture and on the magnitude and direction of the load applied. If the ridge is large and of well-trabeculated bone, the rate of resorption is slow. When only a small and poorly trabeculated ridge remains after the extraction of periodontally involved teeth, there seems to be a more rapid resorption in response to pressure.

The most frequent problem is presented by the patient who cannot or will not tolerate a partial denture to replace the lower posterior teeth. If resorption of the upper anterior ridge occurs in these circumstances, consideration should be given to the provision of a complete lower denture. Otherwise, extensive resorption of the upper alveolar process with replacement by fibrous tissue is likely to occur and result in a 'flabby' ridge. In addition, tongue spread posteriorly into the vacant lower molar areas, together with forward posturing of the mandible to achieve occlusion, will make the prognosis for a lower complete denture at a later date most unfavourable.

ALTERNATIVE TREATMENT
TO COMPLETE DENTURES

Before deciding to render a patient edentulous it should be realized that the masticatory efficiency of a few natural posterior teeth in occlusion with other teeth is often good. In fact, it is probable that the efficiency of four molars in occlusion is better than that of many complete dentures. The position of the remaining posterior teeth in the arch will influence the operator in his decision on whether to extract, assuming of course that their periodontal condition is sound. For example, teeth at the distal ends of the arch will usually provide suitable abutments for tooth-supported partial dentures and help to resist anteroposterior and lateral movement of the prosthesis. Thus, a patient presenting with 8   3 | 3   8 in the upper jaw and 8̲   3̲ | 3̲   8̲ in the lower, might well be advised to retain the teeth and have partial upper and lower dentures to restore aesthetics and function. But if the position of the remaining posterior teeth is such that free-end saddles exist, the problems of restoring these by partial dentures must be borne in mind.

A small group of teeth remaining on one side of the jaw only, for example 4̲5̲6, occasionally contributes to masticatory function without affecting retention and stability of the denture unduly. When they are not in occlusion with opposing natural teeth, however, they should be extracted. The contribution to denture comfort and efficiency of a few unilaterally positioned teeth is less in the upper than in the lower jaw.

RETENTION OF MOLAR TEETH ONLY

The retention of molar teeth at the distal of the arch is an advantage in the lower jaw as they prevent lateral and distal movement of the denture during chewing. In general, the retention of molar teeth in the upper jaw is not so satisfactory since an extension of the denture round the tuberosities usually provides equal resistance to displacement. On the other hand if upper molar teeth on either side are in occlusion with natural lower teeth they may be retained because of their contribution to efficiency in chewing.

RETENTION OF NATURAL CANINES

It is sometimes suggested that canines should be retained because they offer good lateral stability to an otherwise complete denture and may be used to increase retention of the denture and help the patient, particularly the elderly, to learn to control it. This is of especial advantage in the lower jaw. However the retention of the lower canines can present some problems in denture design. The teeth are often supra-erupted and their tips may lie close to the opposing alveolar ridge even when the mandible is in the postural position. The danger here is that a lower denture may be constructed with an occlusal plane that is too high in relation to the resting position of the tongue and that

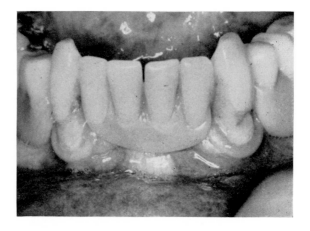

(a)

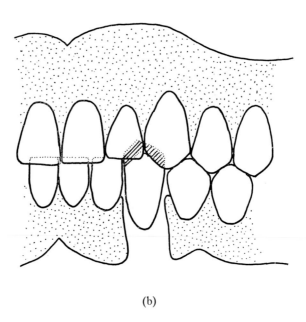

(b)

Fig. 3.4 The problem of retaining lower canines:
(a) the tips of the canines are well above the occlusal plane;
(b) the height of the canines in relation to the denture teeth results in interference on
any lateral movement. They may be ground as indicated in the drawing to allow
lateral excursive movements.

to create sufficient interocclusal space between upper and lower dentures the occlusal face height may be increased beyond the norm for the patient. Alternatively the operator may decide to accommodate the canines by incorporating a large step in the occlusal plane. This will effectively limit any excursionary movements of the mandible (Fig. 3.4) and cause rocking of the upper denture whenever movements are attempted, with subsequent trauma to the supporting tissues and the possibility of fracture of the upper denture base or teeth. Therefore if canines are retained which are supra-erupted or where a large vertical overlap had existed in the natural dentition, the length of the crowns of the retained teeth must be reduced.

A further danger of retaining canines is the probability of deterioration of their supporting tissues caused by the coverage of their gingival margins by denture base material and also by the leverage exerted on the teeth by clasps used to aid the retention of the denture.

However, when the remaining areas of the edentulous ridge have undergone gross resorption, or difficulties of adaptation to dentures by an older patient are foreseen, there are advantages in retaining the lower canines in particular for a few years. The advantages may be greater, however, if a more sophisticated approach is made to their retention and an overlay prosthesis planned.

Chapter 4

Overlay Dentures

Modified teeth or root surfaces may be used for support and retention of an otherwise complete denture. Such a prosthesis is called an *overlay denture* or a *hybrid denture*.

Support from roots reduces the load applied to the soft tissues and can thereby improve the efficiency of complete dentures in mastication. Retention obtained from attachments secured to the roots gives the patient more confidence in the use of complete dentures, particularly in the lower jaw.

The mucoperiosteum covering the denture bearing areas is not designed to accept occlusal loads applied to it by a denture. Nor does the shape of the alveolar ridge always provide sufficient positive retention. Whilst a subconscious reduction of the functional load by the patient assists in limiting tissue trauma, some patients suffer from constant discomfort particularly on the lower denture bearing area. Tissue trauma is increased if there is excessive denture movement or vigorous muscle activity, either during eating, or during 'empty mouth' grinding or clenching. Although muscular control is normally developed and prevents undue or embarrassing denture movement, many patients seek better oral function than that given by a denture that is supported and retained only by the edentulous ridge.

There is still a general tendency for dentists to think that when a patient has only a few teeth left, the best treatment would be to remove these and provide complete dentures. It is not usually possible, however, to predict with certainty whether the patient will have any problems in the future with complete dentures. Once the remaining teeth have been extracted their potential value in support and retention of a denture is lost. For problem cases which arise after removal of all the teeth, attempts are sometimes made by means of implants of various types to provide a denture support which is superior to that provided by the mucoperiosteum alone. It should be appreciated, however, that the periodontal membrane of the natural tooth is ideally suited to give support against occlusal stresses. The root of a natural tooth is therefore superior to any form of artificial implant. If such support is available, it should not be discarded unless one is sure that the patient will be satisfied with a conventional type of complete denture, supported entirely by the mucoperiosteum. In fact there is something to be said for always retaining some teeth in a modified form for use immediately as aids to support and retention, or as an insurance policy to be used at a later date if problems arise with a conventional type of denture.

Apart from providing the possibility of increased support and retention for a denture, the presence of some modified teeth may also give to the denture wearer the advantages of alveolar ridge preservation and better intra-oral discriminatory ability.

Alveolar Ridge Preservation

Extraction of mandibular teeth, in particular, results in a rapid and progressive loss of the residual alveolar process. Studies have shown that, when comparing the anterior part of the lower alveolar process to that of the upper jaw, the ratio of bone loss is 4 to 1. This loss of bone from the lower anterior region has a serious effect on the function and comfort of a lower denture.

There are, of course, marked differences in the rate and amount of resorption of alveolar bone in individual patients in a given period of time. Studies have shown, however, that the retention of modified teeth or roots in the anterior part of the alveolar process prevents alveolar bone loss in the areas concerned, provided of course that periodontal inflammation does not occur. In the first two years of one study, no change occurred in the height of the residual alveolar ridge where roots had been retained, compared with an average bone loss of 4 millimetres in the first year after extraction in a patient provided with conventional mucosa-borne dentures.

Discriminatory Ability

It has been shown that with complete dentures, the ability of patients to perceive small directional lateral forces is reduced. The minimal threshold for perception of force with mucosa-borne dentures is 6 to 10 times that required when receptors in the periodontal membranes of natural teeth are involved. In animal experiments, the natural canines were shown to be the most responsive of teeth to blunt stimulation. Further, the removal of the entire pulpal tissue resulted in no change in the response of their periodontal receptors. Also, if all the crown and even most of the root was removed, only light pressure on the remaining part of the root was necessary to cause a response. Anterior teeth are more sensitive to load than the posterior teeth and they are more able to discern small lateral deflective forces.

There appears to be little doubt that if a denture is in contact with or attached to roots, the patient has a significantly increased ability to discriminate between the size of objects placed between the teeth and to sense the direction and to control the amount of force applied to the denture and its supporting tissues. This ability is reduced markedly when the last tooth or root is removed from the dental arch.

SUPPORT

If root support for a prosthesis is planned, two or more roots should be retained, preferably one on either side of the midline. Although the retention of roots in any area of the mouth appears to offer advantages, this is particularly beneficial in the lower anterior region. As many lower anterior teeth as possible should be retained provided they have satisfactory alveolar bone support and that periodontal inflammation is absent or can be controlled.

To utilize a root for support, the crown is reduced either to a conical form or to a root face slightly above the level of the gingival margin. This reduces the trauma to the gingival tissues by the overlay denture when it is seated. The conical form is used where deposits of secondary dentine in the teeth of an older patient have reduced the size of the pulp chamber so that it may be accommodated within a shorter conical clinical crown. Telescopic crowns may then be fitted, consisting of two gold thimbles which fit one inside the other. The smaller is attached to the tooth and the larger to the denture.

Where this is not practicable, endodontic treatment is carried out, the crown of the tooth removed, and the root face trimmed to a domed or tent shaped form.

Where the root has been trimmed almost to the gingival margin, the root face is covered with a diaphragm which is retained by a short post that extends into the root canal. If adjacent teeth are used, the root caps may be joined together. This requires, of course, that the crown preparations or the root canals are made parallel, a circumstance not always readily achieved. The overlay denture presses on the metal covering when a load is applied to the denture. At rest, there is a small space between denture and root surface. The overlay denture may be located precisely in the case of telescopic crowns, or to a lesser extent by incorporating a hollow or protrusion on the mating surfaces. With less precise methods of location, a number of teeth may be utilized without having to consider their relative angulations.

It is preferable to cover the exposed dentine and so reduce the possibility of carious attack. With good oral hygiene and application of topical fluoride, however, caries may be avoided. Whilst a gold covering reduces caries, its margins may well cause gingival irritation.

Coverage of the gingival margins of the reduced teeth or roots, with consequent stagnation, predisposes to deterioration of the periodontal ligament and bone support. However the ease of cleaning the remaining parts of the teeth together with the reduced crown-root ratio has been found to result in an improvement in the health of the periodontal tissues and a reduction in the mobility of the roots where this had previously been evident.

A similar type of support can be incorporated in an immediate denture by preparation of one or more teeth, construction of the denture, followed by extraction of the non-required teeth.

RETENTION

Retentive devices can also be attached to roots, particularly those which have been root filled. These devices may be of simple construction, such as wires engaging in undercuts on studs attached to the root. Others consist of manufactured components which have two parts. The patrix, or male portion, is attached to the root and the matrix, or female portion, to the denture.

The retentive type of the overlay prosthesis should be considered where the residual ridges are almost non-existent and in cases where for reasons of speech, retching or excessive salivation, a palateless type of upper denture is necessary. The natural teeth intended for use with this type of prosthesis are chosen according to the principles of indirect retention used in partial denture designing. Here, maximum indirect retention is achieved when the clasp line, in passing through the denture base, divides it into two approximately equal parts. Where the alveolar ridges are well formed, teeth on only one side of the arch can be utilized as retainers for the prosthesis using the extended labial and buccal flanges of the denture to provide indirect retention. With low alveolar ridges the flanges will not be of sufficient size and therefore indirect retention must be achieved by using teeth on both sides of the arch as retainers (Fig. 4.1).

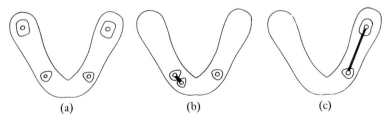

Fig. 4.1 Location of abutments for an overlay prosthesis:
(a) ideal position;
(b) anterior teeth with 32| splinted together;
(c) teeth on one side of the arch only—only suitable where the alveolar ridge is well-formed.

The retainer teeth may be splinted together, thus possibly reducing the rate of bone loss which may take place. Alternatively, roots may be joined together by a connecting bar which itself has a retentive shape.

Simple attachments to individual roots can be made by creating an undercut on a stud attached to the diaphragm on the root surface. The denture has a recess which is spaced away from this stud. Into the sides of the recess are fitted stainless steel wires which engage in the undercut. The attachment is not a precise one and the wires can be adjusted to vary their retentive effect.

More precise methods of attachment are available as manufactured units. These are generally a press-stud type of fitting for use on individual teeth. Some of these locate the denture and roots precisely and firmly, whilst others allow some individual movement between the two.

TYPES OF ATTACHMENT

For use on individual teeth, the Rotherman type of attachment (Fig. 4.2) consists of a circular patrix with an eccentric annular groove, deeper on one side than the other. The matrix is a clasp-like structure retained in a recess

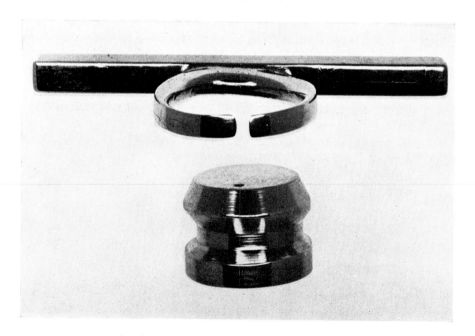

Fig. 4.2 Rotherman eccentric type of attachment.

within the denture. This is pressed over the patrix and fits into the undercut in the annular groove, where it resists displacement of the denture; the deepest undercut being engaged by the tips of the arms of the matrix. This type of attachment is small in height and does not interfere greatly with denture design. It gives good retention, is readily cleaned and can be adjusted for degree of retention.

The Dalbo 604 attachment (Fig. 4.3) is somewhat taller in form and secures retention by the matrix gripping below the equator of a ball-shaped patrix. A spring-loaded form of this attachment, 604P, achieves some occlusal loading of the tooth; the spring allowing for soft tissue compression.

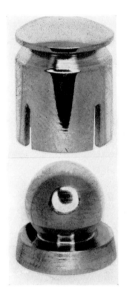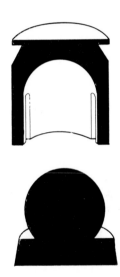

Fig. 4.3 Dalbo 604 attachment.

Where the retained roots are on either side of the mouth, they may be joined and splinted together by a bar. This may be of oval, D-shaped, or rectangular section. A Dolder bar joint of oval section (Fig. 4.4) retains an open metal sleeve attached to the underside of the denture. This type of bar gives good retention which can be modified by adjusting the sides of the metal sleeve matrix. The matrix is positioned so that a space is maintained between it and the upper surface of the bar when the denture is at rest. When locating the sleeve matrix on the cast, a spacer is placed between the matrix and the patrix. The thickness of this spacer should be related to the compressibility of the

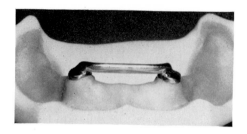 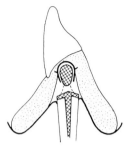

Fig. 4.4 Dolder bar and sleeve.

mucosa. This ensures that on compression of the soft tissues under the remainder of the denture, the load is shared by the roots and the tissues and is not supported only by the bar.

Many of these attachments are soldered to the root diaphragms but some

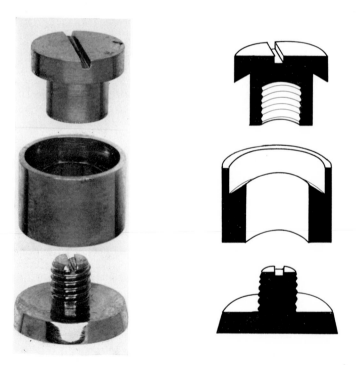

Fig. 4.5 Schubiger screw block attachment. The base is attached to the tooth and the screw retains the middle sleeve section to which a Dolder bar can be attached.

can be screwed into place. With several types of attachment, the thread is the same, so that different attachments can be screwed into the same diaphragm without having to replace the diaphragm and post. For example, the Schubiger screw block (Fig. 4.5) allows the attachment of a Gerber patrix, or the attachment of one end of a Dolder bar, to the same root. This has two advantages. Teeth utilized originally for individual attachments may later be combined for use with a Dolder bar. For example, if $\overline{43|3}$ are used with individual attachments screwed in place on Schubiger blocks, then if $\overline{4|}$ is lost, $\overline{3|3}$ can be joined by a Dolder bar screwed into place. The second advantage of this type of attachment arises if the cementation at one end of a Dolder bar fails. With screwed attachments, it is possible to take the structure apart, to effect repair and then to reassemble it. When soldered joints are used, the entire structure must be removed for any repair.

POINTS IN TECHNIQUE

To accommodate the bulk of the patrix, the upper portion of the root canal may be widened, thus allowing slight recessing of the patrix into the root. Sufficient dentine must be left, however, to give adequate strength to the wall of the canal.

The matrices may be attached individually to the denture or alternatively fixed to a metal sub-base round which the denture is moulded subsequently.

The technique varies from case to case but usually the apex of each root canal is sealed whilst the teeth still have their normal crowns. Good access to the pulp chamber is created. Then the crowns are removed and a temporary denture provided which simply fits over the roots. It is preferable that this denture is not spaced away from the gingival margins otherwise the gingival contour tends to change during the course of treatment.

Impressions of the root faces are recorded with posts in position, using a copper ring to ensure good adaptation of the impression material to the gingival area. To the dies from these impressions transfer copings are made with a projection into the mouth which has an undercut or cube shape. An impression of the entire denture bearing area is recorded and to this, a special tray is made. This should be closely adapted to the saddle areas but spaced away from the root faces. The tray may either allow sufficient space to accommodate the copings or alternatively, holes may be made in the tray through which the copings can protrude. An impression is recorded in a material such as an elastomer or zinc oxide-eugenol paste. When the copings protrude through the tray, they are attached to it by a self-cure acrylic polymer or by the use of impression plaster. To the resultant impression the diaphragms are constructed and the patrices arranged so that they are approximately parallel. Divergence of the angle of the patrices causes difficulties in locating the more precise types of attachment and the use of some form of parallelometer is necessary.

One technique is then to complete the denture on this impression, locating the posts and diaphragms first on the cast and then putting in place the matrices and waxing up the denture. An alternative method is to construct the posts with diaphragm and patrices and then to cement these in place. An impression may then be recorded in a silicone or thiokol impression material, either in the type of tray previously described, or in the denture which is completed except for the attachment of the matrices. A recess is left in the fitting surface of the denture to accommodate the matrix and a small amount of impression material placed in this recess to take an impression of the patrix.

In either case, duplicate male attachments are inserted into the impression and the cast poured. It is then a relatively simple matter to place the matrices in position and to attach these to the denture.

When a Dolder bar is already soldered to the diaphragms and posts, then it has to be cemented into the mouth and an impression recorded of it *in situ*. The space beneath the bar can be filled in with wax or plaster. A detachable bar retained by screws can be removed in the impression and thus located more precisely on the cast.

One of the problems with all types of attachment is their bulk and the effect this has on the shape and size of the denture provided. Speech difficulties may arise from restriction of tongue space. It will be appreciated that dentures must be constructed which conform to the normal principles of denture design. Correct peripheral extension is essential. Anterior and posterior tooth positions, occlusion and the shape of polished surfaces should not be modified in an attempt to accommodate the use of attachments. In particular, the occlusal face height of the dentures should not be increased to accommodate the extra bulk. Attachments should be considered as additions to a normal denture rather than that their presence should create a new denture shape.

Rebasing

Another difficulty associated with the overlay denture arises when one wishes to rebase it at a later date. It is possible to record a wash impression and to place duplicate patrices into the matrices before pouring the cast. However, difficulties often arise due to small technical inaccuracies and frequently, the attachments must later be removed from the denture and relocated with precision in the mouth.

Techniques of construction and rebasing of overlay dentures are developing actively, and the reader is referred to specialist texts and the current literature for details.

CARE OF OVERLAY DENTURES

All patients with complete dentures require regular inspection. Those with the overlay type of denture should be seen every six months. Then the periodontal support of the remaining roots may be carefully assessed, both visually and with the aid of radiographs. Any deterioration of the gingival margins and the periodontal ligament suggests either poor oral hygiene or movement of the denture or both.

Chapter 5

The Provision of
Dentures After Extractions

An immediate denture is one that is constructed prior to the extraction of the natural teeth and inserted immediately after their removal. Such treatment has been practised for at least 50 years. At one time, however, it was an un-common procedure reserved for certain patients who were so treated because loss of teeth was a particular embarrassment to them professionally or socially, or because they were prepared to pay the higher fee that was charged for such treatment. All other patients were rendered edentulous and then, after periods of time varying from a few weeks to several months, dentures were constructed.

Nowadays, there is an increasing 'awareness' of dentistry by the public, and knowledge of the advantages to be gained by immediate insertion of dentures has spread. In fact, today it is usual for a patient to ask for this type of treatment.

There are, however, some operators who still prefer to delay the construc-tion of dentures for weeks or months after extraction.

DENTURES PROVIDED SOON
AFTER EXTRACTION

Impressions are recorded when there is no longer any danger of disturbing the organizing blood clot within the socket. Under normal healing conditions an intact layer of protective epithelium may cover the sockets within a week, and impressions can then be recorded. Some operators may, however, prefer a slightly longer delay before recording impressions.

During the early healing period there are fairly rapid changes in the overall shape of the alveolar ridge due to soft tissue shrinkage and resorptive activity on the bony margins of the sockets. Therefore, the time interval between re-cording impressions and the insertion of the dentures must be as short as possible. A delay of more than a few days will result in poor adaptation of the fitting surface, resulting in diminished retention. In addition the alveolar ridge is often irregular and nodular at this stage. This is particularly so when the teeth have been removed with some trauma as might be the case under an inadequate general anaesthetic. Deformation or fracture of the socket walls produces a poor denture foundation which is slow to heal. The mucoperiosteum may be stretched tightly over the bony prominences and pressure from the denture in these areas usually causes pain. This situation continues until the nodular areas have been rounded by the slow process of resorption. As tissue changes occur, the denture becomes ill-fitting and non-retentive. Therefore, there will be continued discomfort as the denture moves in function and is thrust against the bony prominences.

In contrast, the denture inserted immediately after extraction has greater stability and retention with less movement occurring and consequently less discomfort. This is largely a result of the careful planning of the denture on a cast obtained from an impression recorded before extraction, when the oral tissues are relatively stabilized in form.

Thus, the provision of a 'temporary' denture inserted in the early weeks after extraction is not a procedure to be recommended. In addition to the disadvantages just discussed, there is also the possibility of increasing the amount of jaw separation beyond tolerable limits where insufficient interalveolar space is available. This may occur where the alveolar ridges are bulbous and in cases where there was previously a large vertical overlap of the natural anterior teeth. Even when the patient is able to tolerate the diminished freeway space, the 'bedding in' of the denture may result in an accelerated resorption of bone.

Perhaps the only advantage of this technique is that memory of tooth shape, position and arrangement should still be fairly strong in the minds of both the patient and the dentist in the early weeks after extraction, and therefore a reasonable aesthetic result should be achieved.

DENTURES PROVIDED SOME MONTHS AFTER EXTRACTION

This treatment plan delays denture construction until there is a smooth, rounded alveolar ridge. The major reconstruction of the extraction area takes place during the first 6 months after extractions, and the subsequent tissue changes, although continuing indefinitely, proceed then at a much slower rate. A study of postextraction tissue changes over a $2\frac{1}{2}$ year period revealed that 80 per cent of the change that was observed had taken place within the first 6 months; after 1 year, 90 per cent of the total change had already taken place.

This study gives some support to those who advise their patients to wait for 6 months before construction of dentures so that resorption may be 'complete'. Undoubtedly, at this time the ridges are much more favourable for denture construction, but the delay results in a number of problems for the operator and the patient. Much experienced guesswork is necessary to produce dentures that have an appearance similar to the natural teeth, and which also restore function at the correct vertical and horizontal jaw relations. Over the months, the dentist's memory of the tooth appearance and the correct facial proportions of the patient will become very hazy. By pre-extraction records, attempts are made to keep information concerning the teeth available during the healing period. Photographs of the patient, articulated casts of the dentition, records of the patient's profile and various facial measurements are all used. Not one of these methods, however, is entirely satisfactory.

Although this form of treatment is illogical it is still used. So much of the information required to construct dentures is available from the natural dentition, that it must be appreciated how unintelligent is this method of destroying all the information and then several months later, trying to guess what it was.

Not only is information on aesthetics lost, but, in addition, the patient's mandibular movements become imprecise due to the loss of tooth contact sensation. The muscles no longer move the jaws together in the same movement pattern which was used when the natural teeth occluded and a variety of different closing movement patterns may be developed. In consequence, the dentist may have difficulty in assessing and recording the correct jaw relations.

Tongue and cheeks begin to invade the future denture areas. As a result the patient has subsequently to adjust to the bulk of the dentures suddenly placed in the mouth, after a period of months when there has been a reduction in the volume of tissue between the tongue and cheeks following tooth extraction and bone resorption.

Without an immediate denture, resorption of the alveolar process may be influenced by pressure from the tongue, cheeks or the opposing jaw or teeth. Heavy chewing directly onto the healing ridges tends to mould them to a flat-topped shape, or where natural teeth remain in the opposing jaw, direct trauma to the ridge by the teeth takes place. In an attempt to approximate the ridges for masticatory purposes, abnormal mandibular movements are likely to develop. In some cases this may result in an imbalance of the musculature with the possible development of a pain–dysfunction temporomandibular joint syndrome.

Even in a 6 month period after extraction the mandible approximates to the maxilla and maintains a new relation closer to it. This is possibly associated with a shortening of those muscles controlling the relation of mandible to maxilla. Such a changed relation is difficult to correct with complete dentures and often becomes permanent with loss of face height and consequent adverse effect on apperarance. Whilst some restoration of jaw relation can be achieved when treating a young patient, this type of change is less reversible when treating older patients.

In addition, tonicity of the lips and cheeks of the older patient is likely to be reduced due to lack of tooth support. It must be noted, however, that in the young edentulous patient tonus of the lips is maintained for some considerable time after extraction, and it is difficult to tell from a profile view whether such a patient is in fact edentulous (Fig. 5.1).

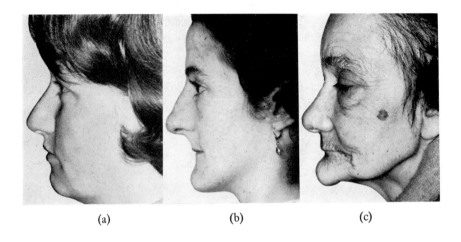

(a)   (b)   (c)

Fig. 5.1 Profile views of edentulous patients:
(a) patient aged 21, edentulous 2 years—lip tone maintained;
(b) patient aged 29, edentulous 6 years—lip tone not maintained;
(c) patient aged 70, edentulous 40 years—lip tone not maintained.

Because a normal lip-tooth-tongue relationship is necessary for correct production of sounds, the absence of teeth affects the quality of speech.

The lack of masticatory function frequently causes gastritis in patients rendered edentulous and this may exacerbate a pre-existing gastric or duodenal complaint.

Thus, immediate restoration of lost natural teeth should be the usual treatment and only in unusual circumstances should the patient have to tolerate an edentulous period. Even when the immediate dentures are worn for only a short period of time, the information transferred by them from the natural teeth is essential and most valuable in the construction of replacement dentures when this becomes necessary.

TREATMENT PLANNING
FOR THE IMMEDIATE DENTURE

As in all forms of dental treatment, the provision of a complete immediate denture requires forethought, so that the best result is obtained with the least inconvenience to the patient.

THE PATIENT WITH DENTAL CARIES

The patient who has been attending regularly for the treatment of dental caries, presents the simpler problem in immediate denture treatment planning. Many of the posterior teeth may already have been lost and a partial prosthesis will have been provided to maintain function. The dental history usually reveals that natural teeth have been extracted singly, and teeth added by immediate replacement, to the existing partial denture. When only a few teeth remain it is necessary to decide whether to remove all the remaining teeth together and provide a complete denture, or to allow them to be lost gradually. Usually a gradual process of replacement of the dentition is preferred, but there are cases where a more radical approach is indicated. For example, when anterior teeth are discoloured as a result of extrinsic or intrinsic staining, or when there are large discoloured restorations, there may be a problem in providing a satisfactory aesthetic restoration. This is often difficult when only one or two stained teeth remain. Again, the difficulties of providing an acceptable aesthetic result by coronal restorations on a number of broken-down anterior crowns, may point towards total extraction and immediate replacement.

THE PATIENT WITH
PERIODONTAL DISEASE

Patients with periodontal disease, require multiple extractions when periodontal inflammation can no longer be controlled. Usually a number of teeth remain both in the posterior and anterior segments of the jaw. Therefore a decision has to be made regarding the order in which teeth should be extracted and the number that are to be replaced eventually by an immediate denture.

GENERAL CONSIDERATIONS ON THE ORDER
AND NUMBER OF TEETH TO BE EXTRACTED

Surgical Problems

Removal of teeth is a relatively minor surgical procedure and therefore it should be possible to extract a large number of natural teeth and to replace them by immediate dentures. Whilst this may be done for a hospitalized patient, it is not advisable for the patient visiting a dental practice. For the ambulant patient, the number of teeth extracted at one time should be limited. When providing upper and lower immediate dentures, the dentist should aim at enabling his patient to resume his normal occupation the day after operation. An important factor to be considered when deciding on the amount of surgery at one visit is the patient's general health and, if necessary, there should be consultation with his physician.

The number of teeth to be extracted in one jaw should not exceed eight, of which up to three may be premolar and molar teeth. Where extractions are to be carried out simultaneously in both jaws, the total number of teeth to be extracted should not exceed fourteen.

It is frequently advocated, when planning an immediate denture, that all the posterior teeth should be extracted and the edentulous areas allowed to heal before the anterior teeth are extracted and the complete denture inserted. It is not so essential that all posterior teeth should be extracted, but rather that the areas of healed ridge should be large enough to resist the forces of mastication. In considering posterior teeth for immediate replacement the possible difficulties of extraction must be assessed. The dentist should inquire about previous extractions; if there is a history of difficulty, radiographic examination is advised. If it seems likely that surgical removal will be necessary, then this should be done some weeks before the immediate denture is to be inserted. Otherwise, because of the amount of bone removed, there will be a lack of adaptation of the immediate denture in the area concerned and prob-able discomfort due to uneven pressure.

A further factor to be considered when deciding on the number of posterior teeth that should be extracted at the time of insertion of the denture, is the distortion of the outer plate of bone which accompanies their extraction. After the removal of molar teeth in either jaw, a bony undercut frequently remains on the buccal or lingual aspect. Increase of this undercut, caused by distortion of the bone on extraction, leads to trauma and discomfort under an immediate denture. Whilst reflection of flaps and bone trimming can be carried out, the authors feel that this type of treatment should be limited to the anterior segment of the mouth when an immediate denture is to be provided.

The number of posterior teeth to be immediately replaced in each jaw should not exceed three. A larger number reduces the possibility of a comfort-able and uneventful healing period after the insertion of the denture. In fact, where there is a history of difficult extractions, it is wise to leave only the anterior teeth for immediate replacement. Certainly all posterior teeth with crowns badly damaged by caries should be removed before immediate denture treatment is commenced.

Maintenance of Jaw Relations

The temporary retention of a few occluding posterior teeth is of advantage in maintaining the present jaw relation and occlusal face height. Where only anterior teeth remain or the posterior teeth are unopposed, there is the possibility of a change in jaw relations in horizontal and vertical planes. As the lower teeth move upwards and backwards over the inclined planes that comprise the palatal surfaces of the upper anterior teeth, a distal displacement of the mandible may occur. Resistance to this displacement may be provided by the presence of well-developed cingulae on the upper teeth, particularly where the incisor tooth relation is Class I. However, in cases with a Class II div 2 incisor relation with a deep vertical incisal overlap and retroclined upper teeth, the possibility of distal displacement of the mandible is much greater.

With continued heavy loading the supporting tissues of the upper anterior teeth may break down causing a progressive splaying of the teeth. The mandible will then tend to take up a more forward position closer to the maxilla. Labial migration of the upper anterior teeth and overclosure are more likely to follow the extraction of the posterior teeth when the anterior teeth have lost bone support due to periodontal disease, or when the anterior teeth are markedly proclined.

When the original incisor relation has been edge to edge, the loss of posterior occlusal contacts does not necessarily result in the mandible being displaced either anteriorly or posteriorly. In fact if some attrition of the incisal edges has already taken place by the time the posterior teeth are lost, the enlarged incisal contact area may provide resistance to mandibular displacement (Fig. 5.2). Alternatively, the mandible may be postured forwards in an effort to gain maximum occlusal contact when some, but not all, of the posterior teeth have been lost.

Clinical examination usually enables the dentist to assess whether a change in jaw relations is likely to occur if all the posterior teeth are removed. When the position and anatomical form of the incisor teeth and the health of the supporting tissues suggest resistance to a change in jaw relations, it is not essential to retain the posterior teeth unless they make a major contribution to masticatory function.

Where many of the anterior teeth have already been replaced by a denture but occlusion of a few posterior teeth maintains the correct jaw relation, an immediate denture is still advisable to avoid the guesswork in determining jaw relations once the vital information given by the occluding teeth has been lost.

Thus, the immediate replacement of $\underline{7\ 4\ |\ 1\ 3\ 5}$ is advisable if $\underline{7\ 4\ |\ 5}$ occlude with lower teeth in the correct jaw relation. There are no advantages in retaining posterior teeth which are out of occlusion and these should be extracted before immediate denture construction commences.

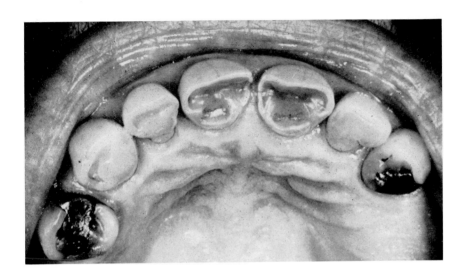

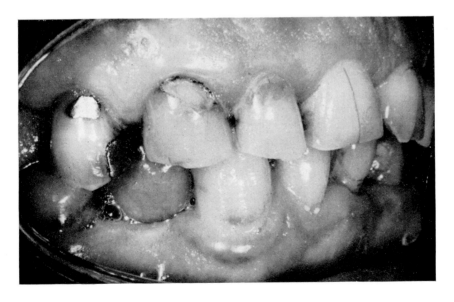

Fig. 5.2 Enlarged incisal contact area preventing distal mandibular displacement.

PROVISION OF A SINGLE
COMPLETE DENTURE

Where there is to be no radical change in anterior tooth position, an immediate denture may be provided in one jaw at a time. The position and form of the teeth in the opposing jaw must be carefully analysed before deciding on their temporary retention. The incisal edges of the natural anterior teeth and the occlusal surfaces of the posterior teeth may require considerable modification if the immediate denture in the opposing jaw is to have any prospect of stability in function. However, the single immediate complete denture should always be considered for patients in poor general health, in preference to immediate dentures in both jaws, as the amount of surgical trauma from multiple extractions is reduced.

CONTRA-INDICATIONS TO IMMEDIATE
DENTURE CONSTRUCTION

There are in fact very few contra-indications to immediate replacement of the natural dentition. In the past it has been suggested that patients with multiple periapical or periodontal abscesses, or those suffering from diabetes, are poor immediate denture 'risks'. Suitable antibiotic cover will, however, usually combat satisfactorily the possibility of postextraction infection in such cases. Again, patients with haemophilia or Christmas disease often have badly broken down or periodontally involved natural teeth which have been retained far too long because of the oft-quoted dangers of multiple extractions in such cases. It is possible to carry out multiple extractions for such patients provided that treatment is carefully planned, and there is cooperation between the physician and the dental surgeon. Patients with haemophilia should be assessed firstly for the degree of haemophilia. In hospital, their Factor D level should be supplemented until healing is satisfactory. The teeth are preferably extracted with local anaesthesia. The immediate dentures act as splints.

Immediate dentures should not be constructed for patients with gross oral neglect for they are unlikely to carry out the home care necessary for the prevention of postsurgical inflammatory sequelae under the immediate dentures. In such cases, acute inflammatory conditions should be cleared up prior to extraction and dentures constructed when healing is well advanced.

Similarly, immediate dentures should not be planned where considerable oral surgery is necessary in the anterior region for the eradication of a cystic condition or for the removal of deeply embedded teeth. In such cases it will be impossible to predetermine accurately the amount of bone removal; also postoperative oedema may prevent the wearing of an immediate denture.

Any patient who has had radiotherapy requires the greatest care when teeth have to be extracted. In fact, extraction of teeth should be avoided as far as possible because of the great risk of an osteo-radionecrosis developing even many years after the radiotherapy. For such patients, teeth should be extracted singly and a denture not inserted in case pressure from it should lead to an intractable breakdown of the healing tissues.

Some patients fear the insertion of the immediate restoration denture and cannot imagine other than acute discomfort to themselves if a denture is placed upon the open socket wound. Uncooperative patients or those of reduced intelligence remove their immediate dentures a few hours after insertion and seem quite happy to await resorption. This is largely a question of patient education and where a good immediate denture service is provided, this prejudice is rapidly overcome. The simile between a cut finger and an open extraction socket is often useful in discussing immediate denture provision with the patient. A cut finger is carefully bandaged, whilst a deep penetrating open wound in the mouth is left completely uncovered. The immediate denture acts as a bandage or splint and in fact gives more comfort than if the area is left uncovered. This argument, plus the advantages of appearance and function, is usually sufficient to obtain the patient's cooperation in immediate denture treatment.

TEMPORARY PARTIAL DENTURES

For patients who are not already wearing partial dentures there are some advantages in providing these approximately 4 to 6 weeks after the extraction of any posterior teeth which are not included in the immediate denture plan. Such dentures are made in acrylic polymer with the addition of simple wrought clasps to give retention. Then, some 3 to 6 months later, these partial dentures are easily converted to immediate complete dentures.

Temporary partial dentures assist in maintaining the jaw relations and also reduce the invasion of soft tissue into the edentulous areas (Fig. 5.3). They help the patient in the transition from the natural to the completely artificial dentition. The patient accommodates to a small denture bulk before being provided with a complete denture. In addition, a pattern for masticatory function is developed with the partial dentures and less adaptation is required when these dentures are converted to complete immediate dentures.

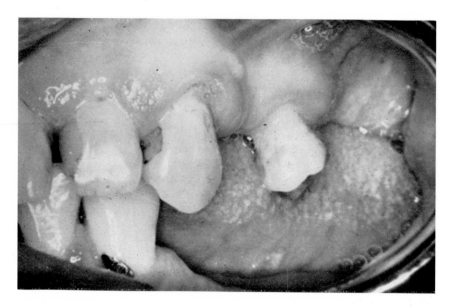

Fig. 5.3 Invasion of the edentulous areas by the tongue.

THE TYPES OF IMMEDIATE DENTURE

There are two main types of immediate denture:
1 The open face denture
2 The flanged denture—with complete labial flange
                        —with part labial flange.

THE OPEN FACE DENTURE

This is the simplest form of immediate denture. The artificial teeth are set either in or close to the sockets of their natural predecessors and no labial flange is added (Fig. 5.4a).

The open face immediate denture is indicated when sufficient retention can be obtained from the rest of the alveolar process. Hence, it can frequently be used in the upper jaw, but is not recommended in the lower.

If the posterior teeth have been extracted within the last few years the ridge shape and size in the upper jaw will usually provide a good basis for retention of an open face immediate denture. A direct assessment of potential retention will be gained if the patient has a temporary partial denture. Where the posterior teeth have been absent for some years, and the ridge shape is poor, the retention of the open face denture may not be adequate and a flanged denture is indicated. In the lower jaw, the retention of an open face immediate denture is always poor and even when the patient has worn a temporary partial lower denture with satisfaction this should be followed by a flanged immediate denture.

THE FLANGED DENTURE

The flange in the anterior region may be either part or complete (Fig. 5.4 b, c). Wherever practicable, the complete flange should be used. Apart from the advantages of superior retention, the presence of a flange gives better protection to the sockets and thus assists more rapid healing.

Whilst ideally, all flanges should extend to the functional depth of the sulcus, difficulties frequently arise in the lower labial sulcus. Here, it is difficult to define the sulcus accurately due to the undercut which is frequently present. Often the impression is overextended and a fully extended flange will cause ulceration in the sulcus.

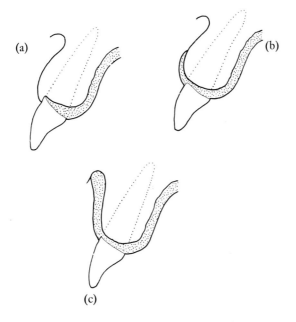

Fig. 5.4 Types of immediate denture:
(a) open face;
(b) part flange;
(c) full flange.

In the case of the lower denture, the flange may result in a poorer appearance than is obtained when an open face denture is used. This is particularly so where a reduction in vertical overlap of the incisors is deemed necessary. The reduction is usually achieved by shortening the lower anterior teeth and the length of the teeth is further reduced in the gingival area when a flange is added (Fig. 5.5). Frequently this appearance of the lower immediate denture has to be accepted. Later, appearance can be improved by the replacement of the lower anterior teeth with longer ones at the rebase stage when additional space will have been created by alveolar resorption.

A flange may often be provided without any bone trimming or alveoloplasty. The temptation to mould the alveolar process surgically for every patient must be resisted, since subsequent bone changes cannot be forecast with accuracy. The surgical removal of undercuts to simplify the provision of a denture with a complete labial flange in the upper jaw is seldom justified.

Obviously the flange must be of thin section or undue prominence of the

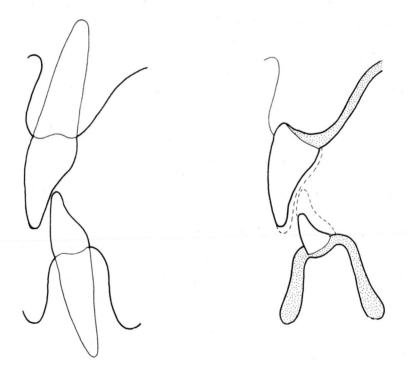

Fig. 5.5 Reduction in vertical incisor overlap at the expense of the lower incisors results in a shortening of the length of the crowns. The presence of a flange reduces their length further.

lips will result. It will be found, however, that sometimes the labial inclination of the alveolar process and the prominence of the canine eminences creates difficulties in achieving a well-fitting thin flange which can be inserted into the mouth easily and without injury to the tissues. It must be appreciated that the difficulties may appear greater on the cast than they are in the mouth. If the undercut areas are small (say up to 2 mm) there should be no problem because the resilience of the mucosa, which has been estimated to be within 1 to 2 mm, will allow the insertion of the denture without trauma. It is when the undercuts are greater than this and in particular when they are diametrically opposed by undercuts in the posterior region that problems arise. Here a detailed analysis of the cast using the surveyor is necessary. Having chosen a suitable path of insertion for the denture it will become obvious whether a complete flange is possible without alveoloplasty.

Alternatively a part labial flange may be used. This type of flange is extended just beyond the maximum contour of the alveolar process, to a point where the undercut engaged can be accepted by compression of the overlying soft tissues. This part flange affords some retention to the denture and avoids the gap between a complete flange and the tissues which is inevitable where a large bony undercut exists.

During the initial postextraction period, patients function quite satisfactorily with a denture that carries only a part labial flange which does not enter all the undercut areas. They are frequently quite comfortable and the appearance, particularly the upper lip contour, is often more natural. As normal postextraction resorption causes a reduction in prominence of the alveolar process, the extension of the flange may be increased.

Whilst most patients can be provided with complete dentures incorporating either a complete or part flange without the need for alveolar surgery, there is a *small* proportion of cases where reshaping of the alveolar process is necessary. Where there is marked protrusion of the upper alveolar process, both appearance and denture function can be improved by reshaping the alveolar bone at the time of extraction. Aesthetic improvement may be advisable when the patient has a short upper lip and displays gingival tissues as well as teeth on smiling. Whilst the patient's facial appearance should not be changed too radically, it may be necessary for denture stability to raise the incisal level and also move the anterior teeth backwards. Unless the shape of the bone is altered there is frequently not room for the position of the anterior teeth to be changed sufficiently.

Before deciding on alveoloplasty, a careful assessment must be made of the bony support of the teeth that are to be extracted. In many cases of superior alveolar protrusion, the outer plate of bone is very thin. This is particularly so where the supporting tissues of the teeth have been affected by periodontal disease. Clinical examination of the depth of pockets, accompanied by radiographs, if necessary, will reveal the extent of the walls of the sockets. Where deep pockets exist, no bone trimming apart from smoothing of the sharp margins of the socket walls is usually necessary. If the labial plate of bone is complete, alveoloplasty will be necessary and may be performed in one of two ways, by either *septal* or *radical* alveolectomy.

In the case of *septal* alveolectomy the interdental septa are removed after the extraction of the teeth and the outer cortical plate is then collapsed lingually onto the inner plate. This reduces the labial undercut, creates sufficient room for a complete labial flange and at the same time reduces the size of the sockets that have subsequently to be filled with new bone. When there is excessive protrusion of the premaxilla a septal alveolectomy will not usually provide sufficient reduction to improve appearance and function. In such cases a *radical* alveolectomy is performed and the outer cortical plate is sacrificed.

At one time the routine removal of the labial plate of bone was recommended in order to create space for a complete flange. However, it is now recognised that retention of as much alveolar process as possible is normally preferred. In particular the labial plate should be retained unless considerable change in shape in the region of the premaxillae is planned. Postextraction resorption appears to be reduced, certainly during the first year, if the labial plate is preserved.

THE IMPORTANCE OF STUDY CASTS

Study casts, mounted on a simple articulator, are essential for correct treatment planning. In association with clinical and radiographic evidence, these casts help in the decisions to be made regarding the order and number of teeth to be extracted. Any aesthetic improvements that might be made by altering tooth form and position are more easily explained and demonstrated to the patient with the aid of study casts. Similarly, the effects on the dentition of any contemplated changes in vertical and horizontal jaw relation are more readily assessed.

The treatment plan should be discussed with the patient and the technician. If changes in shape or arrangement of teeth, or modification to the bone are contemplated, they can be worked out on the casts. Hence, a duplicate set is useful for comparison.

Chapter 6

The Denture Bearing Areas

ANATOMY

UPPER JAW

The posterior border of the denture bearing area is usually defined in terms of the junction of the hard and soft palate. Such a precise anatomical definition distinguishes only between the area of the mucoperiosteum attached to the palatal process and the muscular soft palate with no underlying bony attachment. The periosteal attachment of the mucoperiosteum of the hard palate becomes less firm towards the soft palate and this anatomical outline is masked by the greater thickness of tissue covering the bone. Thus the posterior border of a denture does not often conform to the anatomical extent of the hard palate.

A change in the colour and texture of the mucosal covering indicates the junction between the hard palate and the soft palate. In the healthy mouth, the hard palate has a pale blue-pink colour due to the presence of a stratum corneum. This layer may be totally or partially lost on wearing a denture, particularly if wearing is continuous, and the palate will then appear to be redder in colour. The soft palate however, is yellow-red and often shows injected capillaries on its surface. The surface of the hard palate has sharp detail whilst the soft palate is more roundly contoured due to the presence of glandular tissue. In some patients the palatal foveae can be seen in this area as slight depressions either side of the midline.

It is important that the posterior border of the denture terminates on soft tissue and also that it is extended as far as possible. The posterior border is therefore better defined by function. In some patients, movement of the soft palate occurs at or near the anatomical junction. In others a moderate area of soft palate adjacent to the hard palate does not move and the denture extension can be greater. The slight transverse crease, the 'Ah' or vibrating line, is the only satisfactory means of defining the functional palatal extension of the upper denture.

Posterolaterally the denture bearing area is limited by the hamular notch behind the tuberosity. A fine band of fibrous tissue connects the end of the maxillary tuberosity to the hamular process and, from this, a few fibres of the buccinator muscle spring. The pterygomandibular ligament arises from its attachment on the hamulus of the medial pterygoid plate and passes downwards and slightly laterally towards the end of the mylohyoid line of the mandible. Anteriorly, this ligament provides attachment for the buccinator muscle and posteriorly for the superior constrictor of the pharynx.

Buccally, the maxillary tuberosity extension is limited by the buccinator muscle swinging out to form the cheek, thus closing the space between the maxilla and the mandible. This muscle splits and is attached partly to the pterygomandibular ligament and partly to the upper alveolar process. This often allows a considerable vertical extension of the denture in this region. Laterally the tuberosity area is related to the medial pterygoid muscle and to the coronoid process of the mandible. Both these structures limit the thickness of the denture flange round the tuberosity, since, on lateral movements of the jaw, the coronoid process moves nearer to the upper alveolar process (Fig. 6.1).

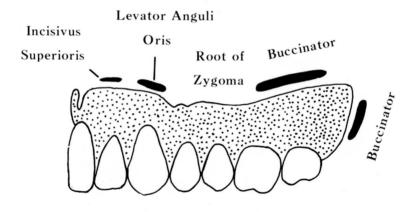

Fig. 6.1 Anatomical structures defining the labial and buccal border of the upper denture.

Mesially, the root of the zygoma presents a large, hard, rounded bony prominence which occasionally offers support for a denture but more frequently must be avoided by a downward sweep of the denture periphery. Slightly forward of this region small frena are frequently seen. These are tendinous attachments of the circumoral musculature, particularly the levator of the angle of the mouth.

Further forward, the upward extent of the denture is limited by the main attachment to the alveolar process of the levator anguli oris and the lateral band of fibres of the orbicularis oris called the incisivus superioris muscle. At the centre of the maxilla, a frenum sweeps down to attach to the alveolar process and thus limits the denture extension in the midline.

LOWER JAW

Starting in the midline labially, the central frenum similarly limits denture extension; then the labial border extends downwards and laterally (Fig. 6.2).

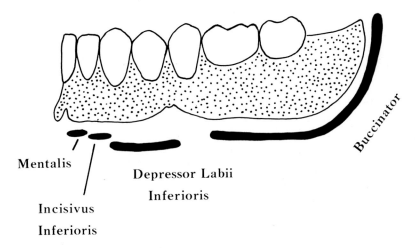

Mentalis

Depressor Labii
Inferioris

Incisivus

Inferioris

Buccinator

Fig. 6.2 Anatomical structures defining the labial and buccal border of the lower denture.

The attachments of the mentalis muscle, the incisivus inferioris and the depressor labii inferioris, control the extent of the denture flange in the incisor region until it passes beyond the second premolar tooth. Then the outline is defined by the attachment of the buccinator muscle to the oblique line of the mandible. Where the fibres of the buccinator decussate with those of the orbicularis oris muscle and the depressors and levators of the angle of the mouth, a hard knot of muscle is found, which is called the 'modiolus' (Fig. 6.3).

Passing backwards, the buccinator often forms a pouch in the cheek and frequently the denture base can be extended laterally to form a pronounced posterior buccal flange. The buccinator thus limits the lateral extension of the denture and, where it swings lingually to its attachment on the pterygomandibular ligament, also limits the distal extension along the edentulous ridge.

Distally the crest of the edentulous ridge bears an elevated soft pad of

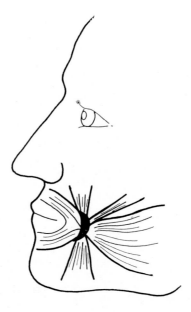

Fig. 6.3 The modiolus. Commencing with the orbicularis oris muscle and moving clockwise, the other muscles are the levator anguli oris, zygomaticus, buccinator and depressor labii inferioris.

mucosa, the retromolar pad. This is oval or round in outline and lies over the retromolar fossa. Just in front of the retromolar pad and often merging with it, there appears in the edentulous mouth a firm fibrous pad (Fig. 6.4). This is often pear-shaped as it arises from the collapse of the distal papilla into the socket when the last natural tooth is extracted. Normally, this papilla behind the last tooth is chronically inflamed due to accumulation of plaque, and this leads to the formation of a pad of fibrous tissue. The pad is not always clearly seen, as forward migration of the third molar tooth reduces the degree of inflammation present and this eliminates the source from which the fibrous tissue of the pad arises. The pear-shaped pad does not move during function but the retromolar pad does so at its distal end, on contraction of the buccinator. Hence, one cannot cover the entire retromolar pad but only its anterior border.

Behind the retromolar pad the buccinator muscle sweeps round the end of the denture bearing area to its attachment on the pterygomandibular ligament. Frequently a denture may be extended distally beyond the attachment of this ligament to run along the inner aspect of the mandible (Fig. 6.5). This postero-lingual extension is halted by the movement of the palatoglossus muscle

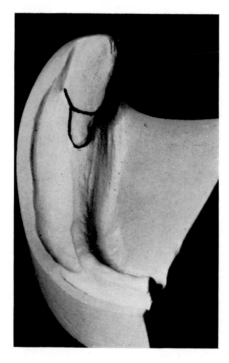

Fig. 6.4 The retromolar and pear-shaped pads marked out. The pear-shaped pad lies anterior to the retromolar pad.

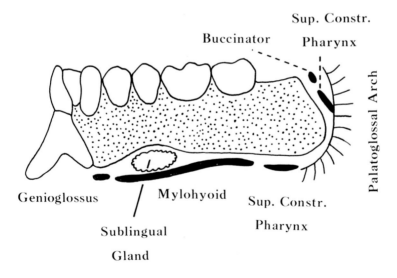

Fig. 6.5 Anatomical structures defining the lingual border of the lower denture.

forming the anterior pillar of the fauces. On swallowing, this muscular sphinc-ter moves forward and brings with it the loose mucosal fold which connects the arch with the lingual aspect of the mandible, thus limiting the distolingual extension of the lower denture. The superior constrictor of the pharynx is attached for a short length to the lingual aspect of the mandible and so defines the denture border downwards into the lingual sulcus. Further forward the attachment of the mylohyoid muscle controls the lingual extent of the denture flange. In the first molar region the sublingual gland lies over the mylohyoid muscle and usually necessitates an upward curve in the denture periphery. Coming to the centre of the mandible the genioglossus muscles spring from the superior genial tubercles and together with the frenum of the tongue produce a marked elevation limiting the extent of the denture in this region.

HISTOLOGICAL STRUCTURE

A knowledge of the histology of the soft tissues of the denture bearing area assists in an understanding of the changes in their shape which can take place on recording an impression.

MUCOSA

The oral mucosa covers the hard and soft palate, the lower alveolar ridge, and is continuous via the sulcus onto the inner aspect of the lips and cheeks. In parts, therefore, it is supported by bone but elsewhere it is a simple lining mucosa related to soft tissues such as muscle and connective tissue. Oral mucosa consists of a surface epithelial layer and a deeper connective tissue layer, the lamina propria or corium.

Oral Epithelium

This is a stratified squamous epithelium arising from a basement membrane (Fig. 6.6). The thickness of the epithelium is made up of cells which change morphologically as they approach the surface. In the middle layers, or stratum spinosum, the cells are separated by intercellular bridges. Tissue fluid circulates between the cells but is prevented from escaping by the closer arrangement of cells in the more superficial layers. These are flatter and show degenera-tive changes. They comprise first of all the stratum granulosum and then most superficially in some areas a stratum corneum or horny layer, without nuclei. The stratum corneum is only present, however, where the mucosa is stimu-lated during function. The tongue and hard palate are used in tactile appreciation of food, and in 'mastication' of softer foodstuffs. The epithelium covering these 'masticatory' areas, together with the crests of the edentulous ridges in the non-denture wearer, show a stratum corneum. Since the non-nucleated cells of the stratum corneum are relatively opaque, they give a lighter appearance to the areas so covered. In the denture wearer a stratum corneum may be seen in some areas. Whilst the edentulous ridges are now protected from direct masticatory stimulation, friction from the denture as it moves slightly against the epithelium in function may produce a stratum corneum.

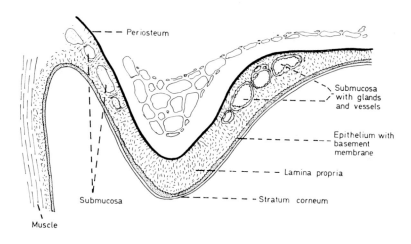

Fig. 6.6 Section of oral mucosa.

Elsewhere, in the sulcus and on the inner aspect of the lips and cheeks, no stratum corneum exists and the stratum granulosum is the most superficial layer. This tissue has a darker colour and the mucosa in these areas appears redder than those with a stratum corneum.

Lamina Propria

The corium or dermis is a layer of dense connective tissue, beneath the basement membrane of the epithelium. It contains a few elastic fibres, blood vessels, lymphatics, nerve fibres and their endings, but is mainly composed of collagen bundles and fibroblasts. In places, it is the only layer between the mucosa and the underlying anatomical structures. The lamina propria is a thin layer on the inner aspect of the lips and cheeks, over the soft palate and on the floor of the mouth. Here it is bound down to the adjacent muscles without a submucous layer.

Mucoperiosteum

Over the crests of the edentulous ridges and in the centre of the palate there is no submucous layer. The mucosa is firmly bound down to the periosteum to form a mucoperiosteum. The original gingival mucosa of the natural teeth grows across the tooth socket to form a firm mucoperiosteal covering. Beyond this gingival mucosa, however, the attachment to the periosteum becomes less firm and there is a thin submucosa which increases in thickness towards the sulcus.

SUBMUCOSA

In the sulcus of both jaws a submucous layer forms a soft cushion between the mucosa and the muscles beneath. Also, in the upper jaw, between the crest of the ridge and the centre of the palate in the molar and premolar regions, a submucous layer occurs, which contains the greater palatine nerves and vessels, mucous glands and fat cells. This submucous layer is not loose as in the sulcus, but is bound to the palatal bone by fibrous strands which pass through it joining its lamina propria to the periosteum. Lying between the fibrous strands in the posterior part of the palate are numerous mucous glands; in the anterior part of the palate there is an accumulation of fat cells.

SENSATION

Nerve endings in the normal gingival mucosa around standing teeth are found in the dermis and also in the epithelium. In the former, they consist mainly of Krause corpuscles. Just under and within the epithelium various types of endings are found. These may be fine, free nerve endings, coils or whorls, varying widely in complexity. On extraction of teeth and healing over of the resultant wound, this pattern of innervation is disturbed. It appears that the innervation of the mucosa covering the normal edentulous ridge is less orderly and less profuse than that found in normal gingival tissue. A plexus of nerves exists in the deeper part of the connective tissue beneath the epithelium. End organs are of the mucocutaneous type. The number of organized endings per unit area is generally greater in the female than in the male and in the older patient than in the younger patient. The distribution varies in the two jaws. In the upper jaw, the nerve network decreases from incisors to molars, whereas in the lower jaw, it increases from incisors to molars. The wearing of a denture may produce a decrease in mean nerve-net complexity.

Local increases in nerve distribution may, however, produce trigger points. In these small areas a biopsy shows an increase in nerve distribution in both connective tissue and epithelium. Fine intra-epithelial nerve fibres may be found passing up to the surface layer of the epithelium. Pressure from the denture on nerve endings situated so superficially in the mucosa not surprisingly evokes a painful stimulus.

THE AREA TO BE RECORDED

The impression should record the greatest possible extent of the future denture bearing area. It may be that the denture eventually will not extend quite as far as some of the limits indicated by the impression but in order to design the denture accurately the whole of the potential area should be included in the impression and reproduced on the cast.

The upper impression includes the alveolar ridge and the hard palate. Although the denture extent is limited posteriorly by the vibrating or 'Ah' line and by the hamular notches, the impression should normally extend some 2 mm behind these limits, unless a major impression technique is used which determines precisely the posterior extent of the denture bearing area. The labial and buccal extent is determined by the *functional* shape of the sulcus.

The lower impression includes the alveolar ridge extending posteriorly to include all the retromolar pad. Labially, buccally and lingually the limits of the impression are defined by the functional shape of the sulcus.

Of particular importance in defining the limits of both upper and lower impressions is the need for an understanding of the term 'functional sulcus' as this determines the extension and thickness of the future denture borders.

The sulcus areas may be subdivided into labial and buccal areas of both upper and lower jaws and the lingual area of the lower.

LABIAL AND BUCCAL SULCI

When the mandible is in the postural position and natural teeth are present, there is little space existing between the mucosa of the lip and cheek and that covering the alveolar ridge. Resorption of the outer alveolar plate of bone following extraction creates a greater potential denture space. In places where the surrounding structures prevent the collapse of the cheek onto the ridge, i.e. in the upper zygoma region, a natural space frequently exists. In the tuberosity region, the space is affected markedly by inward movement of the coronoid process when the mandible moves contralaterally. In all other areas, the potential space is limited by the elasticity of the submucosa in the cheek and lip and also by muscle tone.

The shape and extent of the labial and buccal sulci varies with the position of the jaw. On half-opening the mouth beyond the rest position, there is usually only a small change in the extent or potential width of the sulcus. In the older patient where atrophic changes in the submucosa have resulted in a reduced elasticity, the potential width may be slightly narrowed and the vertical extent of the sulcus may be decreased slightly. In all patients on very wide opening, there is a marked reduction in the potential sulcus width. In the half-open or rest position, the shape and extent of the sulcus is also affected by the state of relaxation of the circumoral and buccinator muscles. Patients frequently tighten up their facial musculature to 'assist' the operator when recording an impression. This presses the lips against the alveolar process and insertion of an impression tray carrying impression material is difficult to achieve. Such a patient should be asked to relax the lips and so enable an impression of the sulcus to be obtained.

Once the impression material is in place, however, its shape is affected by manipulation of the lips and cheeks by the operator, or by the patient pursing and tensing the lips. The actual shape and extent of sulcus recorded depends upon the volume and viscosity of the impression material and the support

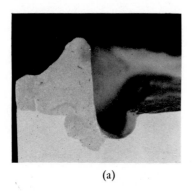   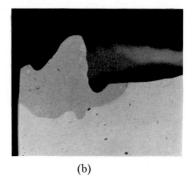

(a)   (b)

Fig. 6.7 Cross-section of lower cast:
(a) from an overextended impression;
(b) from a correctly extended impression.

which it has from the tray or record block. A large mass of viscous impression material displaces the sulcus tissues and causes loss of peripheral adaptation and overextension of the denture. Even if the denture is subsequently made short of the overextended sulcus on the cast, its periphery will not be well adapted in the mouth (Fig. 6.7).

The presence of impression material, correctly supported, results in some of the tissue fluid lying beneath the mucosa being expelled. Compression in one particular direction may be achieved when recording an impression. For example in some techniques, an inward force round the entire border of the impression gives greater compression of the tissues against the ridge and creates greater border or peripheral seal (Fig. 6.8). Whilst the denture made to such an impression presses lightly on the sulcus tissues, the latter do not press back with sufficient force on the border of the denture to displace it.

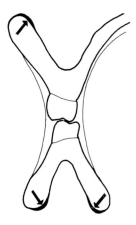

Fig. 6.8 Compressed sulcus shape creating border seal.

The recording of a slightly compressed sulcus shape will result in a denture that has good border seal. When a displacing force acts on the denture, the compressed mucosa by virtue of its elasticity, is able to maintain an intimate seal with the border of the denture. This effect is more readily achieved in the upper denture. With the lower denture, a positive border seal is difficult to achieve. In trying to obtain such a seal, it is important that the border of the denture is not overextended into the area of activity of the environmental musculature, particularly the mentalis muscle. Every effort should therefore be made to ensure minimal distortion of the labial and buccal sulcus tissues during impression procedures in the lower jaw.

The labial and buccal sulci in both jaws are interrupted by frenal attachments. The impressions should record their position so that the denture border can be shaped to receive them without irritation of the frenum or displacement of the denture.

LINGUAL SULCUS

The degree of lingual and distolingual extent which should be recorded in the lower jaw is difficult to define. Much has been written about the extension of the lower denture in these areas, ranging from the underextended to the over-extended form.

The distolingual extension requires a carefully adapted impression tray. Then the fold of the mucosa which joins the palatoglossal arch to the mandible can mould the impression material to indicate accurately the distal extent of the denture. Ideally, this area should be recorded as the patient swallows but this is not possible with all impression techniques and often the effect of tongue protrusion upon this area has to suffice. A similar situation exists when recording the small local effect of the superior constrictor of the pharynx.

In the anterior region the border of the denture is related to an area of mucosa that moves markedly under the influence of adjacent muscles. The level of the floor of the mouth is constantly changing with tongue movement. The lowest level occurs when the tongue is lying in its resting position. If the border of the denture contacts the mucosa with the tongue in this position then a satisfactory peripheral seal is obtained. With movement of the tongue, however, the floor of the mouth rises and a displacing force is brought to bear on the lingual denture border (Fig. 6.9). Therefore, the denture border cannot be extended below the highest level to which the mucosa is raised during function. However, this means that contact is lost when the floor of the mouth drops. Fortunately, this lack of seal in the anterolingual region can be compensated by the surrounding tissues effecting a seal against the polished surfaces of the denture in this area.

It is clear that the correct lingual border of the lower impression is the most difficult to record and must be functional in form. To achieve this the lower impression should be taken with the floor of the mouth raised to the functional position. This is obtained by protrusion of the tongue to the vermilion border of the upper lip, with the mouth half open. Too strong tongue activity, however, can cause folds of mucosa over the mylohyoid muscles to invade the denture bearing area above the functional sulcus depth. The patient should be asked to protrude the tongue in as relaxed a manner as possible. Forceful tongue thrusting against the upper alveolar ridge is to be avoided.

When providing an immediate denture, slight inaccuracies in recording the shape of the ridge tissues may pass unnoticed. Dimensional changes in the soft and hard tissues due to extraction with or without alveolectomy, cannot be forecast with precision. An immediate denture, therefore, is not adapted precisely to the tissues on insertion. Oedema during the first few hours after surgery improves the adaptation, whilst resorption after a few weeks of wear often causes some loss of fit. It is important, however, to define the sulcus extension with accuracy if discomfort and pain for the patient is to be avoided. Even if the denture is not to be fully extended into the sulcus, an accurate record of the entire potential denture bearing area is preferable. Only then can a proper assessment of the use of undercuts be made.

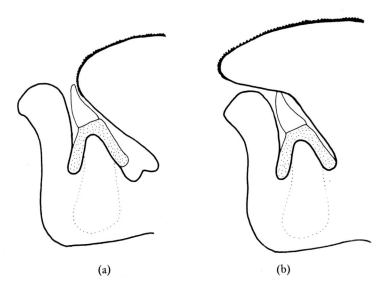

(a)   (b)

Fig. 6.9 The effect of tongue protrusion on the lingual fold:
(a) tongue at rest;
(b) tongue protruded.

Chapter 7

Jaw Relations

It is relevant first to discuss the basic mandibular positions and then to consider the movement patterns. An understanding of both is vital to a true appreciation of many dental problems, particularly in prosthodontics.

TERMINOLOGY

Many generations of students have been confused by the terms used to describe the various basic positions of the mandible in relation to the maxilla. Definitions of such terms as 'centric occlusion' and 'centric relation' often vary in different textbooks. Such confusion together with, in this country, the use of the phrase 'taking the bite' to describe the clinical stage of recording the correct maxillo-mandibular relation, has undoubtedly contributed to the difficulties of teaching; it has limited the student's understanding of this very important stage of restorative dentistry. It has therefore been encouraging to see the acceptance of new definitions of basic mandibular positions and of new thoughts on mandibular movement patterns based on an understanding of neurophysiology. Fig. 7.1 shows the relation between the basic jaw positions and the synonymous terms used to describe these positions.

BASIC MANDIBULAR POSITIONS

VERTICAL POSITIONS OF THE MANDIBLE IN THE SAGITTAL PLANE

(1) POSTURAL POSITION (REST POSITION)

This is the position which the mandible takes up without any conscious control when the patient is standing or sitting in an upright position. This mandibular position is stabilized by the tonicity of the elevators and depressors of the mandible acting synergistically. The weight of the mandible and teeth and the bulk of any appliance placed in the mouth also affect this position.

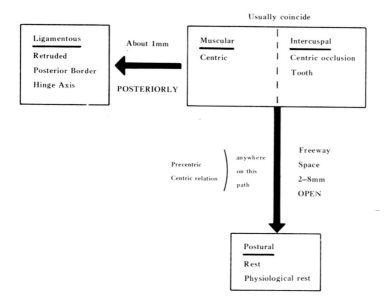

Fig. 7.1 Terms used to describe jaw positions and their relationship. The underlined words are those used in this text.

Neurophysiology of the Postural Position

The fifth cranial nerve has three main nuclei. These are a mesencephalic nucleus, a motor nucleus, and a main sensory nucleus. Efferent impulses from the motor nucleus bring about contraction of the muscles of mastication and therefore control jaw movements. Suitable tonicity of these muscles in the postural position is achieved by the influence on the motor nucleus of impulses from the cerebellum. These impulses not only control tonicity but also ensure muscle coordination, so that a suitable balance of tonicity between the muscles is achieved (Fig. 7.2).

Messages coming into the mesencephalic nucleus from the muscle spindles together with information about joint position which comes to the main sensory nucleus, assist in the maintenance of the correct postural relation of the jaws.

When the mandible is in the postural position the teeth are not together but are slightly apart. The interocclusal clearance is known as the *freeway space*. This clearance is approximately wedge-shaped, being greater in the incisal than in the molar area. Where a large vertical overlap exists, the incisor teeth may not move apart sufficiently for a space to appear between their incisal

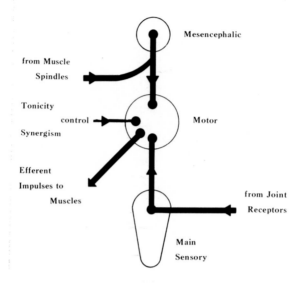

from Muscle
Spindles

Mesencephalic

Tonicity

control

Synergism

Motor

Efferent

Impulses to

Muscles

from Joint

Receptors

Main

Sensory

Fig. 7.2 Main nervous pathways involved in maintenance of the postural position.

edges. The opening of the jaw, however, from the position of occlusion to the postural position reduces the vertical overlap.

The normal freeway space is said to be between 2 and 4 mm but it may vary in the natural dentition from 2 to 8 mm. These distances represent the differences between the postural and occlusal vertical dimensions of the face measured between suitable reference points. Accurate measurements may be made on a cephalograph from nasion to gnathion. Less accurate recordings are made by selecting other reference points on the face.

The postural position is present before the primary dentition erupts—in fact it can be demonstrated in the newborn baby. It is the starting point for some of the early reflex movements of the mandible during suckling, swallowing, coughing, etc. It is probable that this is the first postural reflex fully developed so early in life.

The postural position has a moderate degree of stability. It is impossible to alter it in a short time period by restorative or orthodontic procedures. Its relative constancy can be explained by the stretch reflex—a stretching of the masticatory muscles is followed by a reflexly induced contraction (Fig. 7.3). Therefore, if the jaws are separated by a prosthesis beyond the postural position, muscular contraction results in the teeth being brought into repeated occlusal contact.

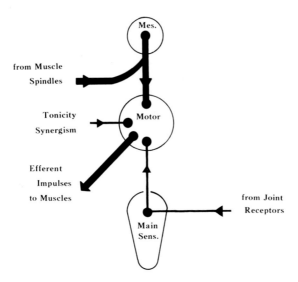

Fig. 7.3 The pathways involved in a stretch reflex.

Variations in the Postural Position

The postural position is, however, subject to variations which may be short or long term. The short term variations occur every day and are related to head posture, breathing and stress. If the patient's head is inclined backwards, for example in a dental chair, the mandible moves away from the maxilla due to an increase in tension in the suprahyoid muscles, and the freeway space is increased. Whereas, if the head is inclined forwards, the reverse occurs as pressure of the throat musculature on the mandible throws the balance in favour of the elevators of the mandible. There is a small increase in the free-way space during inspiration which is greater in a mouth-breathing patient than in a patient who inspires through the nose. When the patient is in a state of stress or intense physical effort, there is increased tonicity of the powerful elevator muscles and the teeth are brought into contact, thus eliminating the freeway space. Pain in the jaw musculature may similarly affect the postural position of the mandible.

Long-term variations may result from a habit of jaw posturing, from a long-standing change in the jaw relation when the teeth occlude, or from age changes. Forward posturing of the jaw may occur in mouth-breathers or where the upper teeth protrude well forward of the lowers. Patients with this type of dentition may adopt a forward posture of the jaw in order to reduce the space to be closed by the lips during breathing and speech.

A reduction of the distance separating the jaw bones with the teeth in contact occurs with attrition, which is uncompensated by further eruption, or from resorption of the alveolar bone under dentures. Then the resting position of the mandible tends to approximate more closely to the maxilla. This is probably an instance of disuse atrophy, occurring particularly with increasing age, and is due to a shortening of the resting length of the muscle.

Even in a young patient, the loss of posterior teeth may allow the mandible to come closer to the maxilla in occlusion. If this state continues for several years, some adjustment of the postural position takes place.

The variations that may be found in the postural position present two facts of practical importance. First, when recording the postural position, the patient must be in a relaxed state with the head held vertically. Secondly, where the acquired postural vertical dimension of the face appears to be too low, it is unwise to attempt a sudden large increase in occlusal face height to improve either aesthetics or the anterior tooth relation. This is particularly so in the older patient. A large increase which eliminates the freeway space, leads to a stretch reflex and trauma to the ridges followed by excessive resorption. By this means the tissues react to restore the freeway space to normal.

(2) THE INTERCUSPAL POSITION

This is the vertical position of the mandible in which there is maximal contact of the upper and lower teeth. It is preferably confirmed by contact of the occlusal surfaces of posterior teeth, though on occasions it may be indicated with accuracy by anterior tooth contact only. The patient always attempts to obtain the maximum amount of contact between units of the dentition whether they be natural or artificial. Therefore the tooth contact position may vary from time to time, depending upon the accuracy with which the occlusal and incisal surfaces fit together.

OCCLUSAL FACE HEIGHT

This is a vertical measurement of the face between two selected points, one above and one below the mouth. When the mandible is in the postural position a measurement taken between the two points will record the *postural face height*. When the teeth are in occlusion, the measurement will record the *occlusal face height*.

HORIZONTAL POSITIONS
OF THE MANDIBLE

(1) LIGAMENTOUS POSITION

This is the most retruded horizontal position of the mandible. It is not a position into which the mandible moves and stays comfortably, but is a position which can be adopted by conscious pull of the posterior and middle fibres of the temporalis, releasing at the same time the pull of the lateral pterygoid muscles. The amount of distal displacement is limited by the relative rigidity of the lateral ligaments of the temporomandibular joint. This is called a border position since it is one of the limits within which mandibular movement can occur.

(2) INTERCUSPAL POSITION

This is the horizontal tooth contact position which coincides with the vertical position previously defined. In only 10 per cent of patients do the ligamentous and intercuspal horizontal positions coincide. In 90 per cent the intercuspal position is about 1 mm anterior to the ligamentous position. The ligamentous position may be passed through during a masticatory cycle but the retrusive facets on the natural and artificial posterior teeth, by the action of their inclined planes, guide the mandible forward (Fig. 7.4). These retrusive facets thus assume a protective role in preventing undue backward displacement of the condyles.

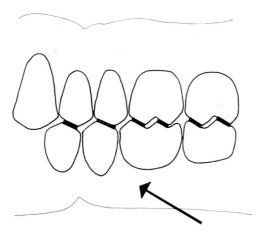

Fig. 7.4 Retrusive facets preventing distal movement of the mandible behind the intercuspal position.

(3) MUSCULAR POSITION

As the term suggests, this is under the control of the musculature in contrast to the ligamentous position, which is controlled by the joint ligaments and the intercuspal position which is controlled by the teeth. It is the horizontal contact position of the mandible determined by an automatic muscle pattern acting as the mandible closes from the postural position.

In most cases with natural teeth, the muscular position coincides with the intercuspal position. In some, however, the two positions do not coincide and the intercuspal position may be posterior, anterior or lateral to the muscular position. Only rarely do the ligamentous, muscular and intercuspal positions coincide.

The Origin of the Intercuspal and Muscular Positions

The first tooth contact relation occurs with the primary dentition. As the teeth erupt and come into contact, impulses from the periodontal receptors are transmitted to the brain through the main sensory nucleus. The joint receptors similarly register and monitor an 'acceptable' joint position (Fig. 7.5). This

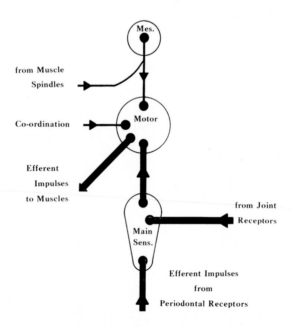

Fig. 7.5 Main nervous pathways involved in maintenance of the intercuspal and muscular positions.

incoming information modifies the motor impulses transmitted to the muscles which control the movement of the mandible. The muscles learn the position of occlusion which provides maximal occlusal contact with even loading on all the teeth and therefore minimal torque on the roots of the individual teeth and an evenly spread output from the periodontal receptors. The cuspal form of the teeth guides the direction of mandibular movement to end in good occlusion.

If the muscles accidentally bring the jaw into a lateral or protrusive position, the periodontal receptors of the teeth in contact in this incorrect position and the receptors in the joints, quickly inform the brain of the unusual occlusal position (Fig. 7.6). Suitable efferent motor impulses then bring about correct jaw positioning which is confirmed by normal impulses from the periodontal receptors.

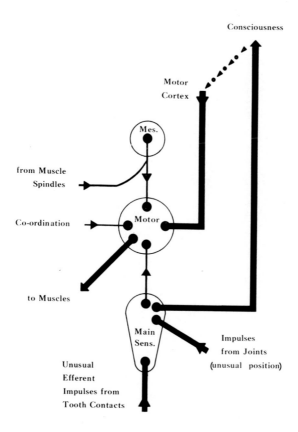

Fig. 7.6 The response to an unusual stimulus causing a change in pattern of movement by a conscious action.

MOVEMENT PATTERNS ON CLOSING

With the full eruption of teeth, therefore, an innervation pattern of jaw movement is developed and because of repetition becomes stabilized. Then, due to familiarity, control over this movement changes from a conscious, thoughtful process, to one without conscious control. Lower centres in the brain take over and control this type of automatic movement and all that is required is a voluntary initiation of jaw movement, a wish to open or close the jaw. Fine control and completion of the movement is then automatic. Tooth contact terminates the muscular closing movement.

This movement pattern remains relatively stable provided that the integrity of the dentition is maintained. Even after loss of the teeth, however, the automatic muscular movement pattern persists for a short time. Muscular control still moves the jaw in the same manner as though the teeth were still there to occlude. But, since this movement does not end in occlusion, there is no reinforcement of its neuromuscular pattern. Consequently, with the passage of time, the precision of movement diminishes.

CHANGES IN MOVEMENT PATTERNS

Like most other reflexes, mandibular movement patterns may be altered or suppressed. The changes may be short term or of longer duration.

Short term changes are frequently the result of tooth or joint pain. For example, if a restoration on a tooth is incorrectly contoured, the premature contact rapidly results in the development of a mild periodontitis. The tooth is painful on occlusal contact and the patient is conscious of the pain. He makes a conscious effort to bring the mandible into such a relation with the maxilla that the involved tooth with its painful stimulus is avoided. He may or may not be successful. If he is, the muscles learn this new movement pattern and eventually the closing movement is changed from one of conscious to one of subconscious effort. Provided that the occlusal disharmony has been of only short duration, however, the removal of the cause usually produces a rapid return to the previous automatic movement pattern.

The long-term variations in reflex patterns are usually associated with a more permanent occlusal disharmony. Probably the earliest examples occur during the change over from the deciduous to the permanent dentition. During the mixed dentition stage there are many occlusal interferences and the muscles are constantly learning new patterns of mandibular closure to avoid teeth which are interfering a little as they erupt. This interference not only affects the movement pattern but also helps to guide the teeth into their correct occlusal relation. The constant adaptation of the muscles to new stimuli is responsible for the difficulties which are encountered when recording the correct horizontal maxillo-mandibular relation in children. With the completion of eruption of most of the permanent dentition, the movement patterns become more firmly established since there is then greater precision of the contact position between the teeth. In this situation the intercuspal and muscular position, as defined earlier, will coincide. A malocclusion of the permanent dentition, however, whether it be developmental, or acquired through early loss of the deciduous teeth, will cause non-coincidence of the new intercuspal and the previous muscular position. The earlier an abnormal intercuspal position is adopted and used, the more difficult it is to break the habit. This is one of the important arguments for the elimination of tooth interferences in the deciduous dentition and for early orthodontic treatment.

In the adult the most common causes of altered reflex movement pattern are the loss of permanent teeth and faulty restorative dentistry. Tilting or migration of teeth into adjacent edentulous spaces creates occlusal interferences and a new intercuspal position. To accommodate this, the patient must learn a new pattern of muscular movement. As more teeth are lost, different intercuspal positions may have to be learned in order to obtain maximal tooth contact or the best interdigitation of the teeth.

If the patient's pain is severe, as may occur with direct or indirect injury to the joint, there may be continuous contraction of some or all of the muscles capable of moving the joint. The muscles then splint the joint and prevent the experience of more pain by limiting its movement. The trismus seen after a difficult third molar extraction is a familiar example of nature's method for resting the painful area.

MOVEMENT PATTERNS OF MASTICATION

Just as the reflex closing pattern is influenced by sensations from tooth contact, the patterns of movement used in mastication are similarly developed and maintained. Most patients chew with greater facility on one side than on the other. From experience they find that the teeth on one side produce more even stimuli from their periodontal receptors than those from the other side. This, the more comfortable side, then becomes favoured and is more frequently used. After a period of use, the chewing movement becomes automatic, varying with the texture of the foodstuffs being eaten.

The extent of lateral and protrusive jaw movements used during mastication is limited by the range of movement possible before uncomfortable tooth sensations are produced. For example, in patients with a large vertical incisal overlap there are limits to the amount of lateral movement which is possible before the canine teeth make a jarring lateral contact. Because this type of sensation is unpleasant the patient avoids this degree of lateral movement and limits the movement to a chopping or sagittal chewing stroke. Patients with an 'ideal' occlusion, however, can use a wider range of lateral and protrusive movement in chewing as they find this possible without discomfort.

As with closing or opening patterns, chewing movements are subject to short and long term variation. A cavity or a poorly contoured restoration in a tooth may cause a change in chewing movement and will probably make the patient chew on the other side of the jaw. If the cause is soon removed reversion to the previous unconscious automatic movement quickly occurs. Long standing occlusal change, however, will produce, first of all, a conscious alteration in the chewing pattern. With passage of time this becomes an automatic pattern of movement.

Thus the receptors in the periodontal membrane control within fine limits the range of movements used in chewing. Occasional heavy contact of one or two teeth is slightly jarring to the patient but causes no serious discomfort. It causes an immediate adjustment back to within the normal comfortable limits.

After the teeth are extracted, receptors in the mucosa have to take over the role of sensing pressures from the dentures. The threshold of stimulus necessary to fire the receptors in the mucosa of the edentulous ridge, is much greater than that required to stimulate the periodontal receptors. Thus, the patient can apply a greater load to dentures before becoming aware of the pressure being applied. Unfortunately, the stimulus at which the pain threshold of the mucosa is reached, is less than that which causes pain in natural teeth. Therefore the range of discriminatory, comfortable loading of the tissues is smaller with dentures than with natural teeth.

There is frequently a change of chewing pattern when a patient moves from the natural to the artificial dentition. The range and sometimes the extent of chewing movements are reduced. On the other hand, the patient who has used a chopping stroke with the natural dentition may find that, at the pressures tolerable with dentures, mastication is inefficient. Then the patient may investigate the possibility of using ruminatory strokes to deal particularly with fibrous foods such as meats, fruits and vegetables.

Chapter 8

Denture Retention and Stability

Various forces maintain apposition between the denture and the tissues. Those forces which function between the fitting surface of the denture and the tissue which it covers and cause them to remain together may be called *retentive forces*. These retentive forces are assisted by pressures from the opposing teeth, and from the tongue, lips and cheeks during function. Any pressure onto the occlusal or polished surfaces should result in a closer adaptation of the denture to the tissues and therefore may be called a *stabilizing force*. If the pressure tends to move the denture away from the tissues either horizontally or vertically, then it is contributing to instability of the denture.

There are limitations to the amount of direct retention available between the tissues and the denture. Retention depends upon the shape of the ridge, its soft tissue covering, the adaptation of the denture to the basal tissues and the viscosity and amount of the saliva. When retentive forces are high, some unstabilizing forces will not be effective in dislodging the denture. When the retentive forces available are low, it is essential not only to use these forces to the maximum but also to make full use of every possible stabilizing force, and to reduce unstabilizing forces.

RETENTION

The forces affecting the retention of dentures are adhesion, cohesion and weight.

ADHESION AND COHESION

When two different substances are in close contact, the molecules of each body attract those of the other. Thus the molecules making up the epithelium and those of the denture base are attracted to each other if denture adaptation is perfect within very fine limits. Since, however, there is a layer of saliva between the denture and the tissue, the effect of direct adhesion between them is probably negligible. The more important effect is the adhesion of the saliva molecules to the denture and to the tissues. On removing a denture from the mouth, a layer of saliva remains on both denture and tissues, so that this adhesive force is greater than the forces holding the molecules of the saliva together.

Attraction between molecules within the same substance is called cohesion. Hence the limiting factor in the retentive effect of adhesion and cohesion is the cohesion of the saliva, as it is this which breaks down on removing the denture.

Whilst adhesion and cohesion are the fundamental intermolecular forces, they give rise to macroscopic properties of the saliva, namely surface tension and viscosity. An understanding of the mechanisms by which surface tension and viscosity produce retention makes their clinical application more readily understood.

SURFACE TENSION

The denture loses retention when the saliva film breaks down into two layers, one on the denture and the other on the tissues. To break down the layer of saliva, air must enter this film between the denture base and the tissues. Resistance to air penetration is provided by the meniscus of the saliva which forms at the line where the denture and tissues are no longer in intimate contact. The meniscus forms due to the surface tension of the saliva as it stretches across the gap. Provided that the gap is small the meniscus remains complete. If the gap widens, the meniscus is stretched (Fig. 8.1). The surface tension forces are then inadequate to keep it intact and the meniscus breaks and allows air to enter.

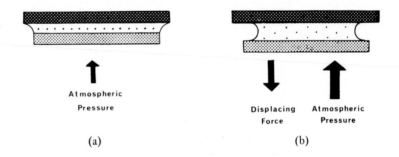

(a)   (b)

Fig. 8.1 The effect of the saliva meniscus:
(a) resting state—slight reduction in internal saliva pressure;
(b) on displacement—further decrease in saliva pressure due to change in shape of the meniscus.

Due to surface tension forces, there is a small reduction of pressure within the saliva film. Consequently atmospheric pressure helps to maintain the denture in position.

Atmospheric Pressure

Apart from the effect of surface tension in reducing slightly the internal saliva pressure, both sides of the denture are subject to atmospheric pressure. Atmospheric pressure or 'suction' as it is incorrectly called, contributes very little to the retention of a denture until an attempt is made to move it away from the tissues. Then, provided that the saliva film remains intact, a reduction in pressure occurs between denture and tissues and atmospheric pressure resists displacement of the denture. If the saliva film breaks down and air enters the space between denture and tissues, the denture is no longer retained. Hence it is important to exclude as much air as possible from the saliva film. Some dissolved air always remains, but if air bubbles are present these expand rapidly and connect up with the atmosphere thus producing a loss of retention. Air pockets remain in areas of poor adaptation, deep relief chambers or places where the denture has been adjusted away from a deep undercut. When only a small space has been created it fills with saliva. A larger space, however, usually contains air and this reduces denture retention.

The total effect of surface tension and atmospheric pressure is related to the area covered by the denture. The larger the area, the greater is the total retentive effect.

VISCOSITY OF THE SALIVA

The relationship between the denture and the tissues is a dynamic one. Whenever the denture tries to move, the viscosity of the interposed saliva film resists or dampens this movement, and thereby provides a retentive force.

Viscosity of the saliva depends upon its mucin content. Parotid secretion is mainly serous and therefore the secretion of the mandibular and the sublingual glands is the more important for denture retention. Mucin is also secreted from the palatal glands and lies between denture and tissues, flowing slowly to the periphery. Here it remains in the sulcus or on the soft palate until it is swallowed.

A thin film of saliva resists flow much more readily than a thicker film. Resistance to flow varies inversely as the cube of the film thickness. Thus by halving the gap between denture and tissues, the retentive force due to resistance to saliva flow is increased eightfold.

If the saliva itself has a high viscosity, it resists flow more effectively. Hence the use of denture fixatives or adhesives which produce a large increase in the viscosity of saliva. Unfortunately with the forces usually generated in the mouth, a saliva of such high viscosity cannot be compressed to a thin film. Therefore a marked increase in viscosity is necessary to produce an effect similar to that of decreasing the film thickness.

The danger of using denture adhesives is that whilst a thin film of saliva is developed initially, this gradually increases in thickness and the patient finds difficulty in reducing it down again to a narrow section. Unless there is plenty of further highly viscous saliva available in the mouth, then as soon as the denture is tilted or is moved away from the tissues, there is a shortage of saliva and the denture falls. This is what usually happens when a denture adhesive is in use as the adhesive-thickened saliva beyond the border of the denture is usually swallowed and does not remain in the mouth.

If a denture is loaded at one side, then the saliva film is thinned on this side and the denture may attempt to move away from the tissues on the opposite side. Here any extra saliva from the sulcus can flow in and so maintain the continuity of the saliva film in the increasing space. Hence adequate saliva volume is necessary and retention is therefore poor in the mouths of patients whose saliva volume is low.

The rate at which displacement of the denture is attempted is also important. To a force applied suddenly, there is little time for saliva flow to occur and the denture remains in place. If a much smaller force is applied continuously, however, flow takes place and the denture is displaced. Barriers to saliva flow in the form of raised bars may be made at various positions along the denture base. These have a minor effect in improving retention of the denture by resisting flow of saliva between the denture and the soft tissues.

Border Seal

The border or periphery of the denture provides ample opportunity for the ingress of air. Correct adaptation of the denture to the sulcus tissues and to the inside of the cheeks and lips ensures a border or valve seal. During a small displacement of the denture, the soft tissues of lips and cheeks move inwards under atmospheric pressure and maintain contact with the denture, thus preventing the ingress of air. Overtrimming of the border to provide relief for frena allows easy ingress of air as does an underextension of the denture into the sulcus.

In the lower jaw there is a relatively long border for a small area. Consequently the potentiality for air leakage is high. Seal of the tissues against the lingual aspect of the lower denture is difficult to achieve as also is seal at the distal end of a lower denture where it covers part of the retromolar pad. Usually, therefore, border seal in the case of the lower denture is poor. Border seal may be replaced partly by a seal between the inner aspect of the lips or cheeks and the polished surfaces of the denture.

In the upper jaw, the posterior palatal border is similarly the weakest part of the border seal, as only a slight movement of the denture away from the tissue allows the ingress of air and breakdown of the saliva film. A correctly positioned and shaped post dam is therefore essential to maintain retention. Increased pressure on the retromolar pads by the lower denture may have a similar effect.

CONDITIONS WHICH INCREASE RETENTION

From an analysis of the effects of the saliva film on retention, there are thus three important factors.

The larger the surface area, the better is the retention. The retentive force is proportional to the square of the surface area. The effective area is not the total denture bearing area, but the vertical projection of this onto a flat plane.

$$retention \propto area^2$$

The thickness of the saliva film. The retentive force is inversely proportional to the cube of the thickness of the saliva film.

$$retention \propto \frac{1}{saliva\ film\ thickness^3}$$

The viscosity of the fluid film. The retentive force is directly proportional to the viscosity of the saliva.

$$retention \propto saliva\ viscosity$$

Hence the best conditions for denture retention are:—

1 A fully extended denture (with border seal, including post dam)
2 A closely adapted denture (minimal saliva film thickness)
3 A saliva of medium viscosity which can be compressed to a very thin film by the normal intra-oral forces
4 A saliva of adequate volume.

WEIGHT

In the upper jaw, the lighter the denture, the less is the gravitational force moving it away from the tissues. Conversely in the lower jaw, extra weight, within limits, is an advantage in keeping the denture in place. Naturally if too heavy a lower denture is provided, the muscles lifting the mandible find difficulty in supporting the additional weight. In addition, the extra weight may accelerate bone resorption. Stretching a muscle causes reflex contraction and this increases the load on the ridges as the teeth are clenched together, increasing resorption of alveolar bone.

Clinically, a patient who has worn a vulcanite denture with porcelain teeth for many years finds difficulty in controlling a lighter all-acrylic denture. The weight of the vulcanite denture might have been double that of the acrylic one. An average all-acrylic lower denture weighs between 10 g and 15 g; with porcelain teeth this may reach 13 g to 18 g. A vulcanite denture however usually weighs 20 g to 25 g. In these circumstances, increasing the weight of the new acrylic lower denture by incorporating amalgam within its mass is advised. The weight of the lower denture, however, should not exceed 30 g to 40 g if discomfort and resorption are to be avoided.

SHAPE OF THE RIDGE

The ideal shape of an edentulous ridge is one which offers maximum resistance to displacement of the denture vertically, laterally, anteriorly and posteriorly. A ridge with almost vertical, parallel sides, extending over a large area produces the best retention and resistance to unstabilizing forces. The shallower the ridge and the more its sides converge the less effective it is in resisting any displacing forces. When the denture is being displaced from a ridge of ideal shape, it maintains border contact during a moderate amount of movement thus maintaining effective retention from atmospheric pressure and viscosity of the saliva. A ridge which by its shape or by its shallowness allows sideways movement of the denture enables the retentive forces to be overcome easily (Fig. 8.2).

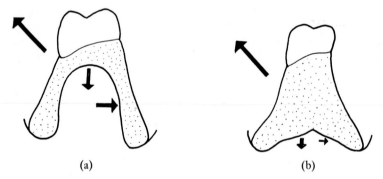

(a)   (b)

Fig. 8.2 The comparative resistance to lateral displacement provided by
(a) a well-formed alveolar ridge;
(b) a poorly formed ridge.

Undercuts of the ridge are acceptable if they can be utilized fully by the denture. Unilateral undercuts can be accommodated by selecting a suitable path for insertion of the dentures. Bilateral undercuts, however, can only be used to the extent by which the soft tissues over them can be compressed. Generally bilateral undercuts of 1 to 2 mm can be used in this way. The actual amount which can be included in the denture depends upon the amount of soft tissue covering the undercut. Where the ridge has only a thin layer of mucoperiosteum a small degree of undercut only can be utilized.

Trimming the denture to fit partly into the undercut area produces a space. If this is filled only with saliva, then little retention is lost, particularly when the denture is extended fully into the sulcus. If the space produced is large, however, an air bubble remains and this reduces the effect of atmospheric pressure in retaining the denture when it tries to move away from the tissues.

POLISHED SURFACES

Since the dentures are in almost continuous contact with lips, cheeks and tongue, the pressure from these structures can be utilized for retention. If the surface of a denture is vertical, then only sideways pressure will be applied to it and this must be resisted either by the ridge or by the pressure from soft tissues on the opposite side of the denture. A sloping surface, however, creates a retentive as well as a sideways component of force. The more horizontal the polished surface, the greater is the retentive component, whilst the more vertical the surface, the less is the retentive force which is achieved. Thus, in general, dentures should present to the soft tissues a surface which faces slightly upwards in the lower jaw thus creating a downward retentive component and slightly downwards in the upper jaw creating an upward component of force (Fig. 8.3).

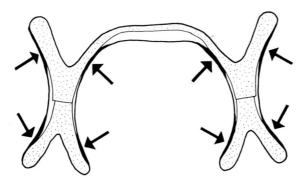

Fig. 8.3 The shape of the polished surfaces of the dentures which allows the adjacent tissues to exert retaining forces.

This general pattern may be modified in certain areas in order to improve the retentive force achieved. The surface of a denture is usually made slightly concave so as to improve the retentive force towards the periphery whilst reducing it at the area nearer the teeth. Since the polished surface near to the edge of the denture has a more continuous contact with the soft tissues the retention of the denture is usually improved slightly by this means. Simply making a denture concave, however, does not produce retention and may indeed cause instability. On hollowing out the lingual flange of a lower denture for example, stability is reduced since the tongue enters the hollow area and, on movement, lifts up the denture. Similarly if the lower posterior teeth are placed too far lingually, the tongue lifts the posterior part of the lower denture upward and forward (Fig. 8.4).

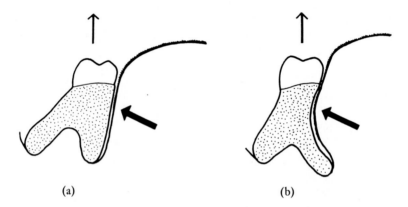

(a)   (b)

Fig. 8.4 Incorrect shaping of the lingual surface of a denture causing displacement by the tongue:
(a) lower posterior teeth placed too far lingually;
(b) hollowing of lingual flange.

In some areas it is impracticable to produce a polished surface of the correct shape. Where there is a bimaxillary protrusion of the alveolar processes, the polished surface of the dentures anteriorly cannot be retentive unless there is considerable thickening of the flange toward its periphery (Fig. 8.5). In general this would lead to instability of the denture on lip movement and so no advantage is gained in attempting to achieve the correct shape of polished surface. In these circumstances a decision must be made as to whether some displacing force from the lip may be tolerated and will be compensated by the retention of the rest of the denture, or whether the anterior tooth position must be changed so that a retentive polished surface can be achieved. The shape of the polished surfaces is most important in those areas which are subjected to considerable muscle pressures. The modiolus, or 'knot' of muscles behind the commissure of the lips is such an area. Here the lower denture must be

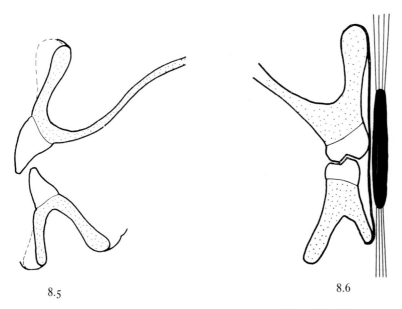

8.5   8.6

Fig. 8.5 The effect of bimaxillary protrusion on the shape of the polished denture surfaces.

Fig. 8.6 The presence of the modiolus influences the shape of the polished surfaces in the premolar regions.

kept to a minimum bulk and should provide a correctly shaped surface. The effect of this knot of muscles on the upper jaw is less marked and the force it applies can be used to retain the upper denture (Fig. 8.6).

In other parts of the denture, particularly in the lower jaw, the shape of polished surface may be modified to produce a more horizontal surface which will give a greater retentive effect. For example lingual tongue rests (Fig. 8.7) provide the patient with a 'shelf' on which to rest the tongue, and thus give a positive downward pressure on the lower denture.

It can be argued that for maximum retention, a denture should fill up all of the space between the tongue on one side and the cheeks and lips on the other. The space available for a denture is defined by the environmental musculature during function. A denture must occupy the zone where the pressures from muscles on either side are more or less equally balanced. This is called the '*neutral zone*'.

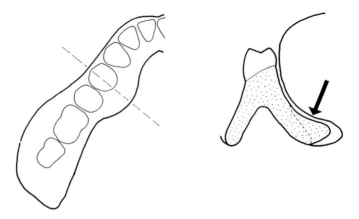

Fig. 8.7 Lingual tongue rest.

Ideally, therefore, we should record an impression of the potential space for a denture as well as the usual fitting surface and sulci. At the impression or trial denture stage it is possible to do this and so determine the denture space available and progress from this to the correct shape of denture to fill this space. The difficulty is one of providing a suitable support and then of getting the patient to perform those motions which will shape the impression material suitably. It is, of course, difficult to get the patient to make a few movements which will copy all the various pressures that will be applied during speech, mastication and deglutition.

In general this technique indicates a somewhat greater space than that which is in fact available. It produces a rather bulky denture which requires some reduction before it is accepted by the average patient. Its shape, however, does not coincide with that already described as being ideal for a denture, particularly in the buccal pouch region. By this technique the buccal polished surface is usually indicated as being convex, whereas normally the denture surface here is made slightly concave. This slight dilatation of the buccal pouch may simply be its adaptation in an attempt to accept a bulk of impression material as though it were a bolus of food. Usually this area is reduced in bulk when making the denture but on all prostheses the concavity must not be made too pronounced. The cheeks are relatively thick muscular structures and they will not conform to a curve of small radius. Consequently if the denture is made very hollow here, the cheeks bridge over the depression which simply collects food whilst the patient is eating. The buccinator is unable to clean out this hollow and often in denture-wearers the tongue cannot move freely into the buccal sulcus without displacing the lower denture. As a result the patient complains of the collection of food within the buccal sulcus.

MUSCULAR CONTROL

Undoubtedly, there is a considerable amount of 'oral gymnastics' in the control of dentures. Even slight changes in shape between successive dentures requires some practice before good control is regained. Many patients present with ill-fitting dentures which have no retention but which can be used by them quite satisfactorily because of the stabilizing influence of the adjacent musculature. Some patients wear dentures broken into two or more pieces and control these quite well, even during mastication.

The importance of muscular control can be shown by applying a surface anaesthetic to all the oral mucous membrane. This eliminates tactile sensation of the dentures which is so important to muscle coordination, and denture control fails.

The precise mechanism by which a patient controls dentures in each case is not at present known. The dorsum of the tongue posteriorly, undoubtedly plays a big part in upper denture retention as do the sides of the tongue in the lower. We do not usually give our patients much advice nor many physiotherapeutic exercises which would help them in learning denture control more rapidly. The tongue is important, however, and the patient should be encouraged to place it gently against the lingual surface of the lower denture as often as possible and so counteract pressures from the lips and cheeks. In this position any polished surface retention is maximal and in addition, by covering a small portion of the occlusal surface of the lower denture some increase in retention of this is achieved. When in this position, the tongue also completes the lingual border seal.

STABILITY

A denture is retained satisfactorily in function when the retentive forces are greater than the unstabilizing forces. Whilst pressure from the lips, cheeks and tongue via the polished surfaces and periphery of a denture may act as a stabilizing or an unstabilizing force, dependent upon the shape of the denture, in general, denture stability during function is related to the occlusion and articulation of the teeth.

OCCLUSION AND ARTICULATION

Occlusion is the static relation of dentures in contact, whilst articulation refers to the dynamic movement of dentures over each other during chewing and sliding movements.

It is important that there should be even contact of the opposing occlusal surfaces in the intercuspal position. Any premature or deflective contacts will cause displacement of the dentures away from the tissues. Hence balanced occlusion or even contact between the two dentures is important.

During chewing movements, the teeth will be separated initially by the food layer, but as mastication proceeds, the teeth may come into contact. It is important that they should be able to glide smoothly over each other so that there will be only a small lateral pressure upon the dentures and the ridges. When the teeth interfere and contact is limited to one or two teeth or cusps, then the lateral pressures in these areas become high. As a result, rotation of the denture about the ridge is promoted. The denture is pulled away from the tissues on the opposite side of the jaw when the retentive forces are insufficient to prevent its displacement. Usually, the lower denture is the first to be displaced.

Attention to the problems of stability is particularly important when a single complete denture opposes natural teeth. The vigour and range of chewing may be greater than that usually employed with upper and lower complete dentures since one half of the masticatory apparatus is fixed. Consequently in these circumstances, it is very important to ensure lack of interference of the posterior and anterior teeth over each other during function. This is particularly so when a complete lower denture opposes an upper natural dentition. Such a situation is usually best avoided at the treatment planning stage as, in the circumstances, a stable denture is often impossible. Difficulties are less when making an upper complete denture to a natural lower dentition, as the retention of an upper denture is usually greater. Modification of the occlusal surfaces of the opposing natural teeth by grinding or by placing inlays or onlays to modify their shape may well be necessary to produce a favourable occlusal surface.

Chapter 9

Mandibular Movements and Posterior Teeth

In the natural dentition, the size, form and occlusal surface of the posterior teeth is genetically determined and then modified by the type and amount of functional use of the teeth. The natural teeth of some patients show little sign of occlusal wear, whilst in others marked occlusal attrition may be seen.

Ideally, during natural function, the occlusal surfaces of the teeth should become worn until they fit closely together and slide smoothly over each other and so perform efficiently the function of mastication. Attrition of the teeth to this extent seldom occurs in the natural dentition in countries where the food is highly refined. Most natural dentitions therefore have a limited range of smooth, ruminatory, masticatory movements whilst some function with only a chopping stroke.

CHEWING MOVEMENTS

The ideal path of movement of the mandible during chewing starts with an opening movement, during which the food is collected and placed on to the occlusal surfaces of the teeth. On the return stroke, the lower jaw approaches the maxilla in a right or left lateral position, so that the teeth are in a cusp to cusp relation. Then the jaw moves medially into the intercuspal position (Fig. 9.1). This cycle may be repeated or may be varied by using the opposite side of the jaw. That portion of the path of movement with the teeth apart is of little interest as far as occlusal form of the teeth is concerned and our interest is centred mainly on the path of movement after the teeth have come near together. They may touch or remain slightly apart with a small amount of food between. The path of movement of the lower teeth into the intercuspal position is, however, similar in both cases.

The direction of movement on tooth contact is influenced by the angle at which both posterior and anterior teeth can move over each other. To reach the position of tooth contact during chewing, the mandible swings to one side. When it moves to the left, the right condyle moves downwards and forwards whilst the left one rotates and moves slightly sideways and backwards (Fig. 9.2).

Condyle Angle

The downward and forward path of the condyles can be considered as a straight line which forms an angle with a reference plane. The two common planes

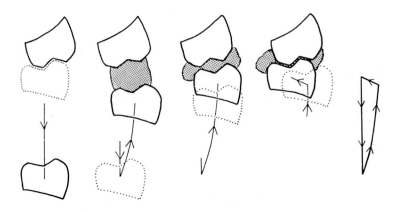

Fig. 9.1 Ideal cycle of mandibular movement during chewing.

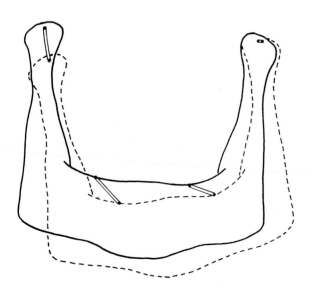

Fig. 9.2 Condylar movements during chewing on the left.

are the Frankfort and the ala-tragus planes (Fig. 9.3). The Frankfort plane passes through each external auditory meatus and the lowest point of the orbital margins. As its name implies, the ala-tragus plane passes through the tragus of each ear and the alae of the nose. The path of movement of the condyle

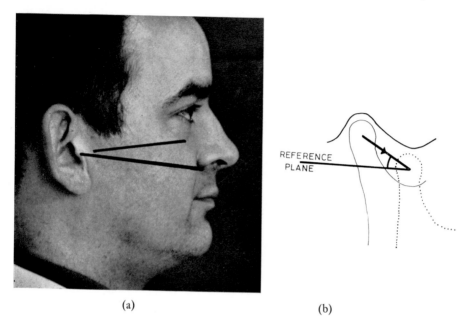

(a)　　　　　　　　　　　　　　　　　　　　　(b)

Fig. 9.3
(a) Frankfort and ala-tragus planes;
(b) the condyle angle.

is restricted not only by the shape of the condyle head, meniscus and glenoid fossa, but also by the attached ligaments and muscles. Thus in this left lateral position the left condyle does not simply rotate, but moves slightly sideways and backwards. This lateral shift of the mandible is called the *Bennett movement*.

　　Thus, when chewing on the left, the right side of the mandible has moved down and forward due to the condyle movement; whilst the left side has been affected only slightly by this movement. If the posterior teeth contact only on the left, the dentures may move away from the ridges on the right. It is preferable, therefore, that the teeth on this side also should meet and thereby provide *balanced articulation* (Fig. 9.4). Since the right condyle has moved downwards, the cusps on this, the *balancing* side must present a steeper slope than those on the left or *working* side. Thus, during a chewing pattern, the path of movement of the teeth on the right is relatively steep but it is shallow on the left. A similar arrangement but in reverse must apply when chewing on the other side.

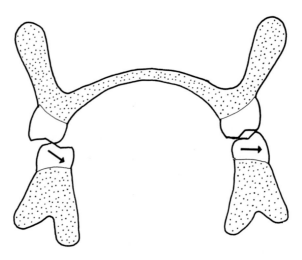

Fig. 9.4 Balanced articulation. As the mandible and the lower denture have moved into a left lateral position, cuspal contacts have been maintained on both sides of the jaw.

To enable these different movements to be accommodated, the posterior teeth in the upper jaw are set facing outwards, whilst the lowers face inwards. This curve of the occlusal surfaces is called the *Curve of Monson*. It causes the angle of the cusps to be made shallow on the side towards which movement of the jaw takes place, the working or chewing side, and increases the effective cusp angle on the side away from which movement occurs, the balancing side. With a steep condyle movement the difference of movement between the two sides of the jaw is greatest and a relatively steep curve of Monson is required together with moderately steep cusps. Conversely with a small condyle angle a shallow curve of Monson is necessary.

INCISION OF FOOD

For the incision of food the lower jaw is protruded, bringing the incisor teeth together. It is then moved backwards usually with a slight side to side motion shearing off a portion of food. With less fibrous and more brittle food, the teeth are used as a point of preliminary indentation and weakening of the food followed by levering against the teeth to promote fracture of the food.

Both on incision and on chewing, therefore, the anterior teeth may come into contact and it can be argued that the occlusal surfaces of the posterior teeth should meet at the same time. The relation of the anterior teeth is decided by the dentist and his technician. The maximum vertical overlap for balanced articulation is of the order of 1 to 2 mm being the height of the cusps of the posterior teeth. With a large horizontal overlap, the vertical overlap can be greater than this, as the possibility of tooth contact taking place decreases. On the other hand a reduction in vertical overlap must accompany a small horizontal overlap of 1 to 2 mm. It is necessary when trying to achieve balanced articulation to keep the path of movement of the incisors over each other fairly shallow and so reduce lateral pressure which may displace the dentures. Thus the anterior path of movement (*incisal guidance angle*) is usually shallow by design, and the path followed by the posterior teeth on protrusion is guided more by the condyle angle. Thus the mandible moves not about a centre of rotation, but slides forward, moving further downwards posteriorly and less anteriorly (Fig. 9.5). In order to accommodate these different movements,

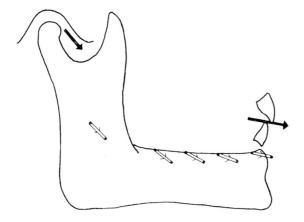

Fig. 9.5 The movement of the mandible on protrusion. Note the progressive decrease in downward movement from condylar to incisor region.

the posterior teeth are set to a curve which increases their effective cusp angle for protrusive movement (Fig. 9.6). This is known as the anteroposterior *compensating curve* and simulates the anatomical '*Curve of Spee*' of the natural dentition. If the incisal angle is made equal to the condyle angle, no curve is necessary but as a shallow incisal angle is usually selected, a curve is common. The steepness of this curve is related to the condyle angle and to the cusp angles of the teeth. The steeper the cusp angle, the less the compensating curve need be, but the greater the incisal angle will need to be, since the steep cusps on the premolar teeth will cause a greater downward motion in the anterior segment.

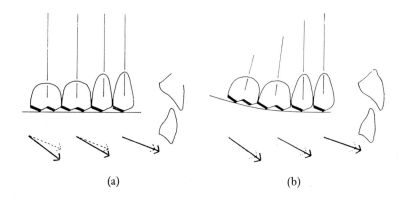

(a)   (b)

Fig. 9.6
(a) Teeth set up to flat plane. On protrusion, the lower teeth move downwards as indicated by the dotted arrows. The mandible, however, moves farther downwards posteriorly (solid arrows) creating a space between the molar teeth.
(b) Teeth set up to compensating curve. The angle of the posterior teeth cusps now increases posteriorly and coincides with the mandibular movement, thus giving balanced contacts on protrusion.

The posterior tooth occlusal surfaces are therefore arranged in two curves —one lateral and the other anteroposterior. These curves are related to condyle angle and to the height and angle of cusps selected. One can therefore argue that to obtain smooth movement of the teeth over each other, i.e. balanced articulation, information on the possible mandibular movements for each patient must be recorded and the teeth arranged to suit each individual pattern.

OCCLUSAL PLANE

The curves to which the posterior teeth are set are usually related in some manner to the flat occlusal plane defined when recording the occlusion. For preference, this flat plane should bisect the inter-ridge space (Fig. 9.7). Then, on occlusion, a retentive force is applied to both dentures. Sloping the occlusal plane up at the back produces a force displacing both dentures whilst sloping it down posteriorly results in more favourable occlusal forces. Unfortunately, such an arrangement is usually incompatible with normal lower

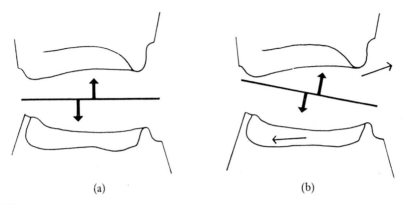

(a)   (b)

Fig. 9.7
(a) Occlusal plane bisecting the inter-ridge space.
(b) Occlusal plane incorrectly orientated. On occlusion, both dentures would be displaced.

ridge shape and with the creation of a suitable compensating curve. The occlusal plane is usually a chord of the compensating curve, meeting it in the canine and first molar regions (Fig. 9.8). Since the occlusal plane is not defined with precision, the relation of the compensating curve to it is subject to various practical interpretations.

Occlusal contact of the artificial posterior teeth should preferably take place at a level similar to that of the natural dentition. Then, the tongue, cheeks and lips may go through the same motions in manipulating the food onto the

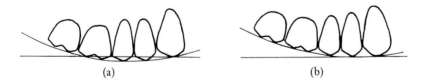

(a)   (b)

Fig. 9.8 The relation of the occlusal plane to the anteroposterior compensating curve:
(a) The occlusal plane is a chord of the compensating curve as may be achieved if the upper teeth are set to a template;
(b) the occlusal plane is a tangent to the compensating curve as will be achieved if the upper teeth are set to the lower record block.

occlusal surfaces of the teeth for mastication. There are circumstances, however, when the occlusal plane is formed nearer the lower ridge in order to improve tongue control of a lower denture.

ARTICULATORS

Various articulators have been designed in order to copy mandibular movements. It is not the intention in this book to discuss techniques of using any one articulator in detail, but simply to discuss their application and accuracy in achieving what they set out to do.

ADJUSTABLE ARTICULATORS

The commonest form of adjustable articulator allows for variations in condyle angles and the relation of the ridges and teeth to them. The nearer the teeth are to the condyles, the greater is the effect of condyle movement on tooth movement (Fig. 9.9). Conversely the further away they are, the less will be the effect. Adjustments are also made for selecting an incisal angle and to allow for the lateral Bennett movement.

Other articulators try to reproduce more faithfully the mandibular movement by allowing for variations in intercondylar widths and for the registration of individual condyle paths. Most articulators assume that the condyle movement is in a straight line, hence the use of the term condyle angle. The actual path of movement of a condyle is, however, more a shallow 'S' shaped curve of which the straight portion is assumed to indicate the condyle angle.

Whilst the condyle path may be determined with some degree of accuracy by several methods, the path along which the condyle moves is not identical

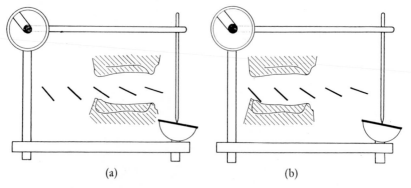

(a)   (b)

Fig. 9.9 The effect of the position of the casts in the articulator on the path of movement of the teeth.

on each occasion. As already noted condyle position and movement are controlled and limited by ligaments and muscles. Fibrous food placed between the teeth causes a small distraction of the condyle on the chewing side. Whilst this affects occlusal balance, it may of course compensate for the bulk of food between the occlusal surfaces of the teeth and thus help to retain balance despite the presence of a thin layer of food between the cusps.

Precise recording of condyle movement may be an unnecessary refinement in view of the variations in path of movement which take place during function. It is also argued that the differences in the path of movement of the posterior teeth with widely different condyle angles are so small as to be negligible when compared with the variation in the actual path of movement during chewing.

AVERAGE ARTICULATORS

Whilst individual records of the condyle angles and tooth to condyle relation may appear to be a precise activity, it is suggested that such precision may not be necessary in practice. Hence, average values for condyle angle and tooth–condyle relations are incorporated in some articulators. These movable, non-adjustable articulators enable a check to be made on the accuracy with which the teeth are positioned so avoiding interference on lateral and protrusive movements and helping to achieve a smooth gliding movement. With a fixed condyle angle and tooth–condyle relation, the anteroposterior and lateral curves to which teeth of a certain cusp angle must be arranged are the same for all cases. Hence, in theory, setting the posterior teeth in contact with the curved template often supplied with such articulators is all that is necessary. Due to the relative inaccuracy of positioning teeth in wax against the template this method alone is not satisfactory and the articulator movement enables the position of the teeth to be checked. Interference of anterior teeth, particularly the canines, can also be checked by movement of the articulator. The limitation of an average value articulator is where the patient's condyle angle differs sufficiently from the average value to cause a practical difference between the articulator movements and those of the jaw.

Other articulators are designed so that after placing the teeth on a standard curve, the lateral and protrusive movement of the articulator is guided by the teeth themselves sliding over each other, controlling their own movement, and not under the influence of a simulated condyle movement.

SIMPLE ARTICULATORS

Plane line or simple hinge articulators record only the occlusal position and do not simulate lateral or protrusive movement. Whilst the articulator has a hinge, its only purpose is to enable the casts to be separated and then returned to the correct relation. The movement of the hinge of the articulator usually bears no relation to the opening and closing movements of the jaw.

When setting up on a hinge articulator, average Monson and compensating curves may be used, together with an arbitrary incisal angle. The average curves may be defined by a template to which both anterior and posterior teeth are set. It may also be defined by a series of measurements referred to a flat plane. On the other hand, it may lack any precise definition, and lie only in the eye of the person setting up. Many technicians, particularly those who have arranged teeth on an adjustable or movable articulator for many years can arrange posterior teeth on a hinge articulator so that they will not interfere grossly during jaw movements. In general, however, freedom from interference and occlusal balance is not achieved by using this type of articulator. Adjustment of the occlusion must be made either at the try-in or finished denture stage by checking contacts in the patient's mouth. Considerable difficulties may arise when trying to check the contacts of trial dentures during lateral and protrusive movements. There is a possibility of distorting the trial base and of loosening the teeth from the wax. If a close approximation to balanced articulation has been achieved in the setting up, then only a small amount of grinding may be necessary. Gross errors, however, may be impossible to rectify by selective grinding.

CONCLUSIONS ON THE NECESSITY FOR BALANCED ARTICULATION

Arguments have swayed backwards and forwards for many years on the necessity for balanced articulation in complete dentures. Exponents argue that dentures will be displaced on chewing if balancing contact is not available on the opposite side of the jaw to that on which the chewing is taking place. It is argued that as many teeth as possible should contact on both working and balancing sides and in protrusion of the mandible. Without such balance, the masticatory efficiency of the dentures and the patient's comfort and confidence with them will be impaired.

A more restricted case is argued for three point contact. This ensures two points of contact on the working side, one anterior and one posterior, and a third on the balancing side. The arguments again are for increased denture stability during chewing and greater comfort to the patient.

Against these arguments is the one that the teeth do not necessarily come into firm contact during mastication. Chewing food requires that a portion of it should remain between the occlusal surfaces. If the teeth on the chewing side are separated, then those on the balancing side will also be separated by a similar amount. Hence the comment, 'enter bolus—exit balance'. In addition, the soft tissues beneath the dentures, particularly in the lower jaw, respond to chewing pressure and are compressed slightly and cause some loss of perfection in any occlusal contact.

Investigations indicate that many dentures are not stable at all during masticatory function. They move away from their basal tissues by as much as 3 to 4 mm and are used in a semi-floating position, being 'juggled' by the complex neuromuscular coordination of tongue, lips, cheeks and of mandibular movements.

Paths of movement during chewing are also dissimilar from the ideal path described earlier. The path may be reversed in direction, that is, progressing from the intercuspal position to lateral excursion, or it may involve passage across the upper tooth from buccal cusp to lingual cusp. Other workers assert that complete denture wearers use only a chopping stroke and that the lateral movement component is non-existent or else extremely small in amount.

Examination of the dentures of some patients shows hardly any signs of occlusal wear after many years, indicating a relatively low level of pressures and jaw movements.

Some patients present, after wearing dentures for some years, with occlusal surfaces which have been ground into perfect sliding articulation. All slightly interfering cusps have been worn away and even the incisal edges are reduced to give the correct incisal angle for balanced protrusive excursion (Fig. 9.10).

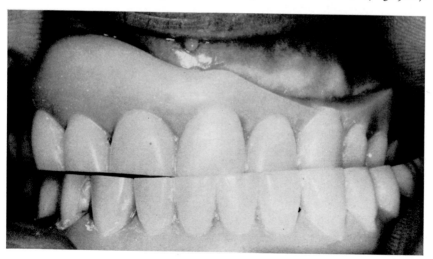

Fig. 9.10 A free-sliding articulation that has resulted from occlusal wear of acrylic teeth.

Other patients produce marked general abrasion of the denture occlusal surfaces, particularly of acrylic teeth. It is suggested that this wear does not take place during mastication but in empty mouth movements. Some patients sit and grind their teeth in moments of stress or simply out of habit. These protrusive and lateral grinding movements may produce surfaces which conform to the normal lateral and anteroposterior compensating curves. In other circumstances, however, most unusual occlusal shapes can be produced. Outside the mouth, these reveal little balanced contact. In use, however, the lack of adaptation of the dentures to the ridges and their consequent mobility enables the patient to manipulate the dentures so that these unusual occlusal surfaces maintain a form of contact during function. It has even been suggested that when a patient has developed such intra-oral skills, discomfort can arise if replacement dentures are made which are very retentive. The patient cannot manipulate the new dentures as he did the old ones.

The dentures of some patients show marked wear of posterior teeth due to chewing sweets. These may have an abrasive or solvent action and produce a gap between the occlusal surfaces of the dentures, usually on one side of the jaw where the sweets are held and sucked (Fig. 9.11).

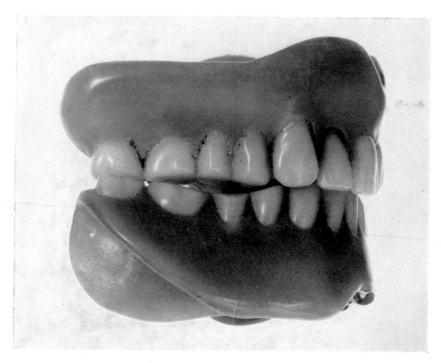

Fig. 9.11 Abrasion of occlusal surfaces of acrylic teeth by sweets.

It is suggested that by giving a patient unrestricted movement possibilities, they will employ these and in doing so, will produce trauma to the underlying tissues from the unstabilizing forces applied. Restriction of the amount of lateral movement by posterior or anterior tooth occlusions (or both) limits patients to a chopping stroke and so causes them to apply stabilizing forces to their dentures rather than movements which might displace them. If such a patient indicates, by producing pressure signs, that they are trying to use lateral movements, then the posterior teeth, if set to approximate compensating curves, can be ground selectively to give a limited range of interference-free excursion.

It would appear from all this conflicting evidence, that there is some argument for providing *the possibility* for a smooth interference-free gliding of the posterior teeth, but not necessarily balanced articulation. If there are obstructions to smooth gliding, then such supracontacts demand a sudden adjustment in the movement pattern of the patient to overcome them. The patient 'chews with a limp'. The provision of dentures with such contacts interfering severely in their paths of movement (Fig. 9.12) would not appear to be advisable. Balanced articulation in the full sense, however, would not appear to be necessary in all cases.

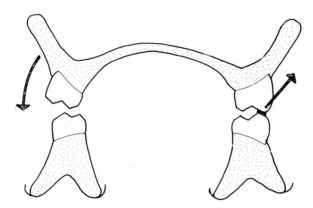

Fig. 9.12 Denture instability caused by cuspal interference.

It is fortunate that the majority of human beings can adapt to whatever movement pattern their dentures dictate, just as everybody has adapted to the various changes which occurred in their natural dentition throughout life. As the permanent dentition erupts, changes in masticatory pattern follow these changes closely. With subsequent tooth loss, further adaptation is demanded and usually is achieved with hardly any conscious effort on behalf of the patient.

Where the necessary degree of adaptation is beyond the patient's capacity, then symptoms arise and the patient requires treatment. In the case of complete dentures, the patient may complain of pain, discomfort or denture instability and then the dentist must try to define the source of the occlusal trauma and eliminate it from his prostheses.

Chapter 10

Selection and Arrangement of Posterior Teeth

There are available a large number of different brands of artificial posterior teeth with wide variations in their dimensions and in the pattern of their occlusal surfaces. Posterior teeth are also available in a variety of materials, i.e. porcelain, acrylic or metal (cobalt-chromium or stainless steel).

The design of artificial posterior teeth tends to follow the form and occlusal surface of the natural dentition. It must be realized, however, that a different set of conditions prevails in the mouth when wearing complete dentures than when the natural teeth were present. Resorption of bone and changes in the tonicity of the tongue, lips and cheeks after extraction of the natural teeth, all affect the space available for artificial teeth. In addition, whilst each natural tooth is individually slung in its periodontal membrane, artificial teeth are but a component part of a single structure. Pressure on one natural tooth is restricted in its effect, whilst pressure on one artificial tooth affects the entire denture.

The variables in posterior teeth are:

    1 Width (breadth) buccolingually
    2 Size, mesiodistally
    3 Length, occlusogingivally
    4 Occlusal surface
    5 Material.

WIDTH

The natural posterior teeth are in a position of equilibrium between pressure from the tongue lingually, and from the cheeks facially. Artificial posterior teeth must occupy a similar position in the neutral zone. If there is delay in replacing posterior teeth after extraction, lips and cheeks move into this zone and reduce its width.

The normal pattern of resorption results in a reduction in the width of the ridge. If a wide tooth is placed over a narrow ridge, forces applied to one side of the tooth tend to rotate both tooth and denture about the ridge (Fig. 10.1). It is preferable therefore for stability on occlusion, that teeth should have a width related to that of the ridge.

In general this means that artificial teeth are narrower than their natural predecessors, even when an immediate denture technique for posterior teeth is followed. Teeth with a narrow occlusal table restrict the bulk of food which can be accommodated between them during mastication. Chewing becomes, therefore, a little tedious and the patient selects a more easily masticated diet or accepts a larger particle size as being suitable for swallowing. On the other hand, narrow posterior teeth exert a larger force per unit area on the food being chewed and this increases masticatory efficiency as compared with broader teeth. Since the load which can be tolerated by the soft tissues under

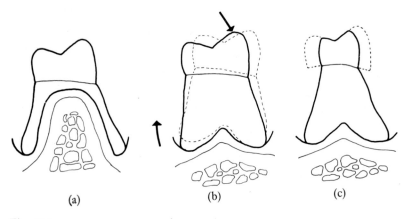

(a)   (b)   (c)

Fig. 10.1
(a) Wide tooth suitable for a broad ridge.
(b) Tooth too wide for a narrow, resorbed ridge. Forces applied to the denture are likely to cause displacement.
(c) More suitable width of tooth for the narrow resorbed ridge.

a denture is only an eighth to a tenth of that accepted by the periodontal membrane of natural teeth, narrow teeth are generally more efficient than broad ones. The upper ridge is usually wider than the lower in a patient who has been edentulous for some time, due to the different rates of resorption in the two jaws. Hence, it is often possible to accommodate wider upper teeth than lowers. It may be necessary to select lower teeth only 2 to 3 mm wide when the posterior teeth have been absent for many years. Here tongue and cheek encroachment may have almost obliterated the neutral zone and the ridge may only be a narrow vestige of its former size.

SIZE

A set of posterior teeth is selected to fill the space between the distal surface of the canine and the mesial of the pear-shaped pad in the lower or tuberosity in the upper. If teeth of too small a size are used, they will not form a continuous guide for the swallowing of food and part of the food bolus may escape laterally into the cheeks. On the other hand by placing a molar tooth over the pear-shaped pad or tuberosity, not only do technical difficulties of setting up arise, but also heavy contact in this area causes some instability of the denture. A denture is most stable to pressure applied in the second premolar and first molar region, as the load is applied more towards the centre of gravity of the denture.

LENGTH

A tooth should be selected which has a length related to that of the canine. If very short teeth are used in order to simplify setting up, the appearance is poor when the patient smiles (Fig. 10.2). Whilst a tooth of suitable length may be selected, it is important to ask the technician to maintain this length, particularly when the inter-ridge space is small, by fitting the tooth carefully to the ridge contour (ridge-lapping).

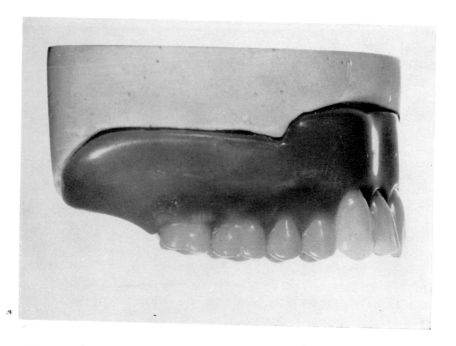

Fig. 10.2 Posterior teeth that are too short in comparison with the length of the anterior teeth.

OCCLUSAL SURFACE

The occlusal surface of artificial teeth evolved first from that of natural teeth. Since these teeth resemble their natural counterparts, they are called 'anatomical', i.e. conforming to the same anatomy. Their surfaces resemble those of newly erupted teeth and little attempt is made to shape the occlusal surfaces to simulate the changes produced by attrition after years of use. The surface of these teeth is ground in, either on an articulator which simulates masticatory movements, or more frequently by the patient during wear. To improve masticatory efficiency and to fit in with various theories of occlusion and jaw movements, many designs of teeth have been produced which have the appearance of natural teeth but whose occlusal surface consists not of rounded cusps but a series of sharply angled cones. Others bear no resemblance occlusally to natural teeth and are designed more for function as components of 'a chewing or grinding machine'. This latter group are called *mechanical* occlusal forms. The subdivision is not precise, as many forms of occlusal surface resemble the cusps of natural teeth but have been modified to function mechanically. An alternative subdivision of occlusal form is into those with cusps and those which have no structures resembling natural cusps but present a relatively flat, grinding surface.

Cusps penetrate food and increase the possibility of a shearing instead of just a crushing action. Therefore they assist in the mastication of fibrous foodstuffs. Cusps, however, need not simulate those of the natural dentition. Provided that prominences of the opposing occlusal surfaces exist which move past each other so that they produce a series of line contacts, they will shear the food like the blades of scissors passing across each other. Such a surface can be produced by cusps similar to those of the natural dentition after attrition or by conforming to a more geometric pattern. Alternatively cuspless teeth may present hollows (inverted cusps) surrounded by relatively sharp cutting edges which shear the food as they pass over each other.

When cusps are present there is a sliding contact between the teeth on passing from the lateral position to the intercuspal position at the end of a chewing stroke. This lateral contact produces a sideways pressure on both dentures which must be resisted by the ridges. If one ridge is resorbed, then the resistance of the teeth to movement over each other may be greater than the lateral resistance offered by the ridge, causing denture movement and pressure and discomfort to the patient. Cusp angle or height of cusp should therefore be related to the height and resistance to lateral pressure of the poorer of the two ridges, usually the lower.

When cusped teeth are used, the patient becomes conscious of a position of maximal cuspal interdigitation. Without this sensation of an intercuspal position, the patient may lose the normal muscular closing pattern. However, when using cusped teeth, the intercuspal position, in which the artificial teeth are set up, and the patient's muscular position, must coincide. Otherwise the inclines of the teeth will direct the mandible into the intercuspal position, i.e. until good interdigitation and maximum occlusion is achieved. In guiding the mandible into this position, pressures on the ridges are set up, since the mandible moves normally into the muscular position. In addition, tension in the muscles controlling the mandibular position may cause muscle spasm and pain.

Some patients have lost definition of their muscular occlusal position. This may be due either to wearing a denture without a correct tooth position, or to partial or complete edentulousness over a period of time. In these circumstances, the difficulty of recording precise jaw relations may be avoided by using cuspless teeth.

The precision of achieving the intercuspal position decreases with age. Jaw movements, in common with all other muscular movements, become less precise on ageing, being subject to less fine control. An *area* in which even contact is possible may therefore be necessary for the older patient rather than a precisely defined intercuspal position.

MATERIAL

In the natural dentition, teeth are worn away gradually depending upon the vigour of chewing movement and the degree of refinement of the foods eaten. Artificial teeth are used much less vigorously. It is preferable that a small amount of abrasion of the occlusal surfaces of the teeth should take place during the life of a denture. This is necessary in the first few weeks of wear to enable small errors or 'high spots' of tooth contact to adjust themselves. At a later date, tooth abrasion allows the occlusal surfaces to adjust themselves when slight changes of jaw relation occur. After a slight amount of ridge resorption, the mandible moves forwards as well as upwards and less damage to the lower ridge occurs if the teeth adjust themselves to this gradual change in mandibular position.

Of the two materials commonly used for posterior teeth, one, porcelain, is too resistant to abrasion and the other, acrylic, may be worn away too readily. Porcelain teeth show signs of abrasion after vigorous and prolonged function, but the degree of wear is only small. If rapid ridge resorption takes place, the rate of self-adjustment of porcelain teeth is too slow. On the other hand, acrylic teeth show a marked loss of both substance and contour after a period of one year or less if subjected to vigorous mastication or a coarse diet. Where chewing function is only light, acrylic teeth are satisfactory, but with vigorous chewers, porcelain teeth are to be preferred. An assessment of vigour of function can be made by examining previous dentures or by palpating the masseter muscles, particularly when the teeth are clenched.

One of the disadvantages of acrylic teeth is that both upper and lower teeth may wear, thus losing all occlusal contour. On occasions, therefore, porcelain teeth are used in one jaw against acrylic ones in the other. Provided that the

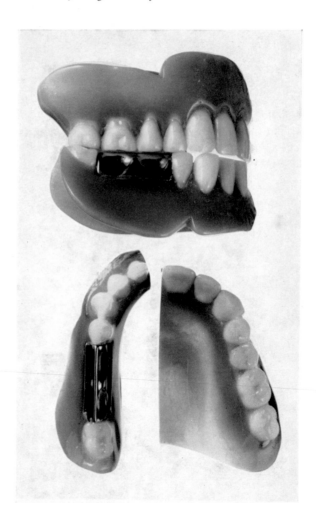

Fig. 10.3 A metal surface in the lower molar region opposing upper posterior teeth of conventional form.

porcelain teeth are not ground but remain highly polished, abrasion is no greater than when using all acrylic teeth.

Perhaps the main reason for the widespread use of acrylic teeth is their simpler technique when setting up. Since it is possible to achieve chemical union between the teeth and the denture base, mechanical retention is unnecessary. Accordingly the teeth may be ground to fit the available space and will still join to the denture base, whereas porcelain teeth require mechanical retention which limits the amount of grinding that is possible. Where there is little inter-ridge space, therefore, acrylic teeth are chosen. In addition any errors of occlusion of the complete dentures are rectified more easily when using acrylic teeth, as their surface may be ground and polished more readily than that of porcelain teeth.

In order to reduce the occlusal table markedly and to maintain a relatively sharp cutting edge, metal is sometimes used to provide a piece of 'masticatory machinery'. This may take the form of teeth which are perforated so that the food passes through them into the buccal or lingual sulcus. In other designs, a single surface of metal in the lower jaw is opposed by normal upper posterior teeth (Fig. 10.3). Metal strips or tubes are also incorporated in acrylic or porcelain teeth so that sharp shearing edges are provided and maintained.

POSTERIOR TEETH FOR THE IMMEDIATE DENTURE

On replacement of a few posterior teeth by an immediate denture, it can be argued that the artificial posterior teeth should conform to the same occlusal pattern as their natural predecessors. Before extraction of the teeth, the patient chews in a series of movements permitted by the occlusal surface of these teeth. To maintain the same chewing patterns this occlusal surface should be reproduced. This argument is valid if the natural teeth are in normal position and occlusion. Frequently, however, the few remaining posterior teeth have migrated and overerupted. Whilst they can be used for chewing in this position the difference in stability between natural teeth and a denture must be remembered. A tooth not in normal position and occlusion will cause instability of the denture.

Acrylic teeth present less technical difficulties where there is a small inter-ridge distance. On removal of the natural posterior teeth from the cast only a small space may remain between the socket area and the occlusal surface of the opposing teeth. Here, acrylic teeth are indicated.

When patients have enjoyed a wide range of mandibular movement as evidenced by marked wear facets on the natural teeth, they should be provided with balanced articulation in the immediate dentures. If it appears, however, that only a chopping stroke has been used, then by setting the teeth to normal curves, it should be possible to grind them into a restricted range of balance later should this be necessary and provided that the anterior teeth allow it to be done.

The posterior teeth are arranged so that occlusal forces applied to them pass through the resorbed ridge areas. Where molar and premolar teeth are to be extracted, the artificial tooth over the socket should be placed in line with the rest of the posterior teeth. In the upper jaw this usually results in the tooth being placed slightly lingual to the socket. However, resorption of bone takes place mainly at the outer plate and then the teeth will be over the edentulous ridge. Usually artificial posterior teeth are narrower buccolingually than the natural teeth. The lingual relation of the tooth is therefore maintained whilst the buccal moves inwards from the cheek. In the posterior area of the lower jaw resorption takes place mainly on the lingual aspect due to the thinner bone in this area. The replacements for lower molar teeth should therefore be placed slightly buccal to the natural tooth position. This not only allows for resorption but also increases tongue space and creates a surface to the denture which is controlled more easily by the tongue.

POSTERIOR TEETH FOR REPLACEMENT DENTURES

Effect of resorption on ridge relations

The alveolar bone surrounding the natural teeth varies in thickness round the tooth sockets. In the upper jaw, the outer plate of bone is generally thinner. Therefore, the upper ridge resorbs mainly on its outer surface, producing a generally smaller arch. Anteriorly, the alveolar bone of the lower jaw undergoes resorption in a similar pattern and usually to a greater extent. The buccal plate in the region of the second and third lower molars, however, is robust, being supported by the external oblique line of the mandible. But the lingual plate is thin and undergoes marked resorption.

Hence, the upper edentulous ridge is smaller than the arch of the natural teeth, whilst the lower ridge maintains its arch width posteriorly, or even appears to become wider as its lingual plate resorbs (Fig. 10.4). If the artificial teeth are to meet despite this changed inter-ridge relation, they must be set to a curve.

The amount of lateral curvature applied to the occlusal surface depends on the condyle angles and on the cusp angles of the teeth being used. With a steep condyle movement, a relatively steep curve of Monson enables a normal tooth relation to be achieved. Where the condyle angle is shallow, only shallow cusped teeth and a large radius curvature is possible. Frequently it is then necessary to set the lower teeth outside the uppers in a reverse or 'crossbite' relation

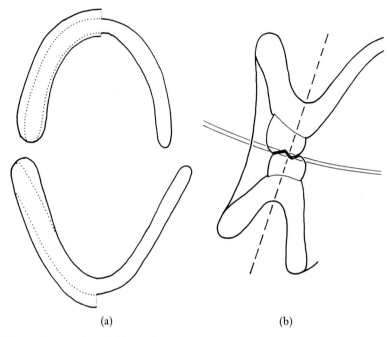

         (a)   (b)

Fig. 10.4 Resorption of ridges after extractions:
(a) the bold lines on the left indicate the original outline and the dotted lines the out-line after resorption. The bold lines on the right illustrate the relation of the upper and lower ridges after resorption;
(b) the lateral curvature to which the posterior teeth must be set after ridge resorption if normal occlusal relations are to be achieved.

(Fig. 10.5). In this position, a reverse chewing movement must be used by the patient. That is, to chew a bolus of food between the teeth on the left, they must move their jaw to the right. Movement to the left simply separates the occlusal surfaces of the molar teeth. Teeth arranged in this relation are there-fore not as efficient for chewing, but this positioning avoids encroachment beyond the neutral zone. On the other hand, this posterior tooth relation fre-quently allows the cheek to be caught and nipped between the occlusal sur-faces, when the patient chews. Reduction of a reverse relation can be achieved by moving the lower posterior teeth lingually or the uppers buccally. The degree of movement of the lowers is restricted by encroachment on tongue

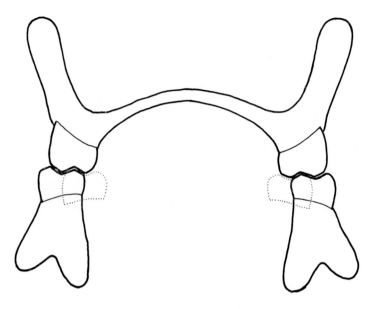

Fig. 10.5 'Crossbite' relation of posterior teeth (the dotted lines indicate the normal position of the lower posterior teeth in relation to the uppers).

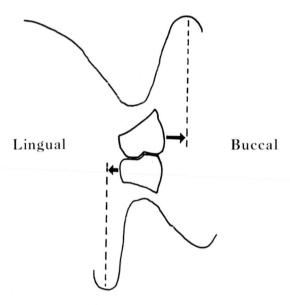

Lingual   Buccal

Fig. 10.6 The lingual aspect of the lower teeth should not encroach beyond a vertical line drawn upward from the lingual sulcus, nor should the upper posterior teeth project beyond a vertical line dropped from the upper buccal sulcus.

space and the creation of an undercut lingual surface to the denture, which will be displaced by the tongue. The lingual aspect of the lower posterior teeth should not encroach further than a vertical line drawn upwards from the centre of the posterolingual sulcus (Fig. 10.6). When the patient has a large tongue and there is relative flaccidity of the buccinator muscles, the neutral zone is found to be positioned towards the cheek and the position of the posterior teeth should follow it. If in doubt, an impression technique as suggested in Chapter 21 is advised to define the neutral zone more clearly.

Outward movement of the upper teeth is restricted by the retention of the upper denture. With a good ridge, the upper teeth are set away from the centre of it, bearing in mind the effect that this may have on midline fracture of the denture. A poor ridge does not allow such great freedom of positioning. In general, the buccal aspect of the upper posterior teeth should not be placed further buccally than a line drawn vertically down from the centre of the sulcus. Beyond this line the dentures tend to be displaced by the buccinator and stability during chewing may be poor.

Chapter 11

Anterior Tooth Position

FOR IMMEDIATE DENTURES

At the treatment planning stage, preliminary decisions were made regarding the type of immediate denture to be constructed. Articulated study casts were used to discuss the treatment plan with the patient, and to illustrate any changes that might be contemplated in appearance by a change in tooth positions, form or shade.

At the trial denture stage the remaining natural teeth are once more carefully examined and final decisions made concerning their artificial successors. If an open face denture has been prescribed, the teeth must be placed near the sockets of their natural predecessors although the inclinations and length of the teeth may be altered. With a flanged denture, however, the operator is free to alter the position of the teeth. In cases where an aesthetic improvement is desired, then discussion with the patient is necessary to discover what ideas he may have on his future dental appearance.

The appearance of the anterior teeth on the denture will be affected by the anteroposterior and incisal relation, the detailed position of individual teeth and the reproduction of individual tooth characteristics.

ANTEROPOSTERIOR POSITION

After loss of bone from periodontal disease, labial migration and spacing of the teeth is often seen. This not only produces an appearance that is displeasing to the patient but, in addition, takes the natural teeth further away from their alveolar ridge support. If this abnormal tooth position is reproduced it may result in instability of the denture as incising forces are directed well in front of the ridge. The artificial teeth should then be arranged in a position palatal to the natural teeth, simulating the appearance before tooth migration took place. Migration of teeth is mainly a rotation taking place about an axis one-third along the root of the tooth. This centre of rotation should be borne in mind when arranging the teeth and the inclination adjusted accordingly (Fig. 11.1).

A more palatal positioning of the anterior teeth may also be necessary where it has been decided to reduce the prominence of natural upper anteriors in Class II jaw relationships.

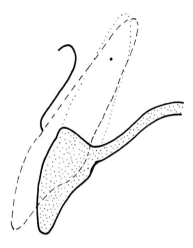

Fig. 11.1 When the natural teeth have migrated forwards, their centre of rotation is approximately at the apical third of the root. This must be borne in mind when adjusting the inclination of anterior teeth.

INCISAL RELATION

An examination of the amount of tooth displayed when the patient smiles, enables the dentist to decide what change in incisal level is desirable for aesthetic reasons. He must also consider whether modifications may be necessary in relation to function. In many natural dentitions, there is a deep vertical incisal overlap. Whilst this tooth relationship can be tolerated by the natural teeth, it may be incompatible with the stability of complete dentures. If the deep vertical overlap is associated with a small horizontal one (Class II div 2 incisor relation), then even a small lateral or protrusive movement of the jaw brings about heavy anterior tooth contact and possible denture displacement.

On the other hand, it can be argued that the artificial anterior teeth should be arranged exactly as the natural teeth. A deep vertical incisor overlap associated with a small horizontal overlap, restricts the patient to certain types of chewing movement. This is mainly a chopping movement with only a small lateral component. In a dentition with a large vertical overlap, the patient is accustomed to the restriction in masticatory movements imposed by the natural teeth. These restricted movements may well be the first that will be employed with immediate dentures. Consequently it is suggested that there is no need to cater for a wider range of masticatory movement than was available in the natural dentition.

The major factor in restricting lateral as distinct from protrusive movements is the relation of the canines. Whilst all the anterior teeth may be considered to present potentially unstabilizing forces when a large vertical overlap is present, the protrusive type of movement is probably used only to a limited extent with dentures. On incision, a large vertical overlap may cause the dentures to be displaced slightly, but tongue control is frequently effective in supporting the upper denture posteriorly and the lower denture anteriorly. Pressure from the hand applying the food for incision may also assist in stabilizing the dentures. In lateral movement, it is mainly the canine relation which controls the freedom of lateral excursion possible. If the canines are in a large vertical overlap—small overjet relation, then ruminatory movement is usually severely limited. Hence if alterations from the natural to the artificial dentition are carried out, the canine guidance (Fig. 11.2) should not be made more limiting than it was in the natural dentition.

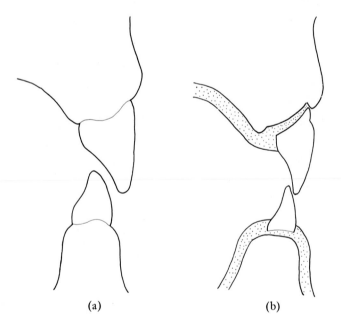

(a)   (b)

Fig. 11.2 Canine guidance:
(a) relation of natural canine teeth;
(b) restriction of lateral excursion on dentures due to reduction of horizontal overlap.

The incorporation of a large vertical overlap produces technical difficulties when setting up, in that a large 'step' appears between the anterior and posterior teeth (Fig. 11.3). This appearance, though common in the natural dentition, offends the trained eye of the technician and frequently that of the dentist. It may also offend the untrained eye of the patient who has never realized that this situation existed with the natural dentition.

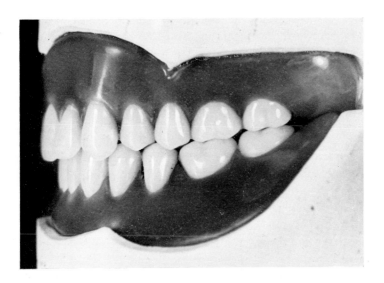

Fig. 11.3 The incisal level and the occlusal plane of the posterior teeth has a marked step due to the large vertical overlap.

Although at first the patient may use chewing movements similar to those possible with the natural dentition, changes in this movement pattern may become necessary due to the inefficiency of dentures as compared with that of the natural teeth. Then a large vertical overlap of the incisors will cause instability of the dentures. In addition, the movement of the dentures may traumatize the healing ridges and bring about accelerated resorption of bone. Where a large vertical overlap is retained for aesthetic or speech reasons, the patient should be recalled at regular frequent intervals after the insertion of immediate dentures. Otherwise resorption, coupled with slight abrasion of the posterior teeth, reduces the extent of ruminary movement available to the patient and causes the anterior teeth, particularly the canines, to come into contact at the intercuspal jaw relation. Attempts to move into even a slight ruminatory excursion then cause considerable trauma to the ridges and further resorption. This only exacerbates the condition and leads to an even more rapid destruction of the underlying tissues.

It would appear, therefore, that where the patient has a large vertical overlap, the amount of freedom of lateral excursion should not be reduced in moving from the natural to the artificial dentition. A reduction of the horizontal overlap to make everybody into a Class I tooth relation should be avoided. Unless the vertical overlap is also reduced, this simply steepens the incisal and canine guidance angle. Where possible, there seem to be advantages in reducing the angle at which the incisors and canines pass over each other. It is impossible to predict whether the patient will utilize the previous masticatory excursions or will investigate new patterns of movement when provided with complete dentures. It is also difficult to anticipate whether the patient will indulge in empty mouth grinding movements after they have been provided with dentures.

In many cases, therefore, it is preferable to modify the anterior tooth relation to one that will not produce great interference even if the chewing pattern changes. Reduction of the incisal guidance angle to give balanced articulation in protrusive movements appears to be unnecessary, but some degree of lateral ruminatory movement should be allowed for when placing the canine teeth.

Marked changes of the order of 2 to 3 mm in the incisal level can readily be made on an immediate denture and generally pass unnoticed by the patient. Fortunately, a patient's memory of his natural dentition is not precise, and provided that a similarity in appearance is achieved, little criticism of aesthetics usually arises. When changes greater than this are necessary, it is advisable to make a major change in the immediate dentures and a smaller one when these are replaced. Unless radical alveolectomy is carried out, a large change in incisal level necessitates considerable alteration to artificial tooth proportions so that they no longer resemble the natural teeth. However, much can be achieved by reducing the incisal height of the lower teeth as these do not contribute so forcefully to appearance.

DETAILED TOOTH ARRANGEMENT

Discussion with the patient reveals his opinion on the appearance of the natural dentition. Frequently there is little or no criticism and the general arrangement of the teeth is copied.

With the patient who 'hates the sight' of his natural teeth, the dentist should decide how deep this dislike is and should modify it accordingly. Sometimes a slight decrease in irregularity is all that is required but in other cases a much more regular arrangement is necessary to satisfy the patient. A patient with moderate irregularity of the natural dentition may state a preference for straight, white teeth. In this case the incisors are arranged in a more regular manner but an appearance of artificiality should be avoided. The dentist may consider that he is pleasing the patient in providing a row of 'piano keys'. This may be so, but if a slight irregularity is introduced, related to the patient's aesthetic comment, not only will the patient still be satisfied, but the dentist's reputation for creating a good cosmetic result will be enhanced.

With an intelligent and cooperative patient there are some advantages in setting up the anterior teeth separately from the trial dentures. Then a more definite discussion can take place. It must be remembered, however, that artificial teeth look both dark and large against a light-coloured cast and some patients will form an unshakeable opinion regarding the anterior teeth based on this extra-oral appearance, despite the change in appearance which takes place on insertion of the teeth in the mouth. This procedure should therefore only be adopted with suitable patients.

INDIVIDUAL TOOTH CHARACTERISTICS

Each natural tooth has its own form and outline. The basic form of the erupted tooth is determined by heredity and due note should be taken of the general convexity of the labial surface and the presence of surface markings. Both these affect the appearance of the tooth.

A set of teeth is selected to match the form of the central incisors. A marked improvement in the appearance of the artificial teeth is obtained by grinding the incisal edges to match the wear facets on the natural teeth. Small changes in outline at the neck are also important in restoring the aesthetic characters of the natural dentition. Frequently the laterals require major modification before they match the natural teeth; it may be necessary to select laterals from another set of teeth. Artificial laterals always seem to be too large, particularly for females in whom these teeth are generally more delicately moulded in the natural dentition. Canines are selected in a darker shade and are similarly ground to match the natural teeth.

ANTERIOR TOOTH MATERIAL

Acrylic anterior teeth are often preferred to porcelain for the immediate denture because of the ease with which they can be modified by grinding to simulate the natural teeth. If the patient has obvious restorations in the anterior teeth then, the reproduction of these in the denture should be considered. Certainly where there are multiple restorations it is inadvisable to provide the patient with 'new' teeth. Proximal fillings of acrylic polymer of a slightly different shade can be inserted in the artificial teeth so that the appearance resembles but does not necessarily copy the natural dentition. Naturally, if the patient had a greatly discoloured restoration in a natural tooth he would ask for it to be replaced by a better filling.

Porcelain teeth generally present greater problems in modification although low fusing stains can be used to modify colour and to create restorations on the tooth. Better quality porcelain and acrylic teeth have some characterization in the form of fillings, opaque areas and staining. Gold restorations can be placed in porcelain teeth but the technique is more difficult than in the case of acrylic teeth.

FOR REPLACEMENT DENTURES

The most valuable method of retaining a record of the natural teeth is by means of an immediate denture. Whilst some changes must be made, this denture generally provides a close aesthetic approximation to the previous natural dentition. Alternatively a cast of the patient's natural dentition, before the teeth are extracted, may be stored, together with details of tooth shade and the position of any particularly large restorations.

When replacing an immediate denture after its period of useful life has passed, care must be taken to reproduce the original tooth shape, shade and arrangement as carefully as possible. This may be done by recording an impression of the denture so that the technician can use this as a guide when setting up. Alternatively, one of the methods for copying a denture, given in Chapter 19, may be used. If this is not done and the tooth position is changed arbitrarily without reference to the previous denture, the patient often reverts to the immediate denture for appearances sake, even though its retention is not as good as the replacement denture.

A patient attending for replacement of non-immediate dentures or who has been rendered edentulous and has been without prostheses, can give little valuable information on tooth size, position and shade. If he is satisfied with the appearance of his present dentures, then this is of assistance when arranging the teeth on the new dentures. The present tooth arrangement may, however, be displeasing to the patient. The dentist may wish to improve the patient's appearance by modifying what he considers to be an unsatisfactory tooth position and arrangement. In these circumstances some guidance is necessary in the arrangement of the upper and lower anterior teeth.

GENERAL TOOTH POSITION

The natural incisor teeth are surrounded by alveolar process. After tooth extraction, a portion of the alveolar bone resorbs. In the anterior region of both jaws, resorption is mainly of the outer plate of bone. The relation between the edentulous ridge after initial resorption and the position the natural tooth occupied is such that the neck of the tooth would be just forward of the ridge. After a greater degree of resorption has taken place, the distance between the natural tooth position and the remaining ridge increases, so that to copy the original tooth position, the artificial tooth would need to be placed further and further away from the residual ridge (Fig. 11.4).

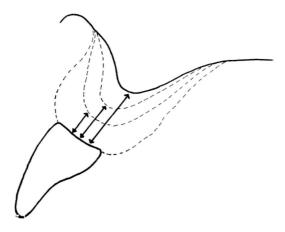

Fig. 11.4 The progressive increase in the distance between the upper anterior ridge crest and the position the natural teeth occupied, which occurs as the result of bone resorption.

It is sometimes stipulated that the distance from the incisal papilla on the palate to the incisal edges of the central incisor teeth is between 8 and 12 mm. This is helpful where little other information is available, but it should be considered as a starting point rather than a precise pinpointing of tooth position.

The advantages of setting the artificial teeth in a position similar to that of the natural dentition are that the dental appearance is maintained, the lips are supported in a similar manner, and the patient can make the same tongue and lip movements in speech. The disadvantage is that as resorption proceeds, the stability of the denture decreases. Teeth placed well forward of the ridge cause instability on incision or on pressure from the lips and tongue during speech and during masticatory movements. For stability during mastication and incision, therefore, teeth should be placed near to the ridge; but for restoration of previous appearance and for speech they should be placed in a position similar to their natural predecessors. The point at which to strike a balance depends upon the prognosis for retention of the dentures, the patient's previous denture experience and development of denture control, and also the patient's desires on function versus appearance. Some patients prefer greater stability and will tolerate some loss of facial support, whilst others will develop suitable 'oral gymnastics' in controlling an unstable denture, provided that their appearance is restored to their satisfaction.

UPPER TEETH

The upper anterior teeth should be placed so that they give support to the vermilion border of the upper lip. The several bundles of muscle tissue comprising the orbicularis oris muscle are not all in line, but curve outwards towards the edge of the lip. Contraction of this terminal muscle band must be resisted by the teeth, otherwise a convex lip shape is produced. Attempts to support the lip by plumping the denture base above the level of the teeth only produce a poor lip shape. This simply makes the lip more convex and the vermilion border rolls under, since it is unsupported by the teeth. In females who use make-up, lipstick is often seen on the skin above the vermilion area in order to produce an appearance of normal lip contour where tooth support is inadequate. It can generally be assumed that the upper tooth position is satisfactory if the philtrum of the upper lip, viewed in profile, is supported so that it assumes a slightly concave shape.

LOWER TEETH

Whilst the lower teeth assist in the support of the lower lip, there is less freedom in positioning these teeth in relation to the ridge. Only when there has been very little resorption and a ridge remains which offers good retention, is it possible to move the anterior teeth very far forward from a position just in front of the crest of the ridge. It is seldom advisable to bring the lower incisor teeth forward of a line drawn vertically upwards from the labial sulcus. On the other hand, if lower teeth are positioned too far lingually there may be difficulties of speech and denture instability due to encroachment on the tongue space. This is particularly marked if the patient has a strong, muscular tongue or is a tongue thruster.

UPPER AND LOWER TOOTH RELATION

Having considered the relation of upper and lower anterior teeth to their respective ridges, then the interrelation becomes important. There is a general tendency to arrange anterior teeth on complete dentures in a Class I incisal relation, that is, with a small horizontal and a small vertical overlap. Such a tendency has arisen from the theories of balanced articulation. Only with small vertical and horizontal overlaps can balanced contact in protrusive movements be achieved.

Three basic types of facial contour can be recognized, straight, convex and concave. These can assist the dentist in deciding upon the incisor relation.

The face with neither concavity nor convexity usually has a normal ridge relation and a Class I (Fig. 11.5a) or a Class II div 2 (Fig. 11.5b) type of incisal relation. The latter usually has very little horizontal overlap but a fairly deep vertical overlap. Usually in this type of case, the development of the lower third of the face is less than that seen in a Class I dentition. The gonial angle of the patient is more square and there is a deep labiomental cleft. The lips show great activity on swallowing and the corners of the mouth are drawn in. There is a small inter-ridge space, unless there has been considerable resorption of bone.

The convex face indicates a prominent maxilla (Fig. 11.5c) and is often associated with a Class II div 1 type of anterior tooth relation with a large horizontal overlap.

The concave face (Fig. 11.5d) usually indicates a Class III incisal relation with the teeth edge to edge or the lower anterior teeth in front of the uppers.

These are the more obvious extremes of facial development and many patients present with patterns in between these. It must also be remembered that, in the edentulous state, the soft tissue profile depends at least partly on the support the tissues enjoy from the dentures both in anteroposterior tooth position and also in jaw relation. Loss of occlusal face height can convert a Class I ridge relation to an apparent Class III. Final assessment, therefore, of the probable incisal relation can only be done when the correct occlusal face height has been recorded.

If it is obvious that the ridges do not approximate to a Class I relation anteriorly, then attempts should not be made to reduce a large overjet in Class II div 1 or to enforce a normal horizontal overlap in situations which were naturally an edge to edge (Class III) incisal relation. Whilst the anterior tooth set-up may not conform to the ideals of tooth placement often advocated, it may well restore the patient's natural appearance and should not create functional difficulties.

The main problems seem to arise when treating Class II div 2 patients who had a deep vertical overlap with little horizontal overlap of their natural anterior teeth. Whilst many of these patients can be 'converted' to a Class I incisal relation, this necessitates a reduction in the incisal level of the anterior

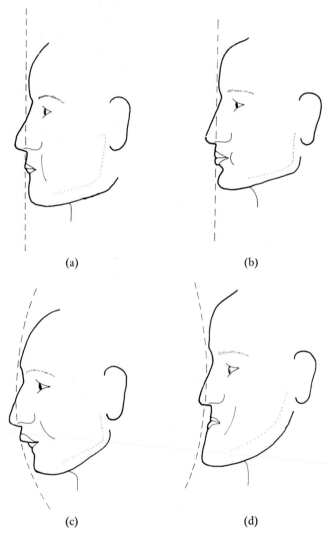

(a)   (b)

(c)   (d)

Fig. 11.5 Facial profile types:
(a) Class I;
(b) Class II div 2;
(c) Class II div 1;
(d) Class III.

teeth. For some patients, a return to a Class II div 2 anterior tooth relation is necessary to give them a satisfactory appearance without increasing their occlusal face height beyond physiological limits.

It has been argued that a large horizontal overlap causes difficulties on incision, since the patient has to move the mandible further forward to make the teeth meet. Biting off food with the incisors is not essential, however, with dentures. It can be done with the canines, or the food can be cut up before placing it in the mouth. If the patient's ridge relation is such that the upper ridge is well in front of the lower, then a large horizontal overlap is indicated in dentures. Difficulties sometimes arise, however, when trying to change an incisal relation from one denture to another. If, despite the jaw relation, a Class I anterior tooth relation has been used in previous dentures, then speech difficulties often arise if reversion to a more 'natural' Class II div 1 relation is attempted. The speech difficulties may be of only short duration or they may persist.

Of course, if the lower anterior teeth are always placed near to the ridge, then the horizontal overlap is increased. Here the balance between retention and stability of the lower denture has to be considered. It may be necessary in some cases to place the lower teeth near to the ridge. If a large horizontal overlap is unacceptable functionally and for speech, then it may be necessary to move the upper teeth back to reduce it a little. Or alternatively, to bring the lower incisors forward and accept a slightly less stable lower denture.

FUNCTIONAL LIP ACTIVITY

Our considerations to date have been in relation to support for the resting lip. It must be realized, however, that lip activity has an important influence on the satisfactory positioning of both the upper and lower anterior teeth. The degree of activity varies between individuals. Observation of the functional activity of the lips is difficult, and even the most careful shaping of the labial surface of the wax rims of the record blocks may not result in the teeth being positioned in a relation which is harmonious with the functioning lip musculature.

However, just as the available denture space posteriorly may be measured by an impression, it is possible to record the amount and direction of lip pressure and thus indicate the anterior tooth position. If the lips act on a mouldable material on the labial surfaces of record blocks, this will be shaped according to the pressures exerted.

Section Two
Immediate Dentures

Chapter 12

Impressions for Immediate Dentures

The philosophy of the operator should be that of making or building the impression rather than taking it. Careful consideration must be given to recording the extent and width of the border of the impression. A single snap impression in a stock tray is unlikely to give the precise definition of the extent of the sulcus which is necessary to produce a denture that will have a satisfactory border seal. The authors recommend a two stage impression procedure. Primary impressions are recorded which indicate fully the possible denture bearing area. To casts made from these impressions, special or individual trays are made which will enable the operator to determine the denture extension with precision.

THE TYPE OF TRAY FOR THE PRIMARY IMPRESSION

A tray should be chosen that conforms reasonably well to the future denture bearing area. An oversize tray is not only difficult to insert into the mouth but, once in, will distort the adjacent tissues. On the cast obtained from such an impression it is difficult to decide where the outline of the special tray should be.

The tray may be of metal or a plastic; both types are available in a range of shapes and sizes. A metal tray may be modified by bending to obtain better adaptation and some of the plastic trays may be moulded slightly after being softened in hot water. The plastic trays are meant to be disposable, so obviating the need for cleaning and sterilizing after use as is necessary with a metal tray. Where only anterior teeth are present, a 'partially edentulous' type of tray should be used to ensure reasonable adaptation of the tray to both anterior and posterior regions, to help in the seating of the tray, and to ensure a fairly uniform thickness of impression material. A 'box' tray may also be used in this situation provided it is modified in the posterior regions by the addition of impression compound (Fig. 12.1). If both anterior and posterior teeth remain, a 'box' tray is used with modification by impression compound where necessary in long edentulous areas.

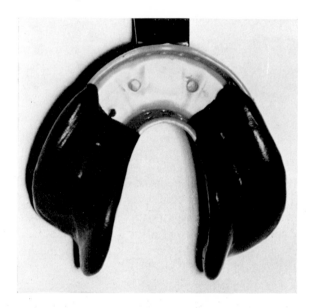

Fig. 12.1 Addition of impression compound to box tray when the anterior teeth only are standing.

The border of the tray should be checked in relation to the functional sulcus. There are three main areas where stock trays are usually underextended.

Upper Jaw

Lateral to the tuberosities. Here complete coverage is essential, as the impression material tends to flow backwards out of the tray rather than sideways into the sulcus by the tuberosities. Commonly, airblows appear in this region of the impression.

Lower Jaw

Distolingually in the lower jaw. Because of the considerable variation in sulcus depth and the distolingual extent, stock trays are invariably incorrectly extended in these areas.

Both Jaws

The anterior segments. If the anterior teeth are at all proclined the flange of the stock tray is unlikely to lie near the sloping alveolar ridge and will not enter the labial sulcus (Fig. 12.2).

This area must always be recorded accurately in the lower jaw, and in the upper if the immediate denture is to carry a full labial flange. Failure to improve the adaptation of the border of the stock tray in the anterior region will invariably result in a recording of the sulcus that is grossly inaccurate both in extent and width.

Improvement of the adaptation of the stock tray border in the areas mentioned may be achieved by the addition of impression or tracing stick compound.

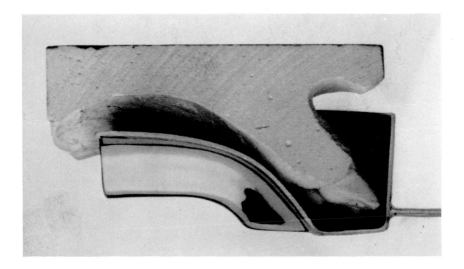

Fig. 12.2 Difficulty of recording the labial sulcus when the anterior teeth are proclined. The tray flange should be modified to fit more closely to the alveolar slope.

MATERIALS FOR THE PRIMARY IMPRESSION

The presence of the natural teeth and the need for accurate reproduction of their contours, indicates an elastic impression material—and the alginates are recommended. The viscosity of the alginates varies and the choice is largely one of personal preference. However, if the only stock tray available is grossly underextended, a brand of alginate should be chosen which when mixed to the manufacturer's instructions gives a mix which is fairly viscous. The higher viscosity will result in extension of the material into those parts of the denture bearing area not covered by the tray. Whereas if an alginate mix of low viscosity is used, the material is unlikely to extend far beyond the limits of the tray and the denture bearing area will not be fully recorded.

Although alginate is generally recommended for the primary impression as a material that will give a satisfactory impression with a simple and quick technique and with minimal discomfort to the patient, there is a particular clinical situation where impression compound is likely to produce a more satisfactory cast on which to build the special tray. When lower posterior teeth have been missing for many years, the adjacent cheek and lingual tissues may have 'folded over' the alveolar ridge. In order to expose the potential denture bearing areas it is necessary to push aside these encroaching tissues. Alginate is not sufficiently viscous to achieve this and all too often a fold of mucosa from cheek or floor of mouth is trapped between the impression material and the alveolar ridge (Fig. 12.3).

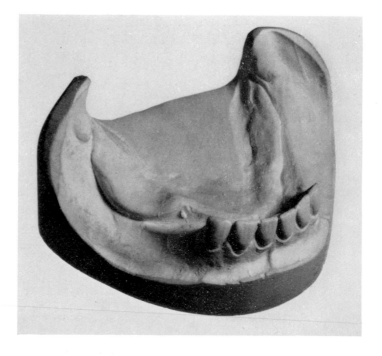

Fig. 12.3 Folds of lingual mucosa trapped between the impression material and the alveolar ridge resulting in an inaccurate cast.

Impression compound suitably softened has sufficient body to push aside the overlapping tissue and to expose the extent of the alveolar ridge. Compound will not, however, record the details of the crowns of the anterior teeth nor record tooth and tissue undercuts. To make use of both the viscosity of compound and the elasticity of alginate in the respective areas where each is needed, a combined alginate–compound technique is used (Fig. 12.4). An adequately extended compound impression is first recorded and whilst it is still soft the compound is removed from the parts of the tray where teeth are standing. The space is then filled with alginate, the tray re-inserted and the impression completed.

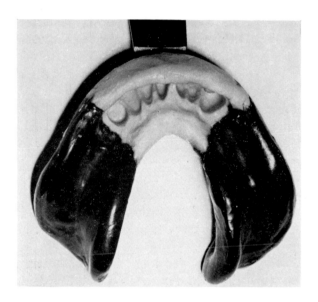

Fig. 12.4 A combined alginate–compound impression.

THE TYPE OF TRAY AND THE MATERIALS FOR THE MAJOR IMPRESSION

The type of special tray that may be used in recording the major impression will be dependent on the impression material that is to be used.

Obviously the material must be elastic and the choice lies between the alginates and the synthetic elastomers. All record accurate impressions with fine tissue detail and the selection is one of personal preference, although the higher degree of elasticity of the elastomers is an advantage where large undercuts are present.

If alginate is chosen, the special tray may be made of shellac or of acrylic and the spacer used on the cast when the tray is being constructed is 3 mm thick.

When using one of the synthetic elastomers, the tray should be made structurally more rigid because of the higher stresses involved in removing the impression. Acrylic is a suitable material. The elastomers are used in thinner section than the alginates and the spacer used when constructing the tray should be 1·5 mm thick. Whilst a rigid tray is essential for accuracy, its use creates difficulties when removing the impression from the cast. Frequently the tray must be destroyed before the impression material can be removed.

Various methods are used to achieve adhesion between the tray and the impression material. At one time, with alginates, perforated trays were favoured, but modern adhesives provide a better bond in some circumstances. The operator should confirm that good adhesion can be obtained with his choice of alginate and adhesive, as some alginates and adhesives are incompatible due to an incorrect pH of the gel and only a poor bond results. In these circumstances, perforations should also be used. Retention of the elastomeric impression materials to the tray may be achieved with one of the special adhesives supplied for use with these materials or by perforating the tray.

As with the stock impression tray so must the border of the special tray be examined carefully in relation to the sulcus. Time taken in adjusting the border of the special tray before proceeding with the major impression is well spent. Also at this time the disadvantages of a hastily recorded and inadequate primary impression are revealed.

The best method of determining and developing the border extent and shape is to add a beading material to the tray periphery and allow the sulcus tissues to mould it functionally. A number of materials may be used for this purpose. Soft wax has the disadvantage that it never reaches a rigid state and is therefore liable to be distorted on removal from the mouth or during the pouring of the cast. Tracing stick is used although its manipulation demands considerable skill and practice. Other border moulding materials are being developed; some are polymers which become rigid after moulding in the mouth whereas others such as the silicone putties are elastic after setting and are specially indicated for use with the silicone type of elastomeric impression material.

Border additions to the special tray for the purpose of ascertaining the correct extent and width of the sulcus should always be made to those areas which are particularly prone to underextension, namely:

1 lateral to the tuberosities
2 distolingually in the lower jaw
3 the anterior segments in both jaws.

In these areas doubt usually exists as to the extension of the tray. In other areas, extension of the tray may be checked visually although some operators prefer to confirm the border extension in all areas by means of a border moulding material.

When an open face denture or a denture with a part labial flange has been prescribed because of a deep labial undercut, it may be an advantage to under-extend deliberately the border of the tray. Removal of an impression from a deep undercut may be difficult because of resistance to displacement. This may also lead to inaccuracies because of tearing of the impression material itself and because of its separation from the tray.

After suitable extension has been achieved, the border of the tray should just contact the sulcus reflection at the same time as the tray also touches the incisal and occlusal surfaces of the teeth and the crest of the ridge. This means that when the impression material is in the tray and acting as a spacer, the border of the tray will be short of the sulcus by the thickness of the impression material. The sulcus tissues then mould the impression material to the correct border extent and form, without interference from the tray, yet with adequate support.

IMPRESSION TECHNIQUE

The operator's impression technique should be similar for both primary and major impressions. With both he should use the greatest care; the more accurate the primary impression, the better adapted will be the special tray which will be used to record the major or 'working' impression. The details of technique will vary slightly according to the impression material chosen but the operator should always pay particular attention to the seating of the tray in the mouth and to recording the extent and width of the functional sulcus with the greatest possible accuracy.

Prior to recording impressions the operator should ask the patient to rinse with a mucin solvent mouthwash such as a teaspoon of sodium bicarbonate in a glass of water. It may also be necessary to wipe adherent mucus away from the posterior part of the palate using a dental napkin.

If there has been recession of the gingival tissues leaving spaces between the tooth contact points and the interdental papillae, it is advisable to block out the spaces with soft carding wax. If this is not done, the impression material will flow into the spaces and make removal of the impression difficult. This is likely to result in a torn and inaccurate impression.

It is recommended that the lower impression should be taken first as the patient is not likely to suffer from the slight anxiety due to fear of retching or of swallowing impression material that may occur with the upper. When the lower impression is taken satisfactorily at the first attempt the patient then has confidence in the operator which overcomes any anxiety they might have over the upper impression.

Using Alginate

Three areas have been mentioned as being likely to cause difficulties. Of these, the upper tuberosity and lower distolingual regions often reveal under-extensions or blowholes in an otherwise perfect impression. This is particularly so when the alveolar processes are pronounced and have not undergone much resorption. To eliminate air and to ensure a good periphery, these areas are prepacked just before inserting the loaded tray, a small amount of alginate being placed in these regions with the finger or spatula. If a very deep palate exists the vault also may be prepacked to reduce the possibility of trapping air in this area.

The volume of impression material placed in the special tray should be related to the thickness of impression required (which is related to the type of impression material) and the area to be recorded. A common failure is to overload the tray and thus prevent it being seated correctly. More care is required in loading the upper tray since it is not as easy for excess material to escape as it is in the lower.

An even more common fault is to push the tray through the material until it presses on the tissues. 'Stops', however, enable the operator to feel more distinctly when the tray is in its correct position. These are small islands of impression compound or wax, of thickness equal to that required in the impression. Wax or compound is applied to the upper tray along its posterior border and to the lower tray over the pear-shaped pads (Fig. 12.5). These areas will all tolerate moderate compression. If the operator presses too hard on the tray in seating it, then pressure falls mainly on these selected areas and is not produced haphazardly over the remainder of the denture bearing area.

Before inserting the tray, the patient should be asked to relax the lips. Access is much easier with a relaxed circumoral musculature, and the impression material will flow more readily into the sulcus.

There are two main methods of inserting the loaded upper tray. In one, the posterior border is applied first to the tissues and then the front of the tray is pivoted upwards. This reduces the flow of excess material over the soft palate and creates slight hydraulic pressure, driving the impression material laterally and anteriorly into the sulcus. A post dam or 'stop' on a tray greatly assists this effect. Unfortunately, this technique tends to trap air, particularly in the posterior sulci and in the centre of the palate. The second method is to place the tray in position anteriorly and then bring the posterior portion up into position. As this movement takes place, the impression material flows along the sulcus and the palate, and drives air before it. Excess material in the tray then flows over the soft palate and more care must be taken in controlling the volume of material placed in the tray.

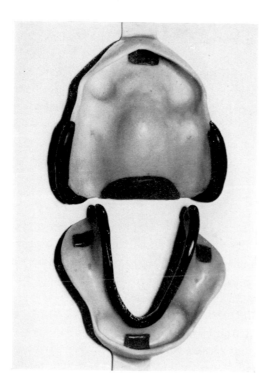

Fig. 12.5 Position of 'stops' in upper and lower trays.

The experienced dentist knows by feel and by visual examination when the impression tray is correctly seated in relation to the sulcus. If in doubt, an examination of the tray border in relation to the sulcus is a clear indication of position.

On insertion of the impression, the lips and cheeks are moved outwards with a finger to release entrapped air and to prevent folding of these structures under the tray. Then the labial and buccal sulcus forms are moulded by the operator compressing lightly the cheeks and lips against the flange of the tray. The patient is then asked to move the lower jaw from side to side. This will bring the respective coronoid processes into a functional relation with the alveolar process in the tuberosity regions and will record the functional width of the sulcus in these areas. During this activity any excess material is moved away from the sulcus area onto the outside of the tray. This prevents sulcus distortion and also assists in retention of the impression within the tray. With alginate, there is no need for very active muscle trimming. Excessive traction upon the muscles of the lips and cheeks only reduces the extent of the sulcus to less than the functional position and so produces an underextended impression.

But there is need for active muscle movement in one area, namely the floor of the mouth. Using the half open mouth technique, the lingual sulcus appears deep because on opening the mouth the tongue moves backwards and the floor of the mouth drops. Therefore, to restore the sulcus to the functional position the patient is asked to move the tongue forwards so that its tip touches the upper lip. It is essential for the patient to maintain the tongue in this position until the impression material gels. If the tongue is retracted while the impression material is still plastic, then an overextended lingual sulcus will be recorded.

The need for careful border moulding of the major impressions cannot be overemphasized. On this depends the comfort of the patient and the satisfactory retention of the dentures. If the tray borders have been adequately checked and corrected, then the impression almost 'takes itself' provided that the tray is not overloaded.

Manipulation of the alginate should be as directed by the manufacturer with the operator paying particular attention to the time advocated by the manufacturer to the various time sequences. After vigorous spatulation the material is inserted whilst the mix is still plastic and before any gelation has taken place. The sequence may be given as:

Mix——Manipulate————Wait————Remove

plastic   plastic–elastic   elastic

It is important that the impression is neither inserted into, nor removed from the mouth during the plastic–elastic state.

With most materials elasticity improves with time as the setting reaction continues. Whilst the heat of the mouth accelerates setting, the thicker sections of the impression are not heated uniformly. That part of the impression round the anterior teeth receives less heat from the oral tissues and is usually the last to gel. When relatively shallow undercuts are present, for example, in edentulous cases, the impression can be removed 30 to 45 seconds after gelation. With large undercuts it is better to hold the impression in the mouth for 60 seconds after gelation to allow greater elasticity to develop.

Alginates are more elastic when distorted suddenly and then allowed to rebound to their original shape. Slow removal causes permanent distortion of the impression. The impression must be removed firmly and quickly. Another effect of slow removal is to tear the alginate away from its attachment to the tray. Should the impression become detached from the tray, distortion occurs, but its effect is often not obvious until a later stage of treatment.

Using the Elastomers

As the special tray for use with an elastomeric impression material is more closely adapted than the tray constructed for use with alginate, perhaps the main indications for use of an elastomer are:
(a) In the lower jaw when the posterior teeth have been absent for many years and where there has been encroachment of the adjacent tissues into the denture bearing area. Here the more closely adapted tray helps to record an accurate reproduction of the denture bearing area.
(b) In cases of microstomia when the small tray will be more easily inserted into the mouth and its relation to the tissues more readily assessed when in position.

It is not possible to prepack areas of the mouth with an elastomer prior to inserting the impression. Consequently even greater care must be exercised when loading and seating the tray. Because the elasticity of the elastomers develops more slowly, an impression recorded in these materials must be left in the mouth for a longer period and the manufacturer's instructions should be followed.

THE CASTS

Dental stone should be vibrated into both primary and major impressions between five and 15 minutes after they have been removed from the mouth and rinsed under cold water to remove adherent mucus and other debris. Where possible the major impressions should be boxed-in prior to pouring with dental stone. If this is not possible the technician must ensure that sufficient stone overlaps the borders of the impression to reproduce their full extent and width.

IMPRESSION PROCEDURE WHEN PARTIAL DENTURES ARE PRESENT

If the treatment plan has included the provision of temporary partial dentures after the extraction of the posterior teeth, these can be converted into immediate complete dentures just prior to the extraction of the anterior teeth. Assuming the border extent is adequate, a box type of stock impression tray is chosen that will enclose the partial denture and the natural anterior teeth. Any clasps present are removed to facilitate the removal of the impression and denture together from the mouth. It is likely that border additions in tracing stick compound will have to be made to correct the adaptation of the stock tray to the sulcus in the upper and lower labial and the lower lingual areas.

The impression should be taken in alginate. On withdrawal, the partial denture will remain in the impression. Stone is poured into the impression and the resultant cast will carry the partial denture in correct relation to the natural anterior teeth (Fig. 12.6).

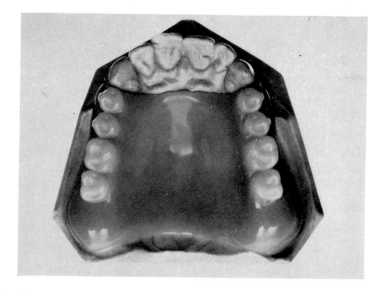

Fig. 12.6 Cast carrying the partial denture in relation to the remaining natural teeth.

Chapter 13

Jaw Relations for Immediate Dentures

One of the main advantages of the immediate denture is that the recording of jaw relations, prior to the construction of the denture, is facilitated by the presence of some of the natural teeth. It is, of course, dangerous to accept without question that the occlusal relation seen when the patient closes the teeth together is correct. It is quite possible that over the years the horizontal and vertical maxillo-mandibular relations have changed from that which existed when the permanent dentition first came into occlusion. Such changes may have been caused by loss of teeth and movement of others into the edentulous areas, attrition of occlusal and incisal surfaces, or drifting of teeth due to loss of periodontal support. It follows, therefore, that there must be a careful examination of the maxillo-mandibular relations that exist in the patient for whom immediate dentures are planned.

The method of approach for this important clinical stage is determined by the coincidence or non-coincidence of the intercuspal and muscular positions, and by the need for any restoration of the occlusal face height.

WHEN MUSCULAR AND INTERCUSPAL POSITIONS COINCIDE

(a) WITH POSTERIOR TOOTH OCCLUSION

Provided that a sufficient number of tooth contacts are present on both sides of the jaw, the correct relation can be obtained without resorting to the use of record blocks. Since the intercuspal position is that of maximum inter-digitation, this position can be discovered from the casts and compared with the patient's intercuspal position. If any doubt exists an intra-oral record can be taken to ensure accurate relation of the casts.

(b) WITHOUT POSTERIOR TOOTH OCCLUSION

Here the casts can only be occluded in the correct relation by means of record blocks (Fig. 13.1). These consist of a base and occlusal rims. The base must have good adaptation to the oral tissues and should not soften or distort in the mouth. Shellac or acrylic are generally more stable than wax and offer a more precise base for record blocks. Rims are made of baseplate wax that will not flow under occlusal loading at mouth temperature. To aid retention of the record blocks, it is sometimes necessary to add simple wrought clasps on the abutment teeth or to use a denture adhesive.

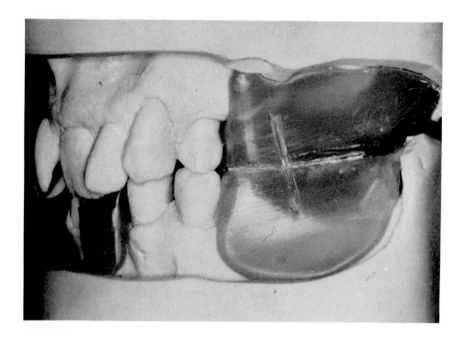

Fig. 13.1 Recording the jaw relations by record blocks in the partially edentulous case.

Accuracy of the Casts

After checking that the bases are well adapted to the casts, the record blocks are inserted and tested for adaptation to the tissues. Finger pressure is applied to either side of the block in turn to determine any rocking. A similar test follows with the fingers placed anteroposteriorly. If a baseplate does not fit accurately, a new impression must be recorded before treatment can continue.

Recording the Jaw Relations

The degree of jaw separation to be used in the dentures is normally that indicated by the contact relation of the upper and lower anterior teeth. All that is required is to establish the degree of separation posteriorly and to record the occlusal plane. However, many patients with only their anterior teeth remaining, habitually posture the jaw forward to obtain good tooth contact. Relaxation is then particularly necessary in order to record the muscular position.

The deep vertical overlap seen with some natural anterior teeth is not always compatible with the retention of complete dentures and sometimes a reduction of this overlap is necessary. A reduction in overlap affects the incisal length of both upper and lower teeth. For maintenance of aesthetics the lowers are usually reduced more than the uppers. At this stage, the position of the occlusal plane must be determined. This can be related to the existing posterior or anterior teeth or may be positioned midway between the two ridges. Where a change in level of the incisor teeth has been decided upon, then this should be borne in mind when deciding the level of the occlusal plane.

The upper rims are trimmed to follow the occlusal plane decided upon. Then the lower rims are trimmed until they just fail to occlude with the lowers when the upper and lower anterior teeth are in contact. In cases of a large vertical incisal overlap it is often necessary to trim away not only the rims, but also a portion of the baseplate, to allow the natural teeth to come into contact. The rims are located using a method that will not cause displacement of the supporting soft tissues. Various methods are available including the use of a thin layer of soft baseplate wax, zinc oxide–eugenol paste or plaster. Alternatively notches may be cut in one rim and small pieces of soft wax added to the other which will flow into the notches when the patient occludes. With all these methods staples may be used in addition to join the rims across the occlusal plane. The operator must observe that the anterior teeth are in contact or in their normal relation.

The upper and lower record blocks frequently stick together and may be removed from the mouth in their correct relation to each other. If they happen to come apart, the method used for their location should ensure that the blocks can be re-located after removal from the mouth.

The casts are placed in the record blocks and the relation of the anterior teeth is again checked to ensure that they contact. If a space exists between them, the most probable cause is that the tissues of the edentulous areas were compressed as the patient closed on wax rims which had not been reduced sufficiently in height. The hard surface of the cast representing the soft tissues is not compressed and therefore the teeth are held out of contact and too great a jaw separation is recorded. A similar error often arises when a 'squash-bite' technique is used; the surfaces of the rims are softened and the patient is asked to occlude. Provided that a sufficient depth of wax is evenly softened, a correct jaw relation *can* be recorded. There is difficulty, however, in softening a large mass evenly and, in addition, it may cool unevenly whilst being placed in the mouth. Then the patient applies a large occluding force not only compressing the mucosa but often distorting the block. In addition, such pressure encourages the patient to protrude the jaw.

A common error in the occlusal relation is caused by a posterior contact of the casts. Suitable trimming of the area behind the retromolar pad on the lower cast, or behind the hamular notch on the upper, enables them to be arranged in the correct relation.

If the teeth on the casts are still apart despite every care in taking the occlusal record, then one or both casts must be considered to be inaccurate.

WHEN MUSCULAR AND INTERCUSPAL POSITIONS DO NOT COINCIDE

(a) WITH POSTERIOR TOOTH OCCLUSION

Here deflective tooth contacts are guiding the mandible into an abnormal intercuspal position. This may be anterior, posterior or lateral to the muscular position. When relaxation is achieved and the muscular position is obtained, there are likely to be only isolated tooth contacts.

Before the jaw relation is registered, these isolated contacts should be stoned to bring about maximal contact between the natural teeth (Fig. 13.2). This occlusal adjustment may take a few visits and usually results in the gradual suppression of the abnormal movement pattern and a return to the original innervation pattern. In some cases it may be necessary to extract a posterior tooth which is preventing the registration of the muscular position.

The casts which have been obtained from impressions recorded *after* the occlusal adjustment may be articulated with or without record blocks.

As an alternative to adjusting the natural occlusion, use may be made of an adjustable articulator which reproduces the hinge axis of rotation of the mandible. The upper cast is mounted using a facebow and the lower cast mounted in relation to it using a wax wafer record taken of the jaw relation just *before* tooth contact. Since the movement of the mandible from the rest position to occlusion is approximately about a hinge axis, the casts may then be brought into occlusion on the articulator. The occlusal surfaces of the teeth are adjusted by trimming away the premature contacts until maximum interdigitation is obtained. This method requires confidence on the part of the operator that he can record a position of the jaw as it follows the correct muscular path to a point at or slightly beyond the postural position. The patient must not wander into the intercuspal position.

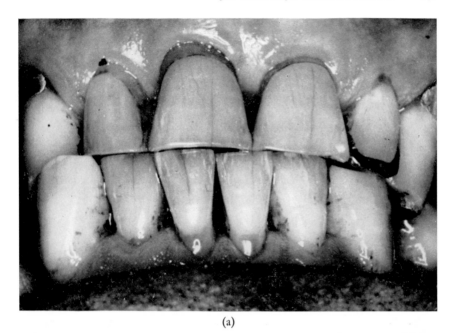

(a)

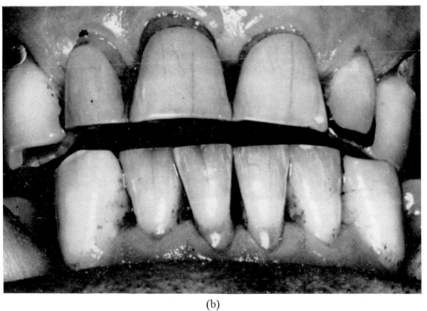

(b)

Fig. 13.2 Non-coincidence of
(a) intercuspal position and
(b) muscular position.
The premature contacts should be stoned before recording the jaw relations.

(b) WITHOUT POSTERIOR OCCLUSION

The abnormal position of the mandible may be anterior or posterior to the muscular position. An anterior positioning (Fig. 13.3) results from a splaying of the upper anterior teeth due to loss of their bony support or when an original edge to edge relation of the anterior teeth has been changed as a result

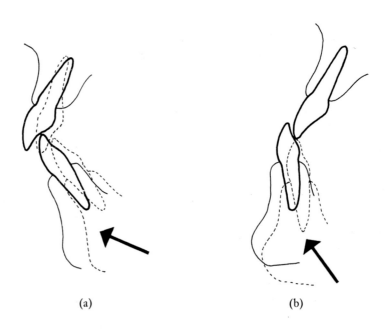

(a)   (b)

Fig. 13.3
(a) Protrusion of mandible to maintain contact of lower teeth with migrating upper anteriors;
(b) Forward sliding from an edge-to-edge contact after loss of posterior teeth.

of loss of posterior teeth. A posterior positioning of the mandible results from a distal guidance of the lower incisors along the palatal surfaces of the upper anterior teeth where posterior tooth support has been lost. It is particularly common in Class II div 2 cases (Fig. 13.4).

With both anterior and posterior mandibular displacement, there is an associated reduction in occlusal face height.

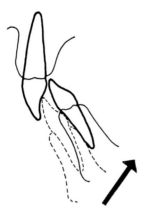

Fig. 13.4 Posterior positioning of the mandible in Class II div 2 case after loss of posterior teeth.

WHERE THERE HAS BEEN LOSS OF OCCLUSAL FACE HEIGHT

If there has been attrition of the incisal edges or if the anterior teeth have splayed forward as a result of loss of bone support, it may be necessary to restore the lost occlusal face height. The methods for ascertaining the correct degree of vertical separation of the jaws are similar to those used with replacement dentures described in Chapter 22. The rule to be obeyed in assessing the required face height is to always have *sufficient* freeway space. Where the increase required is more than 2 mm it may be desirable to construct temporary partial dentures to the newly assessed occlusal face height and to note the response of both the patient and the tissues before providing the immediate dentures.

SHADE OF TEETH

The shade of the natural teeth is recorded by comparison with a shade guide. After moistening the shade guide tooth with the patient's saliva, it is placed alongside the incisors in a gap or, alternatively, it is inverted and positioned with its incisal edge in contact with the incisal edge of a central. In the natural dentition the canines have a greater bulk of dentine, and a thinner enamel covering. Consequently, they appear darker than the incisors. If the shade of the canines differs markedly, then a separate shade should be recorded for them.

PRESCRIPTION

On occasions, it may be possible to record the occlusion and then complete the dentures. In this case, the additional prescription as defined at the end of the next chapter should also be made.

Usually, however, trial dentures are constructed and tried in. The laboratory prescription then consists of:

1 Material, cusp formation and width of posterior teeth
2 Shade of teeth
3 Type of articulator.

Chapter 14

Trial Dentures

The insertion of trial dentures, well adapted to the casts and carrying teeth in occlusion, enables the accuracy of previous recordings to be assessed.

Dimensional accuracy of the casts and correctness of jaw relation are of considerable importance in any denture prosthesis. With replacement dentures, an error discovered after the dentures have been finished can be rectified by a further one or two visits and the patient suffers only a small amount of inconvenience. Errors with an immediate denture that are only discovered after the teeth have been extracted are a major tragedy and may be difficult if not impossible to correct.

In order to check the impressions and jaw relation recorded previously, teeth are set up in occlusion in the posterior edentulous spaces together with any anterior teeth which are absent from the natural dentition. Since the posterior tooth position may well be modified by the subsequent arrangement of the anterior teeth, no attempt is made to fit the teeth accurately to the spaces. They are set up to provide two accurately occluding surfaces.

ACCURACY OF THE CASTS

First, the accuracy of adaptation of the trial dentures to the casts and to the patient's tissues is noted. When record blocks have been used to record the occlusion, any inaccuracy of the casts should have been noted at this earlier stage. When record blocks have not been necessary, it is essential to ensure that the trial dentures fit both the casts and the patient.

JAW RELATIONS

In the mouth, occlusion of the posterior teeth of the dentures is noted and any anterior teeth are compared with the natural teeth for shade, size and position.

If the horizontal and vertical jaw relations, as determined by the remaining natural teeth, have been accepted as correct, then the occlusion of the trial dentures must coincide with the natural tooth contacts. Where a new jaw relation was established at the registration stage the degree of change and the accuracy of its recording is assessed with the trial dentures.

ERRORS IN JAW RELATIONS

It is important to ensure that the trial denture bases are seated on the mucosa. The simplest way of checking this is to insert a small spatula or wax knife between the artificial teeth and to rotate it gently. Alternatively, finger pressure may be applied simultaneously to both trial dentures seating them both onto their respective ridges. If, initially, the trial bases are not properly seated on the mucosa, a space will appear between the occlusal surfaces of the artificial teeth when either of these tests is carried out.

Two main types of error arise. The commoner one is that just described, where there is a space between the occlusal surfaces of the posterior teeth of the trial dentures. This indicates that the distance between the patient's edentulous ridges is greater than the distance separating the same structures on the casts. The latter were mounted on the articulator by using the record blocks and in normal technical work it is difficult, if not impossible, to approximate the casts to a closer relation than that recorded by the record blocks. This type of error, therefore, is of clinical origin.

Record blocks may be regarded as measuring instruments which record inter-ridge distances. To measure accurately, it is essential that the end of the measuring instrument is placed against both limits of the dimension to be recorded. Naturally, if we are measuring a space and do not apply the end of our ruler to one side of the space, we shall record a smaller distance. Similarly, unless the record blocks are touching the mucosa, too small a distance will be measured.

Correction is achieved simply by placing baseplate wax on the occlusal surfaces of the teeth of one of the dentures, softening it and asking the patient to close gently. The operator should take care to ensure that the patient closes into the 'muscular' position. By filling in the gap originally found between the teeth, the wax enables the correct inter-ridge relation to be recorded. The cases are then remounted on the articulator.

A second type of error gives contact of the teeth posteriorly but a decrease in incisal overlap or even a space between the anterior teeth (Fig 14.1). This is commonly called an 'anterior open bite'. Such an error may be either of clinical or technical origin.

If the patient squashes the surface of the wax record rim to any marked extent, a force is applied to the mucosa beneath the baseplate. This soft tissue is compressed, becoming thinner as tissue fluids are displaced, and the inter-ridge distance is temporarily increased. On placing the record blocks on the stone casts, a similar compression is not possible. Thus, the artificial stone casts and the trial dentures record too great a distance between the ridges. Since the tissues are more easily compressed in the distal areas of both jaws, there is a larger increase of dimension distally than in the anterior segment.

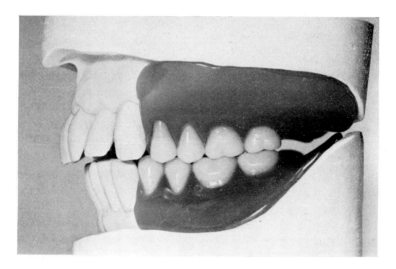

Fig. 14.1 Anterior open bite—note the space between the natural incisors.

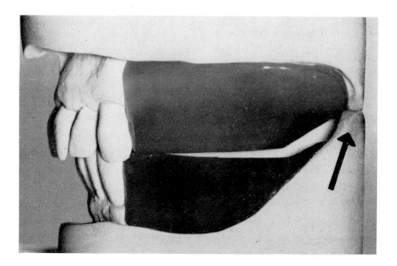

Fig. 14.2 Contact of the casts distally preventing correct location of record blocks.

It is also probable that stress relief in a wax 'squash bite' causes some recovery of the original wax dimension on standing. If a large mass of wax is softened and is squashed by the patient this wax will tend to return towards its previous dimension. Then again, too large an inter-ridge distance will be produced.

In the laboratory, an increased vertical dimension may occur in three ways. First, contact of the casts with each other distally may prevent correct location in the record blocks (Fig. 14.2). This can be avoided if the clinician assumes the responsibility for seating the record blocks on the casts after recording the jaw relation. Secondly, if the casts move within the blocks they obviously move further apart. It is essential when mounting casts on the articulator to seal the record blocks firmly to them. A third laboratory source of inaccuracy is where the technician has failed to arrange the teeth at the correct jaw relation or where movement of the adjusting screw of the articulator has occurred inadvertently.

To rectify this type of error, the posterior teeth must be removed before the correct, smaller, inter-ridge distance can be recorded. Teeth are removed from one denture, generally the lower, and are replaced by a narrow wax rim. The correct relation is recorded by getting the patient to close and make a light imprint of the opposing teeth in the softened surface of the new wax rim (Fig. 14.3).

THE POST DAM AREA

Border seal of the upper denture is achieved by slight pressure along its entire perimeter. In the sulcus, the border of the denture presses lightly on the mucosa but at the posterior border of the palate some extra compression of the soft tissues is made. This latter compression is of particular importance in resisting the loss of seal that may otherwise occur on incision. The position and depth of the post dam must be determined before the trial dentures are prepared for processing. The operator should cut the post dam on the cast whilst the patient is present, so that reference can be made to the oral tissues in the area concerned. All too often, in practice, a line is drawn on the cast and the technician expected to cut the post dam to the correct depth. Even worse, many operators give no guide or instructions to the technician as to its position.

The post dam should be situated just anterior to the axis of rotation of the soft palate and will then lie on non-mobile soft tissue. Its exact position is established by a combination of anatomical markings and a visual assessment of the axis of rotation or vibrating line of the soft palate. The patient is asked to say 'ah' and the vibrating line of the soft palate noted. Using an indelible marker, a line is drawn on the palatal mucosa along the vibrating line from

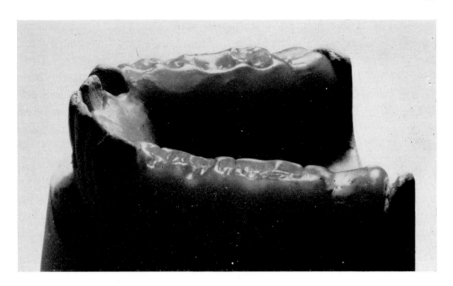

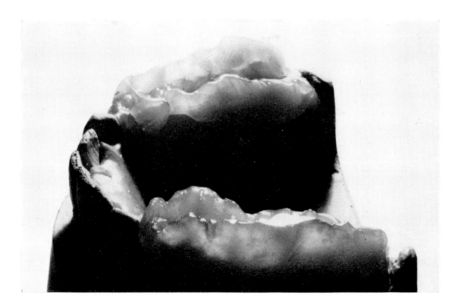

Fig. 14.3 Shallow (correct) and deep (incorrect) indentations in the wax rim when recording the jaw relations.

side to side. The trial denture is inserted and its posterior border adjusted until it coincides with the marked line. The trial denture is replaced on the cast and the post dam marked on the cast at a position coinciding with the posterior border of the trial denture base. A sharp knife is used to make a vertical cut along the marked line. The depth of the vertical cut varies and is determined by the presence, in the post dam area, of submucosa which gives thickness and resilience. Generally the vertical cut will be deeper on the lateral slopes of the palate than in the midline. The vertical cut extends behind the tuberosities to join the distal extremities of the buccal sulcus on each side, thus completing the border seal of the future denture. This initial cut is then modified by scraping away a tapering section of the cast forward of the initial line. Because of the greater softness of the tissue on the slopes of the palate the scraping of the cast should extend further forward in these areas. The resultant modified area of the cast often simulates a Cupid's bow (Fig. 14.4).

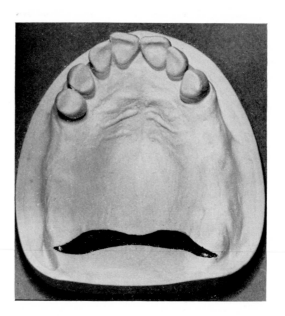

Fig. 14.4 The post dam area.

RELIEF AREAS

Very hard areas in either upper or lower denture bearing areas may be relieved in the finished dentures to prevent excessive pressure. In the upper jaw the median palatal raphé is the area most frequently requiring relief. Recent extraction areas may present bony nodules covered by thin mucosa. These also require relief. The appropriate areas should be palpated and outlined in pencil on the casts. Instruction should be given to the technician on the thickness of relief metal to be used. In very hard areas a combination of gauge 4 and 7 soft metal (tin) sheet may be necessary but gauge 7 alone is satisfactory for most cases.

ANALYSIS OF UNDERCUTS

Whatever type of immediate denture has been planned—open face, complete flange or part flange—it is essential that the prosthesis should go into place after the extraction of the remaining teeth with the minimum of adjustment. Only in this way will there be least disturbance of clot formation and minimal injury to the soft tissues in general.

The operator must not allow himself to get into the position of having to make a number of adjustments to the denture in order to get it seated in the mouth. This can be avoided by a careful analysis of the location and depth of undercuts in the denture bearing areas. The undercuts should be analysed visually and by palpation in the mouth and on the cast utilizing a surveyor.

Frequently, undercuts are pronounced in the tuberosity and canine regions of the upper jaw, and in the lower anterior region. Where the depth of the undercuts is less than 1 to 2 mm no modification of the cast will be necessary because of the compressibility of the soft tissues. Likewise if the undercuts are larger but essentially composed of soft tissues and not bone, no modification of the cast will be needed.

Even when the undercuts larger than 1 to 2 mm are bony in nature, a careful study of the cast on the surveyor may reveal a path of insertion for the denture that will enable all the undercuts to be used. If this is not feasible, the survey indicates in which areas the flange should be shortened or where the undercut on the denture must be reduced.

These decisions are the responsibility of the clinician and he should not delegate them to his technician. If the laboratory is close at hand, there is much to be gained by the clinician and his technician discussing the technical problems in the surgery so that the technician can better appreciate their clinical significance.

The detailed analysis of the cast and of any undercuts will be discussed in Chapter 15.

DEPTH OF THE GINGIVAL CREVICE

The depth of the gingival crevice in the various areas should be recorded on the laboratory card so that reference may be made when the cast is modified. The depth of the crevice should be assessed with a periodontal measuring probe. Radiographs may also be of assistance.

PRESCRIPTION

The additional information to be given in the prescription at this stage of treatment is as follows:-

1 Type of immediate denture
    Open face
    Complete flange
    Part flange
2 Depth of gingival crevices
3 Compressibility of soft tissues over the maximum contour of undercut areas
4 Proposed changes in the incisal level and the anteroposterior position of the upper and lower anterior teeth
5 Proposed changes in the detailed arrangement of the anterior teeth and any 'characterization'
6 Relief areas
7 Colour and thickness of the labial flange, if prescribed.

Chapter 15

Preparation of the Cast

After the trial dentures have been checked in the mouth, they are replaced on the casts and returned to the laboratory. The next stage is to remove the stone replicas of the remaining natural teeth and replace them by artificial teeth. Whatever type of immediate denture is planned it is essential that the dentist and his techician work as a team if a satisfactory aesthetic and functional result is to be achieved. The clinician should not delegate the responsibility of cast modification to his technician. The modifications are based on anatomical factors and the changes that will take place in the gingival tissues after removal of the teeth as well as on the purely technical problems that become apparent on the survey of the cast. It is the clinician who is responsible for the easy and comfortable insertion of the immediate denture and therefore it is he who must prescribe in detail the modifications of the cast and in many instances should do them himself.

THE OPEN FACE DENTURE

With the open face denture, the artificial teeth are usually set in or near to the sockets of their natural predecessors. To do this with accuracy, the stone teeth on the cast should be removed and replaced by the artificial teeth one at a time. If alternate teeth are removed and replaced, the remaining teeth on the cast act as a guide to determine their correct vertical position and inclination. An alternative but perhaps less accurate technique is to prepare a duplicate cast. Then all the teeth are removed and setting up is done, using the duplicate cast as a guide.

Having chosen a mould of anterior teeth that approximates to that of the natural teeth to be replaced, it is useful to reshape the artificial teeth before any of the stone teeth are removed from the cast.

Guide lines are drawn on the casts. First, a line is drawn round the gingival margin of each tooth and secondly, the long axis of each tooth is drawn, extending on to the soft tissue area. Then the incisal level of each tooth is marked on the base part of the cast using dividers (Fig. 15.1). Using a fretsaw

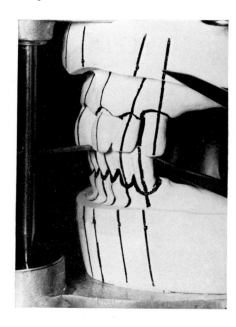

Fig. 15.1 Guide lines drawn on cast, and incisal level measured.

or a fissure bur in a handpiece, a stone tooth is carefully removed. Particular care should be taken to preserve the shape of the adjacent stone teeth. Using a suitable trimmer, a socket is cut which is deeper on the labial aspect than at the palatal or lingual gingival margin. The depth of the socket is determined by the degree of bone loss around the natural tooth which will have been assessed at the previous clinical stage using a periodontal measuring probe. With a normal gingival crevice the labial depth need only be 2 to 3 mm. Where a deeper crevice has been recorded the depth may be 5 mm or more. On the palatal or lingual aspect, the depth required is usually no more than 2 mm and the transition from the socket area to the palatal or lingual aspect of the cast should be made continuous by removing the lingual aspect of the gingival tissues (Fig. 15.2). The interdental papillae on the cast should be preserved intact as the root extensions on the denture prevent the collapse of this tissue into the socket.

The artificial tooth is ground to fit the labial wall of its socket, the remainder of the cavity being filled with wax. Each tooth is treated in the same way and joined with wax to the trial denture already positioned on the cast.

An intelligent and careful approach to the preparation of the sockets cannot be overemphasized. These determine the shape of the surface of the blood clot that fills the socket and are responsible for the ultimate shape of the alveolar ridge after healing. The technique described predisposes to the formation of a well rounded alveolar ridge, whereas haphazard gouging of the cast can only result in a series of indentations in the healed alveolar ridge (Fig. 15.3). Such an irregular ridge is not a favourable foundation for the future replacement denture.

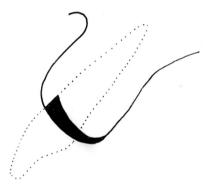

Fig. 15.2 The black area indicates the trimming of the socket and the lingual gingival tissue, for the open face denture.

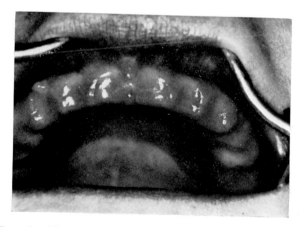

Fig. 15.3 Irregular ridge resulting from incorrect socket preparation on the cast.

THE FLANGED DENTURE

When a complete or part flange has been prescribed, modification of the cast is always required in addition to the removal of the stone teeth, if the denture base is to be closely adapted to the tissues.

Whether an alveoloplasty is carried out or not, there will be an immediate change in the shape and size of the residual ridge because of collapse of the gingival tissues. This collapse is a normal sequel to the removal of teeth and is assisted by the circular periodontal ligament which reduces the size of the wound. The amount of collapse is determined largely by the length of free gingival tissue which is present. When a normal gingival crevice of 1 to 2 mm exists, the collapse will be less than when deep pocketing is present. It must be appreciated that the alveolar bone supporting a tooth does not extend to the enamel–cement junction even in cases which have not been affected by periodontal disease. The part of the root surface not supported by bone supports the surrounding gingival tissues and following extraction these collapse into the socket. Therefore if the cast is not trimmed appropriately, a space will exist between the fitting surface of the flanged denture and the basal tissues.

THE LABIAL FLANGE WITH NO ALVEOLOPLASTY

Guide lines are drawn on the casts as described previously. The stone teeth are removed from the cast singly and alternately as before. The artificial teeth are set up in their place—the fitting surfaces having been ground to fit the unmodified cast. The trial denture with the anterior teeth attached is removed from the cast which may now be further modified.

The trimming of the gingival margins on the cast to allow for their collapse after extraction of the teeth should be done in an orderly sequence. Some authors recommend a useful 'rule of thirds' in which the labial aspect of the cast is divided into three zones between the gingival line and the reflection of the sulcus (Fig. 15.4a). Trimming of the labial surface commences at the centre of the ridge and involves the gingival and middle thirds of the labial surface of the cast with most of it being done in the gingival third.

Step I

The sites of the previously removed crowns are recessed by an amount equivalent to the pocket depth as determined previously by a periodontal measuring probe (Fig. 15.4b).

Step II

Stone is removed from the labial aspect of the cast. A flat cut is made from the depth of the labial aspect of the socket to the line between the gingival and middle third areas. The removal of this stone is equivalent to the change in contour that will occur following collapse of the labial gingival tissues (Fig. 15.4c).

Step III

Another cut is made from the centre of the sockets to the midpoint of the cut made in Step II and completes the contouring of the labial surface of the ridge (Fig. 15.4d).

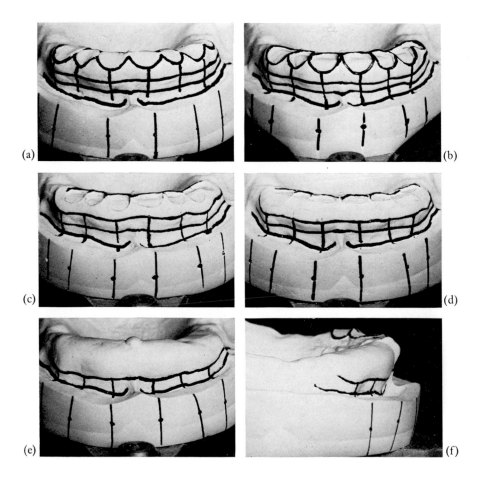

Fig. 15.4 Stages in trimming of the cast for a flanged denture without alveoloplasty:
(a) marking the cast;
(b) preparation of sockets;
(c) first cut on labial surface;
(d) second cut to centre of sockets;
(e) final trimming and smoothing;
(f) comparison between trimmed and untrimmed cast showing amount of cast removed.

Step IV

The lingual gingival margin area of stone is now removed. The future position of the incisive papilla after collapse should be assessed. The cast is built up to simulate the new position of the incisive papilla so that the denture will not place undue pressure on the underlying structures in this area,

Step V

The surfaces of the cast that have been trimmed in Steps I—IV are now smoothed with sandpaper, eliminating any sharp angles (Fig. 15.4e).

During the above sequence of carvings, a moderate amount of stone will have been removed from the cast. The modification of the cast has, however, represented only the change in shape of the soft tissue component of the ridge. Fig. 15.4f shows the comparison between one half of a cast that has been trimmed and the other half before trimming.

The trial denture is now replaced on the cast and a labial flange added. The flange may be complete or part according to the depth and location of undercut areas, the analysis of which will be discussed later in this chapter. The presence of a labial flange and the fact that the artificial teeth need not intrude into the sockets of the extracted teeth means that their position and inclination can be modified more readily in relation to the natural teeth.

THE COMPLETE LABIAL FLANGE WITH ALVEOLOPLASTY

Where a change in shape and size of the alveolar ridge is planned either by transeptal alveolectomy or radical alveolectomy, stone must be removed from the cast equivalent to the change in size and shape of the soft tissues *plus* the proposed reduction in size and shape of the alveolar bone.

Prior to Septal Alveolectomy

The guide lines are marked on the cast as described earlier. The stone teeth are removed singly and alternately, and the artificial replacements are set in their place. The denture is then removed from the cast which may now be further modified.

A pencil line is drawn through the centre of the sockets of the central and lateral incisors and then obliquely to the outer wall of the canine socket, or the premolar if that is the last standing tooth in the anterior segment. On the labial surface of the cast a horizontal line is drawn at the level of the attached gingivae for it is at this point during the operation of transeptal alveolectomy that the outer plate of bone will be deliberately fractured. The stone between the two lines is now removed (Fig. 15.5). This will result in some reduction of the large undercut which was the reason for planning the operation of transeptal alveolectomy. Reduction of the undercut allows the placing of a complete labial flange where this would not otherwise have been possible. As before, the lingual gingival margin area of stone is removed, with care being taken to reshape the cast in the region of the collapsed incisive papilla. The surfaces

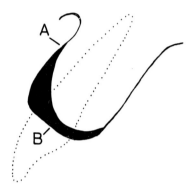

Fig. 15.5 Cast modification for septal alveolectomy. Lines A and B are drawn on the cast and the shaded area removed.

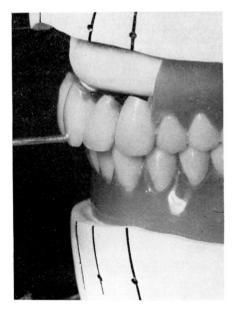

Fig. 15.6 Replacement of the denture after trimming the cast for a septal alveolectomy.

of the cast are smoothed with sandpaper and the denture replaced (Fig. 15.6). The space that exists between the modified cast and the anterior teeth on the denture is now filled with wax and a complete flange added.

Prior to Radical Alveolectomy

Radical alveolectomy is planned where an unsightly premaxillary prominence requires reduction. The amount of stone to be removed will be greater than when a transeptal alveolectomy is planned since there will be a greater change in the height and width of the alveolar process at operation.

As it is likely that the artificial anterior teeth will be placed in a position markedly different from that of the natural teeth, the stone teeth on the cast may be removed together and not singly. The stone cast is now carved until the correct height and width is achieved. During this modification, the casts should be occluded frequently so that the interalveolar space can be assessed. The surface of the cast is smoothed as before and the trial denture replaced. The anterior teeth are set up and a complete labial flange added.

REMOVAL OF POSTERIOR TEETH FROM THE CAST

Any stone posterior teeth that remain are removed from the cast but no sockets are cut. The buccal and lingual gingival areas are reduced, however, because of the tissue collapse that will occur after extraction.

The posterior teeth on the trial dentures were set primarily to achieve positive occlusal contact, so that the horizontal and vertical jaw relations could be checked in the mouth. After the artificial anterior teeth have been set in position and particularly if isolated posterior teeth have now been removed from the cast, it is quite likely that the posterior teeth will have to be reset.

ANALYSIS OF UNDERCUT AREAS

At the trial denture stage, it was recommended that the cast should be analysed using the surveyor so that the clinician and technician should be aware of problems of denture insertion due to undercuts in the denture bearing areas.

After the set up has been completed, the denture is removed from the cast and the surveyor used again for analysis and location of undercuts. The cast is placed on the surveyor table which is adusted to indicate the most suitable path of insertion of the future denture. The cast is now studied for areas that might interfere with the easy and comfortable insertion of the denture in the mouth. As mentioned before, undercuts of less than 1 to 2 mm are of no great significance because of a similar compressibility of soft tissues which should allow the insertion of the denture. Similarly undercuts composed entirely of soft tissue, as sometimes occurs in the tuberosity areas, can be utilized for retention and will not complicate insertion of the denture.

If undercuts of a depth greater than 2 mm are still present, analysis of the cast indicates where the flange should be relieved or shortened.

Vertical relief refers to a shortening of the flange to avoid it entering an undercut area. Horizontal relief refers to a modification of a fully extended flange so that the degree of horizontal undercut engaged is reduced. Examples are shown in Fig. 15.7.

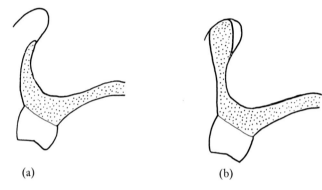

(a)   (b)

Fig. 15.7 Relief of undercuts:
(a) vertical relief;
(b) horizontal relief.

A shortened or part flange is indicated in the anterior region where in the interests of conservation of alveolar bone it is considered undesirable to create room for a complete flange by alveoloplasty. Provided a part flange gives adequate retention of the denture, it is in general to be preferred to excessive horizontal relief of a flange in order to allow the denture to reach the sulcus beyond a deep undercut area. The space between the flange and the slope of the ridge created by a horizontal relief encourages the proliferation of hyperplastic tissue. Further, if as a result of horizontal relief of the flange the border becomes thin and sharp, there is a real danger of trauma to the sulcus. This is particularly so in the case of the lower denture where the foundation is triangular in cross-section and where the denture tends to sink as a result of bone resorption during the first few months after extraction.

To achieve horizontal relief of a denture flange in an undercut area, the technician may be asked to block out the appropriate areas on the cast, after surveying, with plaster. Alternatively he may be requested to thicken the flange near the border so that subsequent relief of the fitting surface will not leave the border of the denture knife-edged.

There is a strong argument to be made in favour of remounting the processed denture on the surveyor. The fitting surface may be reanalysed (Fig. 15.8) and undercuts of the flanges reduced where they would interfere with the easy seating of the denture. Because of the frequency with which irritation occurs postoperatively over the canine eminences, following the insertion of a denture with a complete labial flange, particular attention should be directed to these aspects of the fitting surface of the denture. Here, it is advisable to err on the side of overrelief.

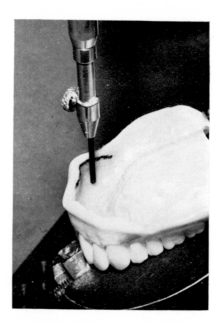

Fig. 15.8 Analysis of the fitting surface of the denture on the surveyor.

There is some advantage to be gained by not extending the labial flange of the lower denture fully into the sulcus as shown on the cast. Despite the greatest care at the major impression stage, an overextended sulcus is frequently re-corded in the $\overline{5 \ | \ 5}$ region because of areas of deep undercut here which make the adaptation of the impression tray difficult if not impossible. A denture fully extended to the impression in this area often causes tissue trauma. It must also be recognised that resorption of bone during the first few months after extraction allows the lower denture to sink a little on its foundation. In this situation even what was originally a correctly extended denture flange will become overextended with resultant trauma to the sulcus.

Therefore a slight underextension of the labial flange by about 2 mm will tend to reduce the incidence of tissue injury. It also reduces some of the difficulties associated with the insertion of a denture into an undercut area.

THE TEMPLATE

Whenever an immediate denture with a complete flange is planned it is recommended that a transparent template or surgical guide be constructed after the cast has been modified. A duplicate of the modified cast is prepared and a clear baseplate made over it either by conventional processing methods or by vacuum forming. The use of the template will be discussed in Chapter 16.

Surgical Techniques
and After-Care

ANAESTHESIA

The selection of either local or general anaesthesia is usually a matter for discussion between the operator and the patient. Systemic disease, however, may indicate a particular method of anaesthesia and it is then essential to consult the patient's physician.

LOCAL ANAESTHESIA

When the operation is to be performed in the dentist's surgery, local anaesthesia is preferably the method of choice. The operator has ample time to work in a careful, unhurried manner. The patient remains ambulant and his occupation should not be interrupted for more than a day unless the operative procedure involves considerable bone surgery. Even then, most patients should be able to follow their regular occupation the day after operation.

There are of course some disadvantages in using local anaesthesia. Highly nervous patients may not provide the cooperation required by the operator when working on the conscious patient. Such patients must be handled gently but firmly and never be allowed to feel any uncertainty as to the success of the anaesthesia or the eventual outcome of the operation. The operator can do much to help by explaining in suitable terms what the operative procedure is to be, so that the patient's fears will be allayed. Naturally, the type of description given must be modified to suit the temperament of the individual patient. The patient may worry about possible after-pain due to the insertion of an immediate denture over recent extraction wounds but he should be reassured that in fact the presence of a well-constructed denture can do much to ensure an uneventful postoperative recovery. After-pain is more commonly caused by surgical trauma, postoperative infection or careless anaesthetic technique. The use of a blunt needle, a careless injection technique or lack of sterility must all be avoided. Rapid injection of too large an amount of anaesthetic solution causes ballooning of the tissues. This not only gives after-pain due to stripping of the mucosa but also creates difficulties in seating the immediate denture. Therefore, by careful surgical technique the dentist can reduce postoperative discomfort to a minimum.

Patients who are very nervous should be premedicated provided that they are accompanied by a responsible person who will take them home.

Although on occasions a patient may be admitted to hospital, it should be emphasized that the minor oral surgery necessary prior to the insertion of the immediate denture, whether under general or local anaesthesia, can be performed quite satisfactorily in the dental chair.

GENERAL ANAESTHESIA

General anaesthesia is often requested by the nervous patient, it facilitates operative procedures and assures painless surgery. Many patients prefer a general anaesthetic simply to avoid the multiple injections necessary when upper and lower teeth on both sides of the midline are to be extracted. When a specialist anaesthetist is available there is no reason why a general anaesthetic should not be given in the dentist's surgery, provided that there are facilities to allow the patient to remain for postanaesthetic care. The specialist anaesthetist will produce the calm and possibly prolonged anaesthesia necessary where multiple extractions together with shaping of the alveolar ridges is planned. However, many dental practitioners who are unable to benefit from the services of a specialist anaesthetist, prefer to use only local anaesthesia in their own surgeries. When a general anaesthetic is specifically requested by the patient or is considered desirable after consultation with his physician, the patient is admitted to nursing home or hospital.

SURGICAL TECHNIQUES

Prior to surgery the remaining teeth should be given a thorough prophylaxis, care being taken to remove all supra- and subgingival calculus. Radiographs should be studied so that the operator will be aware of any difficulties likely to be encountered during extraction and be able to take adequate precautions.

THE DENTURE WITH OPEN FACE
OR PART FLANGE

This entails only the extraction of the remaining natural teeth. However, carelessness at this stage may result in postoperative complications that may make the patient unable to wear the immediate denture. Therefore, the extraction of the remaining teeth must be carried out in as atraumatic a manner as possible. Prior to extraction, it is advisable to insert a sharp-pointed scalpel into the gingival crevice and cut the free gingival fibres which attach the gingival margin to the neck of the tooth and also the transeptal fibres passing from one tooth to another. If the incision is adequate, the tooth will then be attached to the alveolar bone only by the main part of the periodontal membrane. In this way lacerations to the gingival tissues during extraction are avoided. This is particularly important when the gingival tissues still show evidence of periodontal disease since in these circumstances tearing is more likely to occur.

It is also advantageous to pass a straight elevator into the interstitial areas to loosen the teeth prior to the application of forceps. Each tooth should be removed with great care and almost coaxed out of the socket. It must be understood that the greater the trauma, the slower will be the rate of postoperative healing. On careful extraction, most of the periodontal membrane comes away with the extracted tooth. Some damaged remains of periodontium will be found, however, on the socket walls, particularly in the apical region and occasionally towards the margins of the alveolus. More damaged periodontal tissue remains when considerable force is used during extraction and also when the periodontal membrane fibres are very strong. In the latter instance small fragments of dentine and cement may be avulsed from the root and remain in the socket. These degenerating fragments of tissue play no part in the healing process and, in fact, retard the proliferation of connective tissues into the blood clot. In addition, they may provide a nidus for bacteria with the possible development of an infected socket. Difficulties in extraction should therefore be foreseen at an early date and the necessary preparations made for surgical removal of the tooth or teeth with the minimum of trauma.

After the extraction, each socket should be inspected carefully and any periapical granulomatous areas curetted. The alveolar margins are inspected and although no gross bone trimming has been planned, sharp edges or projecting spicules of bone should be smoothed using either rongeur forceps or a sterile bur. It is preferable to elevate the mucoperiosteum from the margins of the sockets. This may be done with a sharp periosteal elevator and avoids undue trauma to the soft tissues on smoothing the socket margins.

THE DENTURE WITH A COMPLETE FLANGE

Often an immediate denture carrying a complete flange may be inserted easily without the need to reshape the alveolar process. This situation arises if the undercuts in the anterior region are minimal in depth or where a path of insertion of the denture can be planned which utilizes the undercuts for retention. In such cases the surgical techniques are as described for the open face or part flange denture.

In other cases, however, where undercut areas are very pronounced or where reduction of prominent premaxillae is planned, surgical reshaping of the anterior part of the alveolar process will be necessary. The reshaping of the alveolar process or alveoloplasty is achieved by septal alveolectomy or radical alveolectomy, according to the degree of change of shape that is necessary.

SEPTAL ALVEOLECTOMY

The stages of this operation are shown in Fig. 16.1.

After careful extraction of the anterior teeth, the interdental septa are removed using a pair of narrow tapering rongeur forceps, thus leaving a gutter between the inner and outer cortical plates of bone. The outer plate must now be collapsed inwards towards the inner plate. To do this it is necessary to weaken it by making vertical cuts at two or sometimes three points.

A fissure bur is placed in the distal part of the last socket and a vertical cut made through the labial plate of bone from the inner aspect of the socket— care being taken not to lacerate the mucosa. If the outer plate appears robust and if the nasal spine is pronounced, a vertical cut is also made in the midline. The labial plate of bone is thus attached only by its edge nearest the sulcus and under finger pressure it is pressed inwards. In most cases a definite crack will be heard as partial fracture takes place and the labial plate can then be moved backwards until it makes contact with the inner plate.

The mucoperiosteum is elevated from the margins of the sockets so that these may be trimmed and made smooth by a bur or rongeur forceps. The interdental papillae and surplus gingival mucosa are trimmed with a pair of scissors to give a straight line of junction. The clear acrylic template which was made on a duplicate of the modified cast, is tried in the mouth to assess whether the change in shape achieved in the mouth is similar to that which was anticipated when trimming the cast. Blanching of the soft tissues as seen through the template indicates excessive pressure; this is commonly seen just distal to the canine sockets. The remedy is to reduce the bone contour in this or similarly affected areas or alternatively to ease the fitting surface of the template and the denture to a similar extent.

When the operator is satisfied that the denture will go into place easily without undue pressure, the wound is irrigated with warm normal saline and the mucosal margins closed by interrupted sutures. These will hold the soft tissue margins together to encourage healing by first intention and will prevent separation of the cut surfaces and delayed healing due to the inevitable slight movement of the immediate denture.

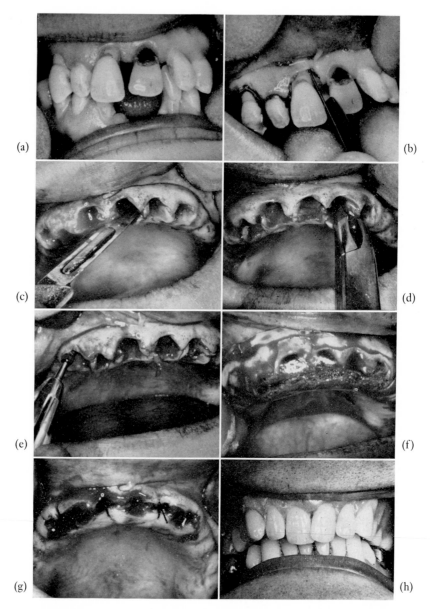

(a)

(b)

(c)

(d)

(e)

(f)

(g)

(h)

Fig. 16.1 The stages of the operation of *septal* alveolectomy.

RADICAL ALVEOLECTOMY

In this procedure the labial plate of bone is removed and therefore a muco-periosteal flap must be raised. This should be done before the anterior teeth are extracted. The incision is as illustrated in Fig. 16.2 and should be made with a sharp scalpel through the mucoperiosteum to bone. The vertical incisions should not extend to the sulcus reflection as this may result in post-operative swelling due to formation of haematoma. The resultant fibrosis may reduce the depth of the sulcus.

The mucoperiosteal flap is raised using a periosteal elevator to expose the labial plate of bone. If the incisions are as shown there will be good access to the surgical area and the base of the flap will be wider than its free end, ensuring a good blood supply. The vertical incisions should be approximately 5 mm behind the most distal teeth to be extracted. This will ensure that the suture lines lie over bone and not over the blood clot.

After the anterior teeth have been extracted, bone is removed with rongeur forceps. This will involve removal of the outer plate, removal of the inter-dental septa and usually reduction of the height of the palatal wall of the sockets. At frequent intervals the mucosal flaps are approximated and the template tried in. Blanching of the tissues or an inability to seat the template properly indicates that more bone removal is necessary. When the template fits, toilet of the area is carried out as before and the mucosal margins trimmed and sutured.

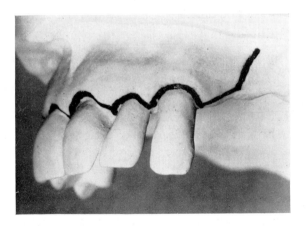

Fig. 16.2 The incision prior to reflecting a mucoperiosteal flap when a *radical* alveolectomy is to be performed.

INSERTION OF THE DENTURES

When local anaesthesia has been used and where there has been no surgery other than extraction of the teeth, the denture is inserted after digital compression of the socket walls. It is important to see that the sockets are filled with blood—if haemorrhage is inadequate after local anaesthesia, a sterile bur should be plunged through the lamina dura of the socket to promote blood flow from the cancellous bone beneath. By pressing the denture firmly into place slight bone displacement due to tooth removal may be reduced without pain to the patient. Where alveolectomy of either type has been carried out, the denture is inserted after the mucosal margins have been sutured.

When a general anaesthetic has been used, the immediate denture may be inserted after removal of the throat pack and just before the patient recovers consciousness. Then, on recovery from the anaesthetic, the patient accepts the immediate denture as a replacement for the natural teeth, and is not so conscious of the difference in sensation between an 'empty' mouth and the bulk of dentures.

It must be remembered that the blood clot is very friable at this time and it is inadvisable to disturb it by inserting and removing the dentures many times in order to make small adjustments. Any gross occlusal errors are noted and their rectification attempted in one stage. Fine correction of occlusal errors should be left until 24 hours have elapsed. If there is a large error, the occlusal surface of one denture should be ground away radically to give some form of contact with the intention of *replacing* this denture and not rebasing it after some initial resorption has occurred.

AFTER-CARE

Most immediate denture patients should be advised not to remove the dentures during the first 24 hours. This ensures that there is as little disturbance as possible of the blood clot. Where there have been only a small number of extractions, however, and healing has proved uneventful on previous occasions, a cooperative patient may be advised to remove the denture and rinse it after meals. All patients should be warned not to do any vigorous mouthwashing at this time. To reduce the possibility of postextraction haemorrhage, instructions are also given to avoid undue exercise, alcohol, or hot food and drink. Analgesic tablets to control any postoperative pain should be given to the patient.

EXAMINATION AFTER 24 HOURS

The patient should return the day after operation when the dentures are removed and the surgical area irrigated with warm saline and examined. On removal of a denture not associated with alveoloplasty, there should be firm, healthy clots in the sockets, with no sign of continuing haemorrhage. Oozing from the sockets indicates delayed clot formation due to trauma from the denture or a systemic cause. In the case of the open face denture, incorrectly shaped 'root' extensions may be traumatizing the surgical area. If so, they should be reshaped. With a complete or part flanged denture, the blood clot may be seen extending from the socket areas. This indicates that the collapse of the gingival tissues after extraction has been greater than the modifications of the cast, and that the denture is not as well adapted to the tissues as it should be.

Where alveoloplasty has been performed, the sutured mucosal margins should be seen to be in close contact. If the change in shape of the ridge achieved by surgery has been greater than planned on the cast, the space that exists between the denture and the tissues will be filled with blood clot. This may come away during irrigation or may disintegrate during the first few days after operation. The denture will therefore be poorly adapted to the tissues in this area and early correction by rebasing will be necessary.

Signs of pressure from the dentures will be seen as areas of inflammation. Adjustment of the fitting surface at this time prevents this progressing to ulceration (Fig. 16.3) and gives the patient greater comfort. A frequent site where inflammation may be found is the canine and first premolar region. Then details of occlusion are checked and corrected where necessary. On this appointment, provided a firm blood clot is seen, the patient is shown how to remove the dentures and is instructed to remove them only for cleaning and otherwise to wear them both day and night.

The patient must be encouraged to use the immediate dentures for mastication. Some are reluctant to do this for fear of pain or damage to the surgical area. Consequently there is a reduction of lip, cheek and tongue movements resulting in oral stagnation. Use of the dentures for moderate mastication increases the blood supply and assists rapid healing. A mouthwash should be prescribed for use three or four times a day. Perhaps the most efficient and certainly the cheapest is a hot saline solution. The tonicity of this should be similar to that of the tissues; one and a half teaspoonfuls in a tumblerful of hot water. A hypertonic solution causes dehydration and shrinkage of the blood clot.

If at the 24 hour postoperative visit the surgical area is clean and the adjustments required on the fitting and occlusal surfaces of the denture are minimal, the patient need not be seen again until 7 days after the extractions. If there are signs of a friable blood clot or considerable adjustments of the denture are necessary, it is advisable to see the patient again 3 days after surgery.

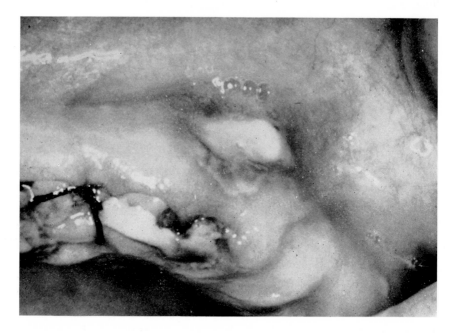

Fig. 16.3 The result of excessive pressure from a denture flange on the labial alveolar slope.

EXAMINATION AFTER ONE WEEK

Seven days after operation further adjustments are made where necessary to the dentures and any sutures that have been inserted are removed. Provided that healing is progressing uneventfully, the next visit may be a month after extraction. Then the adaptation of the denture to the underlying tissues should be assessed with a view to rebasing if there has been much change in the shape of the alveolar ridge.

Unfortunately patients are sometimes encouraged to persevere with an *unmodified* immediate prosthesis for as long as possible. This is usually on the understanding that it is only a 'temporary' prosthesis which will be replaced when the postoperative changes have settled down to a minimum. Such advice is most undesirable as the tolerance of patients to dentures varies so much; the tolerant patient may in fact wear the immediate denture for so long a time that the tissues of the denture bearing area are severely traumatized and may be irreparably damaged. The patient must understand the need for regular servicing of dentures. He must be encouraged to return for regular examination, not only during the early weeks and months after the loss of natural teeth, but throughout life.

HEALING IN THE SURGICAL AREA

The main characteristics of the histogenesis of the reparative processes in the surgical area have been well established by workers using Rhesus monkeys, which have a deciduous and permanent dentition similar to man. Other workers have studied biopsy material from patients who have had immediate dentures inserted. Healing commences with the clotting of blood either in the sockets or, if there has been an alveolectomy, in the reduced socket area.

HEALING AFTER SIMPLE EXTRACTION

After simple forceps extraction and no alveolectomy, the sequence and rate of the reparative processes are probably as follows:

1st Day

The socket is filled with a blood clot; there is a heavy accumulation of granular leucocytes at the surface and the blood vessels around the wound are widely dilated.

After 3 Days

Polymorphonuclear leucocytes, lymphocytes and plasma cells in the fibrin network extend from the surface to just below the level of the alveolar crests. There is an ingrowth of fibroblasts and capillaries into the blood clot particularly at the base of the socket. Epithelial cells are beginning to proliferate from the free edges of the gingival margins that have folded over the alveolar crests.

After 1 Week

Fibroblasts forming young, unorientated fibrous tissue have now penetrated to every part of the socket. The epithelium will be proliferating over the surface of the clot and in some instances there may be a tenuous but complete covering. There are the first signs of bone formation, in that appositional bone appears on parts of the socket walls and trabecular bone in the base of the socket. The bone seen in the socket at this early stage after extraction may be described as immature or young bone; it is very cellular, is less well mineralized and less radiopaque than mature bone. In addition to osteogenesis, there are also signs of osteoclasia on the alveolar crests and the socket walls particularly on the labial aspect.

After 2 Weeks

The socket is filled with young bone except for a cone-shaped area of fibrous tissue extending from the surface of the clot to about a quarter of the depth of the socket. Osteoclastic activity continues on the alveolar crests, on the labial plate and also in the young bone at the base of the socket. This is possibly the beginnings of reorientation of the trabeculae. The epithelial covering of the surface is now complete although varying in thickness.

After 4 Weeks

The socket is almost completely filled with young bone. There is osteoclastic activity in the superficial part of the socket and on the walls, with osteoclasia continuing on the alveolar crests and on some of the newly formed trabeculae. The connective tissue beneath the surface epithelial layers is more mature.

After 8 Weeks

Bone now extends to the level of the alveolar crests which are still undergoing resorption. Bone formation is therefore limited by the original height of the lingual and labial alveolar crests. The original labial plate will, by now, have almost completely disappeared and be in the course of replacement by a newly formed plate of bone. The processes of apposition and resorption on the socket walls makes their demarcation difficult.

Young bone formation is thus probably complete some 8 weeks after extraction.

HEALING AFTER ALVEOLECTOMY

The healing process is similar after alveolectomy. Here there are two possible situations; one where the outer plate of bone is preserved and collapsed onto the inner plate after removal of the interdental septa, and the other where the outer plate is sacrificed.

After a septal alveolectomy the blood clot in the socket area is minimal. Replacement of bone is faster during the first 2 weeks than in the socket after forceps extraction or in the socket area after removal of the outer plate. However, after 8 weeks there is no difference and the surgical areas are filled with young bone. It seems, therefore, that once the blood clot has been completely organized, the rate and mode of bone repair is similar whether the volume of the socket is large or small.

In describing the surgical technique for septal alveolectomy it was emphasized that a mucoperiosteal flap should not be raised. Thus the blood supply and vitality of the outer plate of bone will be maintained despite its relative isolation by virtue of the vertical cuts and horizontal fracture. It will play an important part in the healing process by providing a surface from which appositional bone forms to assist in the filling of the socket area. If a flap of mucoperiosteum is raised there is a danger that the isolated bony plate may degenerate and become infected, with consequent delay in healing.

After radical alveolectomy and removal of the outer plate, the return to normal bone structure is delayed because of the longer time required in the re-formation of the outer cortical plate. The clinical observation of greater postoperative resorption after removal of the outer plate can possibly be explained by the fact that recently formed cancellous bone is exposed directly to the pressure of a denture flange or a shrinking mucosa. Resorption appears to be less when the outer plate is preserved. This may be because the morphology of the compact cortical bone provides greater resistance to osteoclasia than the newly laid down immature fibrillar bone.

In both types of case there follows a gradual replacement of the young, immature bone by a mature bone which is less cellular, more highly mineralized and more radiopaque. There is a rounding of the alveolar ridge achieved mainly by further resorption of the labial alveolar crest and plate. Most of the contour change occurs during the first 6 months postoperative period and it can be said that a relatively stable alveolar ridge form exists after 1 year.

EFFECTS OF IMMEDIATE DENTURES

From comparative studies of patient groups with and without immediate dentures, it is evident that a well-fitting immediate denture does contribute to the healing in the surgical areas after extraction of the teeth and generally results in conservation of the anterior alveolar process, more with respect to height than width, during the first year after extraction. Further, it seems that a closed face immediate denture has a definite effect on the pattern of resorption, the rate of resorption being retarded during the first year compared with the open face type of denture. Apart from the added retention gained by the presence of a complete labial flange on a lower denture, it is possible that the flange contributes to a greater conservation of the lower ridge. Histological studies also suggest that bone formation and repair in the surgical areas proceeds more rapidly when an immediate denture is fitted.

SUBSEQUENT CHANGES

After healing, one might expect that the shape of the alveolar bone would remain the same during the rest of the patient's life. In all bone there occurs continuous repair and reconstruction due to the relatively short life span of the bone cells. Normal bone physiology is dependent upon a balanced activity of three types of cell, namely the osteoblasts which form bone, the osteocytes which maintain its vitality and the osteoclasts which are associated with bone resorption. A balance of activity between osteoclasts (resorption) and osteoblasts (apposition) results in a gradual renewal of the components of bony tissue but without any radical change in the outer shape of the bone. For example, an adult femur is basically the same shape throughout life, yet all of its structure has probably been renewed several times.

Control of balance between apposition and resorption is complex, being partly general and partly local. Of the general factors, the one most intensively studied has been the action of parathyroid hormone. It seems, however, that the resorption incident to the remodelling of bone is only partly under the influence of this hormone. Current thinking is that various hormones do not initiate metabolic processes, but influence them by regulating the rates of specific reactions. The endocrine control of bone is the result of more than eleven simultaneously operating variables and is at present not sufficiently understood, particularly in relation to alveolar bone. In fact this type of bone, in the edentulous patient, may no longer be biologically normal.

Local factors are related to the stresses to which the bone is exposed. It is suggested that the osteocytes act as strain gauges or mechanoreceptors which stimulate either bone apposition or resorption.

The alveolar ridge usually undergoes resorption throughout life. It is often said that the alveolar bone is superfluous once the natural teeth have been extracted, and that subsequently it is gradually resorbed until basal maxillary or mandibular bone is reached.

Unfortunately it is not possible to predict at what rate the alveolar process will be lost after healing. After the marked changes that occur in the shape of the alveolar process during the first few months after extraction, there is a subsequent retardation in the rate of change in the years that follow. In general the changes that occur in the years after extraction tend to be more rapid and more extensive in the lower than the upper alveolar process. In some cases the lower alveolar process appears almost to melt away. There are, however, considerable individual variations and in other cases little change in shape of the alveolar process takes place during one or two decades.

Postextraction reconstruction in the alveolar bone is influenced by the change in functional stress that occurs when natural teeth are extracted. If there is subsequent lack of function (as will be the case if a denture is not fitted) the bone is likely to undergo a disuse atrophy. There is an analogy in the atrophy found in bone stumps after amputation. Here the peripheral end may atrophy until the shaft of the bone tapers to a point. The cortex is thinned by internal resorption and the trabeculae of the cancellous bone are reduced in number and are thinner. The loss of muscle function acting on the bone results in a change in the external shape. It is interesting to note that the wearing of an artificial limb results in less change in external contour although there may be signs of osteoporosis. Similarly, the wearing of a well-constructed and well-maintained denture frequently appears to retard further reduction in ridge size once the major postextraction changes have taken place. The functional forces transmitted by the denture may promote sufficient osteogenesis to compensate for bone lost by the normal rate of resorption. Conversely with lack of function there is insufficient formation of new bone matrix so that resorption proceeding at a normal rate results in a negative bone balance and a state of atrophy and porosis.

Three factors of considerable importance in the future of the alveolar ridge are pressure, the climacteric in women, and age.

THE EFFECT OF PRESSURE ON ALVEOLAR BONE

Bone tissue is resistant to both pressure and tension. It has been suggested that the resistance to tension is from the uncalcified fibrils whereas the resistance to pressure is the property of the calcified matrix. In the natural dentition the force of occlusion is received by the supporting alveolar bone as tensile forces, by virtue of the arrangement of the fibres of the periodontal membranes. With a complete denture the forces directed onto the alveolar ridge are compressive in nature—a type of loading not experienced by the alveolar bone with the natural dentition *in situ*. It is well known that compressive pressure on bone from an arterial aneurysm or a growing tumour can lead to rapid resorption. Why then does alveolar bone not resorb rapidly under the compressive loads from dentures? Obviously there must be considerable variation in the reaction of bone under pressure of different amounts, direction and duration (continuous or intermittent). It is possible that the explanation is to be found in the effect of pressure on the blood supply of bone. If this is interfered with or destroyed then rapid bone resorption is likely. For example, in the case of an expanding aneurysm against a vertebral body or a growing tumour against the femur, pressure is directed to the bone via the periosteum. This will compress many of the blood vessels which send and receive branches into and from the bone. As a result resorption occurs.

Alveolar bone, however, receives its main blood supply from the interdental arteries within the bone. These pass through the canals in the interalveolar septa which persist after the extraction of teeth. In the case of the edentulous ridge then the major part of the blood supply is internal and is only in part obtained from periosteal vessels. This double supply may account for the *relative* resistance of the alveolar ridges to pressure.

The properly fitting denture, by transmitting a well-adjusted intermittent pressure to the alveolar process, should provide a beneficial stimulus to the bone. It is perhaps significant that the loss of the alveolar process is usually greatest on the sides of the ridge. The bone trabeculae, having been orientated satisfactorily to accept vertical loading by the natural teeth, may be able to resist, and in fact be stimulated by a loading of similar direction from a denture. They may not, however, be able to resist horizontal forces although a well-fitting denture with a complete flange may help to reduce or modify these potentially destructive forces.

Differences in pressure and the rate of resorption in the denture wearer are associated with factors such as musucular force, masticatory and denture wearing habits, bruxism and other oral parafunctions. Bruxism and clenching may be particularly important factors in bone resorption in denture wearers. Such parafunctions are often noted in patients who have problems of denture retention or in whose denture there are incorporated errors in occlusion and face height.

Excessive pressure from a denture, particularly if it is localized, often results in rapid resorption of the affected part of the alveolar process. A common example is found in the upper alveolar region when a complete upper denture is opposed by lower anterior teeth only. Pressure on the anterior part of the upper ridge may be excessive and that, together with the adverse direction of the loading, often results in rapid loss of alveolar bone (Fig. 16.4).

Where properly constructed complete upper and lower dentures are provided, the alveolar ridges are apparently able to withstand the compressive forces of mastication. This does not mean that there will be bone apposition, for unfortunately gradual reduction of contour appears to be inevitable. If the fitting surfaces of the dentures are periodically re-adapted to the slowly changing foundation and the occlusal relation is correctly maintained, the rate of loss of bone will be minimized. If the fitting surfaces of the dentures are not corrected, a vicious circle will be established whereby the dentures load tissues with forces of increasing size in adverse directions, resulting in further resorption which in turn increases the traumatic effect of the dentures.

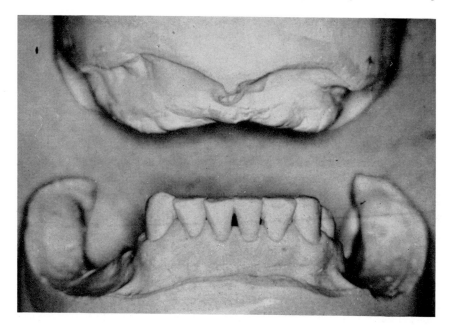

Fig. 16.4 Severe resorption of the upper anterior alveolar ridge caused by six natural lower anterior teeth opposing a complete upper denture.

THE EFFECT OF THE CLIMACTERIC ON ALVEOLAR BONE

It is not uncommon to observe a marked loss of alveolar bone in women at the climacteric, particularly in the mandible. This may be associated with bone changes elsewhere in the body known as postmenopausal osteoporosis. There is a loss of bone mass, increased porosity and a decrease in the thickness of the cortex but a normal ash content. Much work has been done on the relation of reduced postmenopausal output of oestrogen to osteoporosis. The available evidence supports the thesis that postmenopausal osteoporosis is a disorder of osteoclastic activity, though the precise cause of this is unknown. Whilst oestrogen is not a stimulator of bone formation *per se*, it may be to some degree an inhibitor of the resorptive phase of an osteoporosis. Therefore, with a postmenopausal decrease in oestrogen output, osteoclasia becomes more pronounced.

Marked postmenopausal loss of alveolar bone does not occur in every case and this illustrates further the complexity of the endocrine control of bone turnover. Men appear to be spared much of the process of decreasing bone mass as their gonads continue to produce androgens for most of their lives.

THE EFFECT OF AGE ON ALVEOLAR BONE

With increasing age the positive or anabolic phase of growth of tissues is superseded by the negative or catabolic phase which leads to atrophy of all body tissues. Bone in general becomes rarefied and on histological examination reveals lacunae that are increased in size and have the appearance of 'pores' in macroscopic specimens. They are present in the deepest layers of compact bone in the typical picture of senile osteoporosis. In old age there is evidence of extensive bone resorption with little indication of increased bone formation. It is likely that the osteoporosis results from a reduced supply of materials to the structurally and functionally well-organized storehouse which is formed by the bones.

It is reasonable to expect that the alveolar bone will be affected as other bones by a senile osteoporosis although an accelerated loss of the alveolus is not inevitable in the aged. There are many examples of aged patients with well-formed alveolar ridges particularly if they have been rendered edentulous at an early age because of caries. There is no evidence that porotic alveolar bone is more likely to undergo rapid resorption but the reduced bone density together with the reduced bone turnover that occurs with age, may render it more susceptible to functional forces directed from a denture. In the ageing patient where the emphasis is on resorption, more rapid reduction of the ridge may occur than would be the case with similar loading in a young patient.

At present the clinician is unable to predict the subsequent amount and rate of loss of alveolar bone once the immediate postextraction changes have occurred. It has been suggested, however, that people with densely calcified bones in early life have some protection against severe osteoporosis in later life. The distribution of areas of osteoporosis appears to be the result of the inbuilt pattern of remodelling within a bone. In the case of the mandible, areas of marked porosity are more likely in situations where the bone was formed endosteally than periosteally. Endosteal bone encloses vascular networks and marrow and is inevitably more porous than bone formed periosteally. Such bone is more susceptible to haversian remodelling, and once remodelled is more susceptible to the resorptive changes that occur with ageing.

The literature often separates postmenopausal osteoporosis in women from senile osteoporosis. However, there is little justification for the assumption that they are separate entities. In fact, the one may lead inevitably into the other as they are both ageing phenomena.

Section Three
Replacement Dentures

Chapter 17

Rebasing or Replacement of Dentures

At some stage during the life of any denture, consideration must be given to whether its deficiencies should be corrected by modification of the existing denture or whether it should be replaced by a new denture. The same considerations apply whether the denture is a recent immediate prosthesis, or a non-immediate denture which has been worn for some years.

The postextraction changes result in a reduction in ridge size in and near the surgical area. The rate and amount of change varies greatly with the individual and also to some extent with the surgical technique adopted. Investigations have shown that the greatest change occurs during the first 6 months after extraction, with the denture bearing areas becoming relatively stabilized after one year. However, remodelling of the alveolar ridge, with the emphasis on resorption, continues indefinitely.

Thus, during the first 6 months, an immediate denture may quickly lose its adaptation to the tissues beneath it. This is more likely with a lower immediate denture which may be no longer adapted adequately only a few weeks after surgery. On the other hand, an immediate denture in the upper jaw may still be well adapted after 3 or 4 months or even longer. After the early rapid resorption, the subsequent change in contour of the alveolar bone will necessitate correction of the fitting surface of the denture at intervals, but the frequency will vary from case to case. In some it may be necessary every few months, but in others a year or more may pass without the need for correction.

Regular examination of all patients who have received dentures is therefore essential frequently during the first year and at less frequent intervals afterwards. Correction of the fitting surface and selective grinding of the occlusion will then return the prostheses to their former level of function and prevent undue damage to the remaining alveolar bone.

Correction of denture base adaptation is necessary for the following reasons:

TO RESTORE DENTURE RETENTION

There will probably be a complaint of increasing looseness of the dentures although in younger patients it is likely that the environmental musculature will have become an effective retaining force enabling even badly adapted dentures to be reasonably controlled. Reduced retention may make itself particularly obvious during mastication. This is more likely in the case of the open face upper immediate denture where adequate retention may not be obtained until sufficient space has been created by resorption to allow the addition of a complete labial flange.

TO AVOID TISSUE DAMAGE

An ill-fitting denture may damage the tissues of the denture bearing area. The soft tissues will be affected first and later possibly the underlying bone unless the situation is corrected.

After a period of wear, abrasion of acrylic posterior teeth results in a loss of occlusal contacts in the muscular position. Such wear may be caused by coarse foodstuffs and may be accentuated by tooth clenching and grinding. In an effort to gain greater occlusal contact the mandible often assumes a marked protrusive relation to the maxilla. Since abrasion of the incisal edges of the anterior teeth is usually less marked, the lower incisors press heavily against the palatal aspect of the uppers, displacing the lower denture backwards. Consequently, resorption of labial bone takes place in the lower jaw and the condition continues to deteriorate due to further loss of occlusal face height.

Denture malocclusions are also seen where porcelain teeth have been used on the previous dentures. Assuming the original cuspal relations to have been correct, malocclusions arise as a result of alveolar resorption. The mandible moves upwards and forwards and the patient cannot occlude the posterior teeth correctly. Contact of the anterior teeth then occurs particularly when there is a large vertical overlap. The upper denture is displaced forward and an apparent contact of the posterior teeth seen—a contact that can be separated easily by interposing a spatula. The backward pressure on the lower ridge and heavy pressure in the anterior region of the upper, causes bone resorption in these areas. The lower denture is driven backwards causing resorption of the labial aspect of the ridge as it goes (Fig. 17.1). Frequently after several years, such tooth relations are not adequate for satisfactory function and the patient often achieves a more comfortable occlusal contact by protruding the mandible with or without lateral deviation (Fig. 17.2). The lower anterior teeth now lie in front of the uppers and may be chipped as a result of the 'jumping' that is necessary to achieve the protrusive mandibular relation. This new protrusive relation is still uncomfortable, however, often being too far forward to accommodate the change in jaw relationship. Consequently, the lower denture is now driven forwards to try and achieve good interdigitation of the cusps of the porcelain posterior teeth, and also to allow the lower incisors to lie in front of the uppers. As the lower denture moves forward it directs heavy pressure on the lingual remnant of the lower ridge causing its resorption. The result is that little or no alveolar ridge remains.

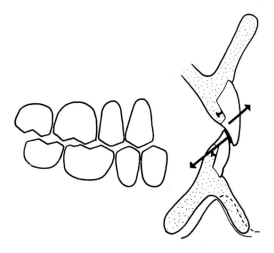

Fig. 17.1 Backward displacement of the lower denture causing labial alveolar resorption. The excessive pressure in the anterior region follows alveolar resorption and loss of occlusal face height.

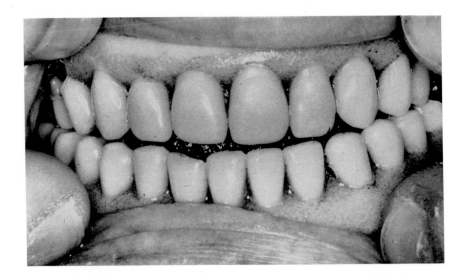

Fig. 17.2 Protrusion of the lower jaw to obtain more comfortable occlusal contacts after posterior alveolar resorption.

REBASING

Correction of defective adaptation of a denture may be achieved by rebasing or relining. The terms rebasing and relining are used loosely. Strictly speaking, rebasing refers to the replacement of all of the denture base by new material with only the teeth in their original arrangement remaining. Relining refers to the procedure of adding new base material to the fitting surface of the denture. In this text the term *rebasing* will be used to signify the correction of adaptation of the fitting surface of the denture either by adding new material to the old base or by replacing the entire denture base. The clinical indications for using either of these two laboratory techniques are the same.

INDICATIONS FOR REBASING

Rebasing should only be carried out when the vertical and horizontal relations of the dentures are approximately correct and the patient is satisfied with their appearance. If the occlusal face height has been reduced by 3 mm or more as a result of tissue change, and there is also an error in the horizontal relation of the dentures, rebasing is not likely to be successful. Such a situation occurs when the patient has not attended for routine and regular examination.

If the immediate dentures have been comfortable and the patient is tolerant, many months may elapse before he attends for treatment. There may now be a considerable discrepancy between the fitting surface of the dentures and tissues and an attempt at correction of such a denture by simple rebasing will usually fail. A similar situation exists when non-immediate dentures have been worn without attention for many years. Again, rebasing will only improve the adaptation of the dentures to the tissues and will not eliminate the occlusal errors.

During the period of rapid tissue change, a number of rebasings may be necessary in order to maintain immediate denture comfort and efficiency. This is to be preferred to the provision of replacement dentures at an early date after extraction. The immediate denture is not a temporary denture but just one of many the patient may have during his edentulous life. The well-planned and well-maintained immediate denture is usually so well accommodated by the adjacent soft tissues that it is frequently difficult to achieve the same success with a replacement denture which does not duplicate the shape of the original. Therefore the ideal sequence will be a number of rebasings followed eventually by the provision of replacement dentures which follow closely the design of the immediate restorations.

The main limiting factor to the number of rebasings that are possible is the deterioration in the aesthetic qualities of acrylic anterior teeth that may result from repeated curing procedures and also from abrasion and attrition of these teeth during use. Likewise much of the occlusal form of acrylic posterior teeth may be lost by attrition and by the selective grinding necessary to accommodate small changes in the relation of the jaws. When porcelain teeth have been used, loss of tooth shape is less marked and the occlusion is better preserved.

THE DIFFICULTIES OF REBASING

Largely because of bad planning and poor clinical and laboratory technique, rebasing has been considered to be a treatment of dubious outcome. Unfortunately, it is commonly believed that the necessary result can be achieved simply by taking a wash impression inside the denture and subsequently rebasing the denture to the new cast. The dentist must be aware of the limitations of such a technique, and of the errors that may be introduced during rebasing.

These are:

1 A disturbance of the occlusal relations of the dentures to each other by the use of too much impression material, or one of high viscosity, or by incorrect positioning of the dentures whilst the impressions are being recorded. The subsequent error in occlusion is an increase in occlusal face height. A careless, hurried laboratory technique has a similar effect.

2 A change in the relation of the upper anterior teeth to the upper lip. Improper seating of the denture or the presence of an undue amount of impression material results in a forward and downward displacement of the denture (Fig. 17.3). As a result the upper anterior teeth are more obvious than before the denture was rebased, and, in addition, the upper lip is made more prominent.

3 Distortion of the tissues or the impression. The former is caused by a localized overcompression of the mucosa. This is shown by exposure of areas of the denture base through the layer of impression material.

Uncorrected disturbances in the vertical and horizontal occlusal relations due to rebasing result in a more rapid resorption of the alveolar bone. Such errors are responsible for the vicious circle that is commonly set up (Fig. 17.4).

As the occlusal face height becomes greater, the freeway space is lost; the dentures become more uncomfortable and valuable alveolar bone is lost.

Whilst the denture is being rebased, the patient has to be without it for a few hours. An alternative is to rebase the denture directly in the mouth with a self-cure material—a technique not recommended except for very minor corrections.

If planned beforehand, the impression may be recorded early in the morning and the rebased dentures inserted later the same day. But in leaving the patient without his dentures even for a few hours, one of the advantages of immediate replacement is lost. The answer is, of course, to have provided the patient with duplicate immediate dentures. These should have been made either when

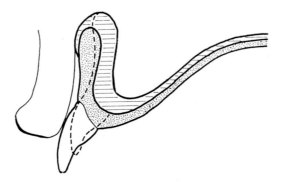

Fig. 17.3 Improper seating of an upper denture when recording a rebase impression. The shaded area represents the impression material.

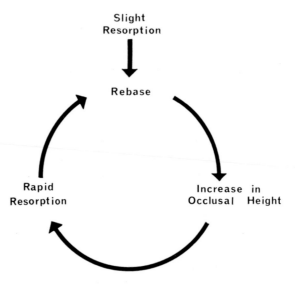

Fig. 17.4 The effect of repeated rebasing.

the original dentures were constructed, or subsequently using a denture copying technique. This may be considered by some to be an expensive luxury—but not to the immediate denture patient. To be deprived suddenly of his artificial dentition may be a major blow to the patient who has satisfactorily changed from the natural dentition to the artificial one. The suggestion of being without the dentures for a few hours may have the effect of keeping the patient away from the surgery until the dentures are so ill-fitting that they are uncontrollable. The sequelae of a patient trying to ware such dentures have already been discussed.

REBASING METHODS

The soft tissues of the denture bearing areas must be examined carefully. If there is denture irritation, attention should be directed to resolving this before rebasing the dentures. This is an important part of mouth preparation. If monilial infection is a contributory cause of the condition, antifungal treatment should be instituted.

PREPARATION OF THE DENTURE FOR REBASING

Correction of Occlusion

Whilst the occlusion of the rebased denture will be checked later, it is preferable to correct a malocclusion before rebasing. Frequently, one finds that occlusal equilibration is difficult to achieve. Then, a decision must be made whether to rebase or replace the denture.

An even contact at the muscular position is first obtained, followed by the removal of contacts causing interference within the paths of movement that the patient is using.

Removal of Undercuts

Since a denture is relatively rigid, it is important that no undercuts remain to lock the denture to the new cast poured into the impression. Otherwise, fracture, particularly of a lower ridge, will occur when trying to separate the denture and impression from the cast.

Border Extension

The border areas of the denture should be examined carefully in relation to the functional shape of the sulcus. Knife-edged borders may have resulted from overenthusiastic polishing of the denture or by reduction of undercut areas of the fitting surface at the time of insertion of the denture. Where the borders are underextended in width or extent, they should be corrected by the addition of a border trimming material which has the requisite physical properties to record the sulcus shape (Fig. 17.5).

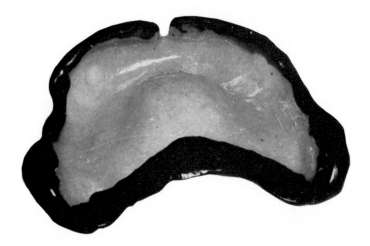

Fig. 17.5 Addition of tracing stick compound to the border of a denture before recording the rebase impression.

Post Damming

A posterior seal is obtained by a functional compression of the palatal tissues at the vibrating line of the soft palate. The relation of the posterior border of the denture to the vibrating line is checked and, where necessary, adjusted. Tracing stick compound is added, the denture inserted in the mouth and pressure applied. The softened impression compound flows under this pressure and selectively compresses the palatal tissues.

The Addition of a Labial Flange

Where an open face immediate denture was provided, a space will have developed between the anterior teeth and the basal tissues during the first few weeks or months after extraction. To restore aesthetics and to improve retention, extension of the denture border in this area is necessary. The pattern of bone change in the labial segment will usually allow the addition of a labial flange (Fig. 17.6). Likewise where the immediate denture carried only a part labial flange because of a deep labial undercut, the progressive reduction of the undercut by resorption will often permit the extension of a part flange so that it becomes complete.

Softened impression compound is added to the anterior part of the denture which is then inserted in the mouth. The patient is asked to contract the lip so that the correct labial shape and border extent may be obtained.

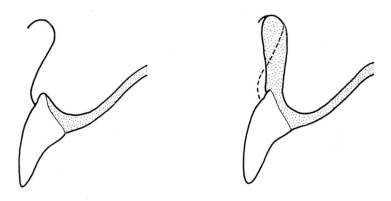

Fig. 17.6 Resorption of bone in the anterior region permitting the addition of a labial flange to an open face denture.

Other Preparations

It is sometimes advocated that the palate should be perforated when rebasing the upper denture. This is aimed at relieving excess pressure as the impression material flows in the small space between the denture and the palatal tissues. Such pressure may distort the soft tissues.

THE IMPRESSION MATERIALS USED IN REBASING

The impression material selected should have a high degree of flow at mouth temperature to allow excess material to escape to the periphery of the impression and so avoid tissue distortion. In addition, it must reproduce fine surface detail and, preferably, should be suitable for additions to be made to it.

If trauma to the soft tissues has occurred, due to prolonged wearing of an ill-fitting denture, a tissue conditioning material may be used. The impression surface is moulded gradually under functional stresses. Impression material is applied to the prepared fitting surface of the denture, it is inserted in the mouth and the patient wears the denture for 1 or 2 days. Then the denture is rebased to the new surface.

Probably the most commonly used materials for recording rebasing impressions are zinc oxide pastes, waxes and self-cure acrylic base—the latter being used as a direct rebasing material.

The viscosity of zinc oxide paste varies according to its basic constituents, mixing time, room temperature and relative humidity; in addition the effective viscosity of a particular paste will be that at the time it is brought into contact with the tissues. This, of course, is true of all impression materials that change from a plastic to a rigid or elastic state as a result of chemical action or temperature change. If a zinc oxide paste is used, one of a low viscosity should be chosen. It is essential to allow sufficient time for the material to flow between the denture and the tissues.

An extra soft wax is also recommended as an effective rebasing impression material. This type of wax has a marked degree of flow (about 90 per cent) at mouth temperature, indicating that the chances of tissue distortion are minimal as the impression is recorded. Obviously such a wax, because of its inelastic properties, is unsuitable for recording undercut areas. Having no setting phase, the wax flows continuously at mouth temperature away from the area of greatest loading, namely, the crest of the ridge, towards the periphery. This flow takes place under a physiological occlusal load and therefore it may be assumed that a selectively compressed impression is recorded.

Self-cure acrylic has been advocated as a direct intra-oral rebasing material. One recognized disadvantage is that its use may lead to a sensitization of the mucosa as a result of the free monomer present during and after polymerization. A further criticism is that lack of compression of the dough usually produces a porous fitting surface. Also, it cannot be said that the compression of the tissues is wholly under the control of the operator, as the consistency of the material at the time of insertion in the mouth is fairly critical, being determined by the stage of polymerization.

RECORDING THE IMPRESSION

In order to reduce the possibility of a denture malocclusion developing during rebasing, upper and lower dentures should be preferably rebased at separate visits. The occlusion is then adjusted before the second denture is rebased. This prolongs the clinical procedure and may be unacceptable to some patients. However, provided the amount of correction required with both dentures is small and provided the operator is experienced in recording a rebase impression, both upper and lower impressions may be taken at the same visit. Whilst it is possible to record both upper and lower rebase impressions simultaneously, this practice does not allow the clinician either time or opportunity to seat the dentures correctly, nor to perfect the moulding of the border areas of the impressions. The impressions should therefore be recorded separately. Which is recorded first is largely a matter of personal preference but in this text the procedure of the upper first will be described.

The upper denture, with a layer of impression material inside, should be carefully seated with a firm upwards and backwards pressure continuing for 30 seconds or longer. If the denture is not correctly seated and if the layer of impression material is too thick, the denture will be positioned downwards and forwards of its original tissue relation. There is some advantage to be gained by asking the patient to close gently into occlusal contact with the lower denture. The patient must not be allowed to clench or there will be the danger of the upper denture being carried forward. Therefore if the teeth are brought into contact it is a wise precaution for the operator to exert a balancing finger pressure against the labial and incisal surfaces of the anterior teeth on the upper denture.

Heavy occlusal pressure, or a change in occlusion away from the intercuspal position, due to patient fatigue, all cause distortion of the impression.

Before the lower impression is recorded the upper denture should be removed and the impression surface inspected. If the denture base shows through the impression, a thin layer is trimmed away, further impression material added, and the denture reinserted to correct this area of the impression. Similarly, any defect in the border areas should be corrected.

The lower rebase impression is now recorded. The lingual areas must be moulded by the patient's muscle activity, before the teeth are brought into occlusion. If occlusion of the teeth is maintained whilst the impression material sets, it is again important that the pressure applied is only light and is constant at the intercuspal position.

THE BASE MATERIALS USED IN REBASING

The base material used to replace the impression material will usually be an acrylic or other polymer unless clinical assessment of the denture bearing area indicates that a soft lining is necessary.

A soft lining to a denture may be indicated when the mucosa of the denture bearing area has undergone atrophic changes. These occur naturally with increasing age although they may be apparent as a pre-senile atrophy in the female at the climacteric. The lower denture bearing area is the one most likely to require coverage by a soft lined denture. The thin and relatively incompressible mucosa is not able to absorb the energy applied by a complete denture in occlusion. The stresses of mastication are not widely distributed and localized areas are overloaded with consequent pain. The rationale behind the use of a soft lining in such cases is the replacement of the missing resilient tissue by a soft material of similar resilience on the base of the denture. Part of the energy that is transferred to the denture during occlusal contacts is used in deforming the denture base. Consequently the loading of the atrophic tissues is reduced.

With increasing age, resorption of the alveolar ridge may cause bony land-marks such as the mylohyoid ridge, external oblique ridge and the superior genial tubercles to become more prominent. These are usually covered only by a thin mucosa and are liable to be overloaded by a hard denture base. For elderly patients, an alternative treatment to surgery is usually required, and a soft lining in a denture covering such areas is frequently successful in making the denture tolerable.

If a soft denture base is prescribed it is preferable to rebase the denture initially in hard polymer and to perfect tooth contacts in occlusion and articulation before the soft lining is applied. It may be difficult to assess tooth contacts accurately when the soft lining has already been applied; local com-pression of the elastic material creates the appearance of apparent equilibra-tion of tooth contacts when they may not in fact exist.

At the present time the heat-cured silicone rubbers are recommended for use, although improvements in other materials may provide a more suitable soft liner. A *uniform* thickness of 2 mm of silicone rubber proves adequate in most cases. Because of the relatively low bond strength of silicone rubber to acrylic base, the soft liner should whenever possible be 'boxed in' (Fig. 17.7) to reduce the possibility of bond breakdown.

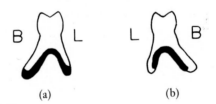

(a)   (b)

Fig. 17.7
(a) The resilient material (shaded black) forms the border of the denture;
(b) The material is 'boxed in'.

REPLACEMENT OF IMMEDIATE DENTURES

Earlier in this chapter, deterioration of the shape of the acrylic teeth on the denture was mentioned as a limiting factor as to the number of rebasing procedures that may be done. When aesthetic qualities have obviously been lost and where gross discrepancies exist between the dentures and the tissues and there are errors in vertical and horizontal jaw relations, replacement dentures should be prescribed in preference to rebasing immediate dentures.

Replacement of immediate dentures may also be necessary in the following circumstances:

WHEN A GRADUAL CORRECTION OF MALOCCLUSION HAS BEEN PLANNED

When a gross malocclusion existed in the natural dentition, the treatment plan with the immediate dentures is sometimes to effect a gradual correction. A particular example of this is the patient who presents with habitual forward posturing of the mandible as a result of earlier loss and non-replacement of posterior teeth. In older patients particularly, the correction of this occlusal malrelation should be gradual and therefore earlier replacement of the immediate dentures is necessary with the new dentures carrying the correction a stage further.

BECAUSE OF ERRORS IN TOOTH FORM, POSITION AND ARRANGEMENT

Anterior Teeth

The appearance of the dentures may not be to the satisfaction of the patient or dentist, or both. When the natural teeth are of satisfactory form, position and arrangement it is easy to obtain a successful result in an immediate denture by placing the artificial teeth in positions almost identical to their natural predecessors. But when the position of the natural anterior teeth necessitates an alteration in their position in the immediate denture, it is frequently difficult to decide with certainty just how much change should be made. It is also difficult to assess the patient's reaction to changes in appearance. Much will depend on the personal attitude of the patient and the ability of the environmental tissues to adapt to the new tooth positions. There may be dissatisfaction with appearance if the anterior teeth differ too markedly or too little from the originals. Similarly, a large change in vertical and horizontal alignment of the anterior teeth may be criticized by the patient. Much can be done to reduce the impact of this change by early discussion with the patient aided by casts set up on the articulator.

Again, because of lack of space between the ridges, teeth shorter than normal may have been used on the immediate restoration denture, particularly in the lower jaw. A large vertical incisor overlap in the natural dentition may be reduced in the immediate dentures. To achieve this, the upper or lower teeth (or both) may be made shorter than their natural predecessors. After alveolar resorption, more space becomes available and teeth of normal size can be used on a replacement denture.

As the rate and amount of alveolar resorption is unpredictable there will be some cases when little resorption occurs. An alveoloplasty is now necessary in order to set teeth of the right size in a correct relation to the adjacent tissues on replacement dentures. The experienced dentist will have recognized during his planning the possible need for surgery before replacement dentures may be constructed and will have warned the patient accordingly.

An error may have been made in the position or inclination of the anterior teeth relative to the ridge crest, causing instability of the denture. This occurs if the teeth have been positioned or inclined too far labially and the retentive potential of the denture has proved to be poor.

Posterior Teeth

Reduced stability of the dentures results if the upper posterior teeth have been placed in the position of their natural predecessors. After resorption of the outer plate of bone, masticatory loads will be directed more to the tissues of the sulcus than to the crest of the ridge, and the opposite side of the denture will be displaced during chewing.

If, on the other hand, the lower posterior teeth have been positioned too far lingually, the reduction of space causes displacement of the lower denture by the tongue.

The patient may complain of instability of the dentures on chewing due to cuspal or incisal interference. Uneven pressure from the interfering tooth contacts may result in damage to the underlying soft tissues and alveolar bone. In many cases careful selective stoning of the interferences will enhance the stability of the dentures during masticatory and empty mouth tooth contacts.

In Chapter 9 it was suggested that it was important to provide the possibility of a smooth interference-free contact of the posterior teeth. Examination of the basal tissues and the surfaces of the teeth may reveal that an immediate denture patient, who was originally provided with a relatively locked occlusion, has started to experiment and to use more extensive, excursionary, functional movements. Provided that the posterior teeth had originally been set to approximately suitable anteroposterior and lateral compensating curves, selective grinding will often provide the patient with the freedom of movement he desires. However, when the posterior teeth have been set to completely incorrect curves, this may not suffice and replacement either of the posterior teeth or of the dentures may be necessary.

ON COMPLETE FAILURE

On occasion, the immediate restoration may prove to be completely unsatisfactory because of gross errors in the various clinical and laboratory stages. Errors at the jaw relation and try-in stages may result in such inaccuracies in the vertical and horizontal relations of the denture, that they cannot be corrected by grinding. Technical faults affect the physical properties and appearance of the denture base material. Increased occlusal face height also follows improper laboratory technique. Where these clinical or technical errors are gross it is necessary to make replacement dentures.

Again, the value of the prescription to the technician cannot be overemphasized. Unless the dentist is prepared to prescribe in detail on the laboratory card exactly what technical work he requires at each particular stage, then failure is likely. Teamwork between dentist and technician is essential.

Failure of immediate dentures may occur because of lack of cooperation and tolerance on the part of the patient. Complete immediate dentures replacing only a few natural teeth for a patient who has never worn partial dentures may fail because of a general lack of interest in dentistry on the part of the patient.

Another cause of failure may be an error of judgment on the part of the dentist when planning the type of immediate denture. For example an open face upper denture might have been prescribed in the case of a prominent upper alveolar process in preference to a septal or radical alveolectomy, in anticipation of rapid postextraction resorption. If the bone subsequently shows little postextraction change, the patient may become dissatisfied with the appearance.

Failure of immediate dentures may also occur due to their removal a few hours after leaving the surgery. Some patients are apprehensive of the idea of placing a denture over an extraction socket. To their mind it can only be very painful; to avoid this pain the dentures are removed. An explanation of the effect of wearing immediate dentures on the rate of healing and on comfort during healing will allay any fears, except those of patients of low intelligence.

REPLACEMENT OF NON-IMMEDIATE DENTURES

Up to now this chapter has been concerned with the indications for the rebasing or replacement of *immediate* dentures. It is now pertinent to consider the patient who presents for replacement of complete dentures which were not immediate in type.

DENTURES PREVIOUSLY SUCCESSFUL

Patients are frequently seen who have continued to wear the same dentures for far too long—sometimes the period has extended into several decades. In many instances this has occurred simply because the patient had not been told of the importance of regular inspection of the dentures and their supporting tissues. With others, the cost of replacement dentures may have acted as a deterrent. In either event, the philosophy of the patient is likely to have been 'why interfere with something that is comfortable?'. The dentist must therefore educate the edentulous patient to the need for regular inspection of the dentures and supporting tissues. Because patients so often fail to attend regularly, cynical prosthetic specialists have been known to wish for the development of a denture base material which would fracture both spontaneously and irreparably after 5 to 6 years thus forcing the patient to seek treatment. The patient should be warned that the continued wearing of dentures which have become ill-fitting is likely to result in considerable damage to the supporting tissues with consequent difficulties in wearing dentures later in life. He must forewarn his patient of the necessity for eventual replacement of the dentures due to long-term changes in the jaws and in the dentures themselves.

However, it is not possible to state a definite time after which a denture must be replaced, because the two most important indications for replacement —those of tissue change and denture deterioration—vary with each case.

If the dentures are not maintained by regular correction of the fitting surface and occlusal adjustment, then replacement is usually necessary after a 5 year period. With regular maintenance, however, dentures may last for upwards of 10 years and only require replacement because of deterioration of the tooth material.

Some patients may, because of illness, business commitments, etc., miss a number of routine recall visits. It could be that during this unavoidable absence, considerable tissue change has occurred. If the intermaxillary relations and occlusal contacts are severely deranged, rebasing has a doubtful prognosis and replacement dentures should be prescribed. Again, if a denture has been badly damaged for some reason, replacement may well be preferred to repair.

It is inevitable that some patients will not respond to recall appointments as the dentist's advice regarding regular examination is not always heeded. On presentation after perhaps many years, one is often confronted with the irritating spectacle of dentures once satisfactory but now hopelessly inadequate. There may be inaccuracies in occlusion and probably evidence of severe trauma to the supporting tissues. If there has been considerable ridge resorption it is almost impossible to site the denture properly on the ridge and therefore rebasing procedures are very likely to result in further inaccuracies in vertical and horizontal relations. Replacement is therefore indicated.

DENTURES PREVIOUSLY UNSUCCESSFUL

Where a patient has been dissatisfied with previous dentures the most careful examination of the mouth and the dentures is essential.

Some patients requesting replacement dentures will be presenting to a particular dentist for the first time. They may or may not have been regular patients of their previous dentist and are frequently attending a new dentist simply because they have moved to a new district. There are, however, certain patients who trek from dentist to dentist without getting satisfactory oral rehabilitation and who hope that their current choice of dentist will succeed where others have apparently failed. In this situation everything depends on the ability of the dentist to recognize the problems that exist in the mouth and in the patient in general.

Before the dentist undertakes to construct new dentures for a patient who has been dissatisfied with the previous ones, he must satisfy himself that he can recognize why the dentures have failed, and also, that bearing all considerations in mind, he can improve on them.

Many dentures fail in mouths where there are no real obstacles to successful denture construction. A careful examination usually reveals certain errors in denture design which, if corrected, will do much to ensure success on the next occasion. These are usually the simpler cases to treat.

However, dentures may be unsatisfactory because of problems inherent in the oral cavity that lead to poor retention and contribute to instability. There may be reduced tissue resistance to trauma and a low pain threshold to occlusal loads. There may be psychological problems. In many cases where these inherent problems exist, successful dentures can be constructed if the dentist is aware of the problems, if he plans his treatment carefully and if he prepares the patient and the mouth beforehand.

On the other hand, oral conditions may preclude other than a very minor improvement in denture comfort and appearance. The most difficult cases are those in which the oral conditions are unfavourable and, in addition, the patient is not aware or will not accept the limitations of complete dentures. The point of balance between appearance and function is often a fine one and it varies between different patients. Some are willing to tolerate slight discomfort for appearance. A smaller number are willing to tolerate poor appearance for comfort. It is difficult to predict accurately the outcome of prosthetic treatment in the edentulous patient, who presents with both dental and personality problems. But patients usually wish to know what the chances of successful rehabilitation are, particularly after a succession of unsatisfactory dentures. After examination of the patient the dentist should explain in simple terms the problems of the case and the probable outcome of the treatment. The experienced dentist can also recount to his patient the results of treatment of similar cases. Emphasis must be placed on the need for the fullest patient cooperation both during the weeks after the insertion of new dentures and also during the follow-up period. Without this cooperation success cannot be achieved.

If the dentist, after his examination and assessment, finds the patient's demands to be excessive and unattainable, then he is well advised not to treat the patient. Due consideration must be given to the patient cooperation to be expected during treatment and also for the human frailty of both dentist and his technician. An assessment of prognosis should always allow for a small margin of human error and in discussion with the patient any promises made should cover only a half to two-thirds of the improvement to be expected.

It is very easy to criticize dentures constructed by other practitioners and care should be taken that prognosis is made on the facts presented rather than on the basis of one's own ego.

REFERRING PATIENTS FOR CONSULTATION

Because of the consultant dental services now available in general and dental hospitals, it is a normal procedure for general dental practitioners to refer patients for specialist consultation. The edentulous patient may be referred for diagnosis of oral lesions, for investigation of previous dentures that have proved unsatisfactory, or for assessment of the practitioner's treatment plan. On occasion the patient may be referred for specialist treatment that might include both surgical preparation of the mouth and denture construction where complex problems exist.

There is much to be gained by consultation with one's colleagues. The dental practitioner should benefit from a study of the consultant's report on the patient he has referred and the patient should appreciate that the dental practitioner has taken sufficient interest in his case to see that the best treatment is obtained.

There is a routine to be followed when referring patients. An appointment should be made with the consultant and he should be supplied with a case history and any relevant study casts and radiographs before the patient attends. The consultant will subsequently communicate his findings and recommendations to the practitioner. Where a practitioner has had problems associated with treatment of the case he is referring and when he wishes to pursue the consultant's recommended line of treatment himself, there is much to be said for the practitioner attending the consultation with the patient. Details of treatment can often be explained better verbally and by demonstration than by letter.

Chapter 18

Examination of the Edentulous Patient

Diagnosis is the identification of a disease by investigation of its symptoms. To diagnose is to identify by careful observation.

Although in the edentulous case the examination is concerned mainly with recognition of the possible problems associated with complete denture construction, the dentist must assume responsibility for the diagnosis of localized lesions of the oral mucosa, the underlying bone, the lips and the tongue. He must recognize the early symptoms of the common degenerative diseases and nutritional deficiencies and the lesions of the oral cavity which are manifestations of systemic disease. The dentist plays an important part in the early detection of oral cancer, as most edentulous patients are in the older age group. He must also familiarize himself with the normal tissue changes which are characteristic of the climacteric and of old age.

Probably the main cause of failure in the prosthetic treatment of the edentulous patient is the *inadequacy* of the initial examination and failure to formulate and follow a treatment plan related to the clinical situation presented.

The examination and diagnostic procedure with any dental patient consists of (1) recording the patient's history; (2) extra- and intra-oral examination; (3) the use of additional or special investigations. Where a disease or lesion is present, a diagnosis may then be made and treatment instituted. For edentulous patients where there are no pathological abnormalities or when such a lesion has been treated, a treatment plan is evolved to ensure satisfactory rehabilitation of oral function by the construction of complete dentures.

THE CASE HISTORY

The dentist should establish a routine for recording the patient's history. In this way important facts are not likely to be omitted. The data should be recorded legibly and concisely, and with sufficient thoroughness that on any future date their interpretation will be clear. The time spent in recording the history is not only most valuable in future treatment planning but also in establishing a good patient–dentist relationship. This is an opportunity for assessing the patient's personality, his attitude towards dentistry and the probable degree of cooperation to be expected towards the future plan of treatment. At this initial visit an effort should be made to gain the patient's confidence and to get him to relax.

During the questioning of the patient, whilst taking the case history, the examiner can often make an initial assessment of the proportions of the face. The lip position and movement during speech, together with the amount of tooth shown are valuable aids in ascertaining whether any dentures present are at a normal, increased or reduced occlusal face height.

ROUTINE DATA

These are recorded by an assistant and include the patient's name, address, phone number, date of birth, nationality, marital status and occupation. The name and address of the patient's physician should be obtained so that consultation and cooperation in treatment may be sought when necessary. Most of these personal data are for purposes of filing records and identifying and contacting the patient.

The date of birth is particularly useful in treatment planning in the edentulous case. The dentist should attempt to relate the chronological age of the patient with the apparent biological age of the tissues. Tissues still young in a middle aged patient respond more favourably to the presence of dentures than do prematurely old tissues.

THE COMPLAINT (C.O.)

The patient should be encouraged to express in his own words the main complaints. Much information may be gleaned from the patient's comments on the present dentures although these may be confirmed or contradicted during the subsequent oral examination.

PAST DENTAL HISTORY (P.D.H.)

Knowledge of previous treatment of the natural dentition indicates the patient's general attitude to dentistry. It is also important to know when and why the natural teeth were extracted.

Details of the patient's previous experience with either partial or complete dentures are invaluable. This is particularly so in a patient who has been provided with many dentures, all of which have been unsatisfactory. Only by careful questioning and comparison of complaints with the errors in the various prostheses can a true picture of the problem be obtained. Tactfully, patient–practitioner relations during previous treatment should be ascertained, together with any comments on the care with which the treatment was given.

GENERAL MEDICAL HISTORY (G.M.H.)

The past medical history is not as important in dental diagnosis as in medical diagnosis. The relevant medical history however, includes facts regarding the general physical condition of the patient, particularly concerning disorders of the alimentary tract. Chronic gastritis is a condition that is particularly common in patients of middle age. Predisposing causes are faulty feeding habits and hurried meals which may be related to defective mastication caused by absence of dentures or, where they are present, by their inefficiency. Where there is a history of denture intolerance with evidence of reduced soft tissue resistance, inquiries should be made regarding the patient's diet.

Dietetic surveys indicate that most older people are in a sound nutritional state. Some, however, are prone to take only a borderline amount of potassium, vitamin D, vitamin C and iron. Potassium deficiency may manifest itself by such signs as apathy, muscle weakness, depression or mental confusion. It has been shown that there is some correlation between intake of potassium and muscle power, and possibly muscle control. Vitamin D deficiency is apparently common among older women who live alone and who go out infrequently. The combination of a borderline intake and lack of sunshine may precipitate the onset of osteomalacia. This condition is difficult to diagnose and the symptoms are such that the patient may be thought to be hysterical or imagining complaints. Occasionally scurvy due to lack of vitamin C is seen but haemorrhage from the tissues of the edentulous areas is most uncommon. Many older people seem to suffer from an iron deficiency and yet are not anaemic. It is still uncertain whether an iron deficiency contributes to the tiredness and apathy commonly found among older people.

Thus although it has not yet been proved that imbalance in the ingestion or metabolism of vitamins, carbohydrates, proteins, minerals and electrolytes is specifically related to a patient's ability to adapt to and tolerate dentures, a dietary investigation may prove useful in patients presenting with problems of denture tolerance. Correction of dietary deficiencies where they exist may be a very simple matter. For example potassium and vitamin D deficiency would be overcome if the older person could be encouraged to consume a pint of milk regularly each day.

In the female patient over 35 years of age information should be obtained about the cessation of menstruation. The menopause is one landmark of the period of transition from maturity to senility known as the climacteric and which covers approximately the 15 years between the ages of 45 and 60. During this time the metabolic processes and the functions of other glands are becoming adapted to the cessation of ovarian function and women may experience a variety of metabolic and neurologic upsets which constitute the postmenopausal or climacteric syndrome. It should be noted that these arise some months or years after the interruption of normal menstruation and never whilst menstruation remains regular.

Two types of women at the climacteric have been described. In one there is a sudden and complete deprivation of oestrogen and this usually leads to severe metabolic and neurologic upsets. In the second type, although menstruation ceases, there remains an adequate submenstrual level of oestrogen for 10 or 15 years resulting in an asymptomatic climacteric period (Fig. 18.1).

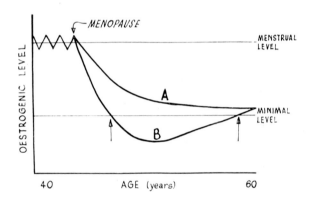

Fig. 18.1 Difference in levels of oestrogen after the menopause. Curve A: adequate, curve B: inadequate.

In the past, the variety of the symptoms presented by the climacteric woman, together with a paucity of information about their aetiology, has led clinicians to label all the complaints as emotional. Although some of the symptoms may have an emotional basis, they do in general have their origin in metabolic, endocrinal and structural changes. The immediate cause of the symptoms is believed to be the compensatory activity of the anterior lobe of the pituitary gland. Seventy-five per cent of women experience some disturbance at the time of the climacteric but only 25 per cent require medical advice and of these, not more than 5 to 10 per cent need more than reassurance.

Information should be sought about current medical treatment with particular reference to the taking of steroids and anticoagulants; any history of an allergic response to antibiotics is noted. Such information is essential if any surgery is contemplated during mouth preparation for dentures.

SOCIAL HISTORY (S.H.)

The effect of modern life with its pressures and rapid pace may cause some patients to find difficulty in tolerating or adapting to a new prosthesis. Home and working conditions play a major part in determining a patient's reaction to treatment. A few discreet questions will enable the dentist to gain some idea of the patient's general living conditions and whether he is under particular stress at this time. In dental practice the services of an experienced dental nurse are often invaluable for obtaining this type of information as the patient will feel more relaxed when talking to her away from the dental chair.

The experienced dentist also assesses the social status of his patient and knows how to gain the confidence of patients who come from widely differing social conditions. He also relates his treatment plan to the working and living conditions of the patient. The mental attitude of the patient is a most important consideration and the classification of the patient, referred to in Chapter 2, is useful in assessing the probable emotional response to treatment.

THE CLINICAL EXAMINATION

This is the second stage of the diagnostic procedure. As examination is both visual and by palpation, good illumination is essential. The order of examination is a matter of personal choice but a systematic routine should be followed. A suggested sequence is: general appearance; the face; the lips; the cheeks; the vestibular sulcus; the soft palate; the tongue; the sublingual areas; the saliva; existing dentures; the denture bearing areas.

The dentures should be examined both in and out of the mouth and any effect they might have had on the oral tissues noted. The examiner should be alert for the possible problems to be encountered in the construction of new dentures. These may be biological or mechanical, or both. Unfortunately, all too often in the past, the biological factors have been ignored and only mechanical factors considered. The systematic noting of the influencing biological factors, favourable and unfavourable, their interpretation and relation to treatment planning is essential if a successful result is to be achieved.

GENERAL APPEARANCE

Much information can be obtained from observations of the general appearance of the patient and of the uncovered parts of the body—the face and hands. The basic physique of the patient should be noted. He may be asthenic, plethoric or athletic. Both the asthenic and athletic types are likely to have a good tissue resistance to intra-oral prostheses whilst plethoric individuals tend to exhibit a less favourable reaction.

Observations of the general cleanliness of the patient will usually give some indication as to oral hygiene habits.

THE FACE

Much can be learnt from a careful examination of the patient's face—both full and in profile. The texture of the skin helps in an assessment of the probable biological age of the patient in comparison with the chronological. When age changes, such as wrinkling, are observed in the skin as a result of the atrophy of the underlying fatty tissues and muscles, it is likely that atrophic changes affecting mucosa, submucosa, musculature and bone will also be noticed when the oral cavity is examined.

The important landmarks used in assessing occlusal face height and the adequacy of intra-oral support of the facial tissues are shown in Fig. 18.2.

The labiomental angle or sulcus runs between the lower lip and the chin and gives an indication of the relationship of mandible to maxilla. This angle is obtuse in the Class I and Class II types of case, acute in Class II div 1 and

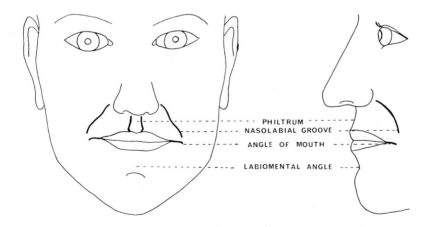

Fig. 18.2 Facial landmarks used in visual assessment of the occlusal face height.

negligible in Class III (see Fig. 11.5). When overclosure is present the sulcus is deepened and the angle is made less, whilst an opposite effect is achieved with too great an occlusal height.

The commissure or angle of the mouth is supported by the arch form of the upper teeth. After loss of the natural teeth the corners of the mouth droop and fissures develop if similar horizontal support is not given by a denture together with a satisfactory restoration of occlusal face height. Saliva collects, there is maceration of the tissues and infection may develop. These painful fissures extend laterally and downwards over the skin (Fig. 18.3), and constitute a condition known as *angular cheilitis*. This condition has a multifactoral etiology. It is caused not only by lack of support from dentures, but also by vitamin deficiency, particularly of the vitamin B complex. It may also accompany an intra-oral mycotic infection.

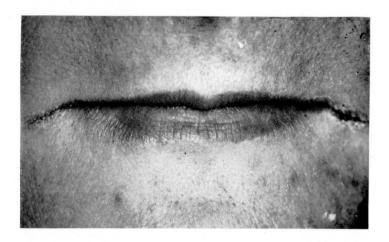

Fig. 18.3 Angular cheilitis.

The philtrum is the diamond-shaped depression which is normally seen in the centre of the upper lip and below the base of the nose. If this is flattened it also indicates poor denture support of the upper lip.

The nasolabial groove extends laterally and downwards from the side of the nose. It becomes more pronounced with age and also with loss of occlusal face height and horizontal support from the teeth. The patient's initial complaint may concern this accentuation of the nasolabial groove. It is not easy to eliminate these folds by prostheses and the dentist should be guarded in his comments on what improvement in appearance there is likely to be.

Prognosis for cosmetic improvement is even more doubtful when severe folding of facial tissues is accompanied by poor alveolar ridges. The temptation is to position the teeth too far forward in the field of activity of the lip and cheek muscles. The musculature then acts as a strong displacing force on the dentures. The ridge shape is unable to combat this force, and retention of the dentures is inadequate. When there is an intractable angular cheilitis and deep nasolabial fissures associated with gross alveolar resorption, sufficient cosmetic improvement cannot be achieved by dentures. There may then be an indication for consultation with an oral surgeon. A facial operation designed to elevate the corners of the mouth and eliminate the tissue folds may be the only satisfactory way of treating the situation.

THE LIPS

These should be examined first with the mandible in the postural position. Normally the lips are in light contact; if they are separated this may be due to mouth breathing because of nasal obstruction, or it may be the normal posture of the lips.

Incompetent lips are those unable to produce a labial seal with the mandible in the postural position without a conscious contraction of the circumoral musculature. There may be incompetence because of shortness of the upper lip, or obtuseness of the angle of the mandible, or both. Incompetence of the lips may continue into the edentulous state and therefore must be noted, as the lip relation is one of the aids at the stage of occlusal registration.

Potentially competent lips are those which, but for the protrusion of the upper incisors between them, would be able to make an anterior seal. Therefore, on extraction of the natural teeth a normal lip relation will be achieved.

With the dentures *in situ*, the lips can be used as a guide to the assessment of the occlusal face height. The patient should be asked to close the teeth together and the lips studied both from the front and in profile. Separation of the lips with the mandible in the occlusal position occurs in patients with dentures at too great an occlusal face height or if the anterior teeth are positioned too far forward. If the vertical dimension is too great, the lips will also appear tensed as the patient tries to keep them in contact. The contact may be partly or completely broken as the operator watches. Contraction of the fibres of the mentalis muscle pulling upwards on the lower lip is seen by the typical 'orange peel' surface over the chin. With a considerable increase in vertical dimension the lips may be constantly apart.

If the occlusal face height is too small there will be a pursing of the lips. With greater degrees of overclosure the lower lip will be unduly prominent and the approximation of the nose and the chin noticeable. The hidden red border of the upper lip, the pursed lower lip and the prognathic mandible—all features typical of overclosure, are particularly obvious in profile (Fig. 18.4).

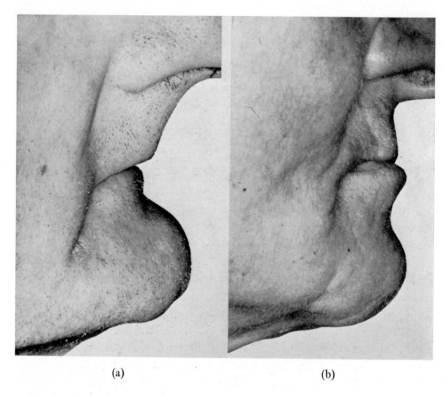

Fig. 18.4 The effect of overclosure on profile in
(a) an old patient—lips inverted;
(b) a middle-aged patient—lower lip pursed.

The lips should be palpated and their relative thickness, tonicity and mobility noted, bearing in mind the relation between these factors and the stability of complete dentures. The thick lip with a good layer of resilient submucosa between the mucosa and the muscles usually allows a more forward positioning of the anterior teeth for aesthetic purposes without sacrificing stability than does the thin lip. A thin lip usually results from atrophy of the submucous tissues and necessitates a more lingual positioning of the teeth if adequate stability is to be achieved.

In the young patient it is not usually possible to recognize the edentulous state if the lips are in light contact. The lips are full and everted despite the lack of support from teeth. The labiomental angle is maintained and the vermilion borders of the lips completely visible. In old patients there is a different picture. Due to atrophy, the skin and submucosa of the lip is thinner and it leans into the mouth. The vermilion border is reduced to a line and the oral opening appears to be constricted (Fig. 18.5).

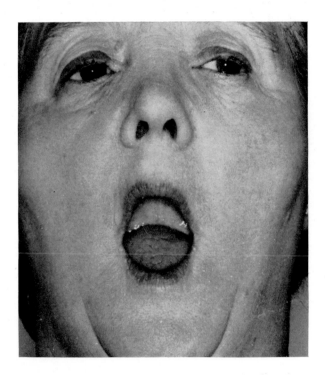

Fig. 18.5 Constricted oral opening.

The patient is now asked to open the mouth. In the young patient the lip remains everted but in the older patient the thin atrophic lower lip falls farther lingually like a curtain and is obviously a potential displacing factor for the future lower denture (Fig. 18.6).

A finger inserted behind the lips enables their resistance to forward movement to be assessed. Lips that offer little resistance are likely to develop a good seal between lips, mucosa and denture. There is less favourable prognosis if a marked resistance to finger pressure is felt either because of a marked muscular contraction or because of the lack of elasticity found in the thin lip.

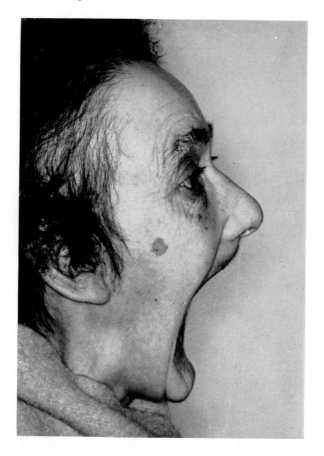

Fig. 18.6 Marked falling in of the lower lip on mouth opening in an old patient.

THE CHEEKS

The age changes described in the lips occur also in the cheeks. The examiner feels the resistance offered by the cheeks to displacement. He must note their encroachment over the alveolar ridges, particularly the lower. As with the mentalis muscles in the case of the lower lip, so there may be an inward displacement of the buccinator muscles reducing the available denture space. A loss of elasticity of the mucosa of the cheek in the old patient may predispose to cheek biting; if this has already occurred with previous dentures a white line of keratinization may be seen on the mucosa opposite the occlusal surfaces of the posterior teeth.

THE VESTIBULAR SULCUS

The reflection of the mucosa away from the alveolar ridges to form the lining mucosa of the cheeks and lips is at varying distances from the crest of the ridges. A note is made of the relation of the resting sulcus form to the crest of the ridges. For example, where gross bone resorption has occurred in the lower anterior region and there has been an inward migration of the origin of the mentalis muscle, the shallow form of the sulcus is evident, with the muscle active beneath (Fig. 18.7).

The fibrous attachments of the cheek and lip muscles to the alveolar ridges form the buccal and labial frena. If these are attached near the ridge crest they interfere with denture retention since excessive relief for them in the flanges of the denture reduces border seal and in the case of the labial frenum predisposes to midline fracture of the denture, particularly in the upper jaw.

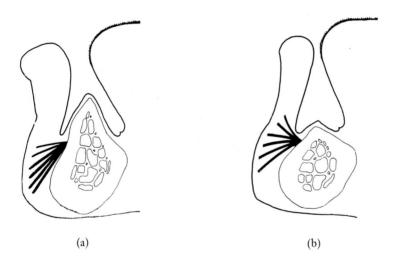

(a) (b)

Fig. 18.7 A diagrammatic illustration of the effect of age changes in the lower anterior region:
(a) the ridge is well formed, the lip is supported and the origin of the mentalis muscle is low;
(b) the ridge is resorbed, the lip inclines inwards and the origin of the mentalis muscle is near to the crest of the ridge.

THE SOFT PALATE

It is important to appreciate that the soft palate has both resting and elevated positions. Two main types of soft palate can be recognized (Fig. 18.8). One is fairly horizontal and moves but little. The other is more vertically positioned and has a definite axis of rotation. In the first type of palate, it is relatively easy to get an effective post dam seal; in the second it is more difficult.

If there is a history of nausea and retching with the present dentures, the posterior palatal areas should be palpated to assess the validity of the complaint. It will generally be found, however, that the dorsum of the tongue is the more sensitive receptor for the retching reflex.

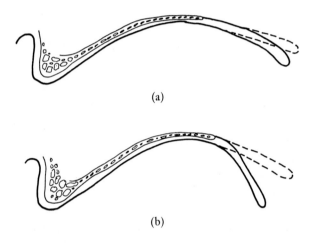

(a)

(b)

Fig. 18.8 Two types of soft palate:
(a) horizontally positioned with little movement;
(b) more vertically positioned with considerable movement and a definite axis of rotation.

THE TONGUE

The shape, size and tonicity of the tongue is of particular interest to the dentist. The tongue fills much of the oral cavity when the jaws are at rest and it is in close apposition with the lingual area of the lower denture and the palate of the upper. The tongue is an essential organ for lower denture control but if the denture violates the space normally occupied by the tongue, the latter can have a violent displacing effect. If posterior teeth have been lost and not replaced, the tongue will have spread laterally and so reduced the width of the neutral zone. In cases of macroglossia there may be constant irritation of the tongue by dentures, and in such circumstances surgical reduction of the size of the tongue is to be considered.

The shape, size and colour of the tongue are important. Extreme deficiencies particularly vitamin B complex and iron may produce surface changes which are more obvious in the tongue than in other mucosal areas.

THE SUBLINGUAL AREAS

These are best examined using a tongue spatula to deflect the tongue. The depth of the lingual sulcus is noted and an attempt made to assess the probable distolingual extent of the future denture and its effect on retention.

THE SALIVA

By questioning the patient and by observation, the quantity and viscosity of the saliva can be assessed. An intact thin film of saliva between the denture and tissues is essential for retention and comfort.

Lack of saliva on first examination may be due to nervousness of the patient and flow will become normal when the patient becomes relaxed. Resting saliva volume may be determined by noting the amount absorbed by two cotton wool rolls placed in the sublingual areas for two minutes. Weighing gives an accurate assessment but the degree of wetness of the rolls on removal affords an approximation.

Viscosity may be assessed by wetting the finger and thumb with saliva and rubbing them together. The amount of mucin is related to the relative quantities of parotid and submandibular secretion. The latter produces mucin together with the palatal glands.

Dryness of the mouth (xerostomia) may be permanently present after irradiation of the head and neck area or after surgical removal of one or more of the salivary glands. A permanently decreased salivary flow also accompanies vitamin B and iron deficiencies, diabetes mellitus and diabetes insipidus. Decreased salivary volume is often noticed during the climacteric. Xerostomia leads to generalized discomfort in the mouth which is frequently aggravated by dentures. All dentures move to a greater or lesser degree in function and if the mucosa is insufficiently lubricated it is likely to be abraded with consequent soreness.

Persistent and excessive flow of saliva (sialorrhea) may occur in certain diseases of the nervous system, such as Parkinsonianism, epilepsy and in mentally retarded patients. The main problem is of drooling at the corners of the mouth. Every effort should be made to keep these areas well supported by correct tooth positioning. Usually sialorrhea is temporary and caused by the presence of a foreign body in the mouth. Impression material, record blocks, the finished denture—all may result in excessive salivary flow. At the impression stage the surface of certain impression materials (e.g. plaster) may be washed away and therefore this fact must be borne in mind when choosing the impression material.

Sialorrhea also occurs in association with oral ulcerations, particularly those malignant in nature and the examiner should be alert in the older patients as he may occasionally be able to detect an early oral cancer.

EXAMINATION OF EXISTING DENTURES

So much can be learnt from a systematic examination of the existing dentures and yet so often they are completely ignored in diagnosis and treatment planning. It is usual to divide previous dentures into two categories—those that have proved successful and those that have failed.

SUCCESSFUL DENTURES

These may be successful in the opinion of both the patient and the dentist or of the patient only, for there will be instances when, although the patient believes the dentures to have been very successful, the dentist will consider them to have many shortcomings. This is particularly likely when the effect of the existing dentures on the basal tissues is being assessed. The dentist will often find that some correction and alteration is necessary to preserve the oral structures. Due to gradual changes in the supporting tissues and wear of the occlusal surfaces of any acrylic posterior teeth the vertical and horizontal jaw relations change. When the patient has attended regularly for periodic modification of his dentures the amount of correction necessary with new dentures will be small. When he has not attended for some years marked changes may have occurred in the relation of dentures both to their respective basal tissues and to each other. It is indeed amazing how some patients are able to tolerate, control and be perfectly satisfied with the most ill-fitting dentures. A denture that has been worn for many years often fits only at the border as resorption of bone from the alveolar ridge has destroyed the original adaptation of the remainder of the denture base. The forces of mastication are resisted by the border tissues, and retention and control is entirely by the environmental musculature.

In cases where the existing dentures are assessed as successful by both patient and dentist and only require replacement because of deterioration of the teeth, a denture copying technique should be prescribed. This will ensure maximum patient comfort, and satisfaction with the replacement dentures and will obviate the need for the guesswork normally necessary with conventional replacement denture techniques.

When the dentures are assessed as unsuccessful by the dentist but successful by the patient the dentist must be wary about his comments on the dentures and must also be conservative in his suggestions for alterations in the replacement dentures. This is particularly so with elderly patients where marked modification in denture form may cause difficulty in adaptation and so produce an unhappy patient.

UNSUCCESSFUL DENTURES

Under this heading will be considered those cases where both patient and dentist agree on the failure of the existing dentures.

A careful examination of unsuccessful dentures in and out of the mouth usually reveals certain errors which, if corrected, will do much to ensure success with the replacement dentures.

The commonest errors are:

1 *Underextension of the Denture Bases*

In the upper jaw there is frequently incomplete extension round the maxillary tuberosities and over the posterior part of the palate. The retromolar and distolingual areas in the lower jaw are similarly often neglected. Lack of extension contributes greatly to poor retention in a denture and also reduces the possibility of correct shaping of the polished surfaces.

2 *Upper Anterior Teeth Wrongly Placed*

Often the upper anterior teeth are set directly over the crest of the ridge. In this position there is restriction of the tongue which then displaces the denture in a forward direction. Lip support is inadequate and appearance is poor. On the other hand, anterior teeth set too far forward can cause instability on incision and also create a non-retentive polished surface.

3 *Premature Contacts or Unbalanced Occlusion*

When the lower denture comes into contact with the upper, premature contacts may be seen which affect both the stability and the comfort of the dentures. These have often arisen from the difficulty of getting the patient relaxed before recording the horizontal jaw relation, with the result that there has been a failure to register the muscular position of the mandible.

4 *Unbalanced Articulation*

Chewing movements may be restricted by too great a vertical overlap in relation to horizontal overlap of the canines and incisors. The use of acrylic teeth predisposes to the gradual development of a deeper vertical overlap of the anterior teeth as the result of wear of the posterior occlusal surfaces. The horizontal overlap is decreased by the forward movement of the mandible. These changes combine to restrict attempts at lateral chewing movements.

5 *Increased Occlusal Face Height*

One of the cardinal rules of complete denture prosthetics is to ensure that there is sufficient freeway space. Frequently one finds this is reduced and sometimes obliterated. The patient's complaints are both many and obvious to the examiner. There is excessive bulk of denture material in the mouth leading to difficulty in speech and mastication. The diminished freeway space restricts the amount of room between the teeth on upper and lower dentures for a bolus of food, and reduces the speaking space. Since the teeth come into very frequent contact the ridges are subjected to repeated overloading with resultant pain, often burning in nature. There is likely to be muscle pain particularly in the masseters and possibly pain in the temporomandibular joint areas which may be referred, via branches of the fifth cranial nerve, to other areas of the face and neck.

6 *Inclination and Level of the Plane of Occlusion*

Ideally the occlusal plane of the posterior teeth should be parallel to both upper and lower alveolar ridges. If it lies at an angle, occlusal contact on an inclined plane causes movement of the dentures during function. If the occlusal plane is placed too high, the tongue displaces the lower denture by pressing hard against its lingual surface.

7 *Lower Posterior Teeth that are Too Wide*

Natural teeth lie in a neutral zone of muscle activity between the buccinator and the tongue. With loss of teeth there is a reduction in the width of the neutral zone as the tongue spreads outwards and the buccinator moves inwards (Fig. 18.9). As the alveolar ridges resorb, the attachments of the buccinator muscles move inwards and reduce further the space available for dentures. The teeth on many complete lower dentures are too wide buccolingually. This leads to poor stability of a lower denture, as the adjacent musculature attempts to displace an object that encroaches upon its area of activity. The tongue is more vigorous in this respect than the cheeks. Even if narrow teeth are used and are positioned too far lingually, the tongue pushes this area of the lower denture upwards and forwards and causes denture instability.

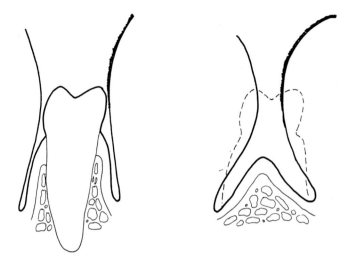

Fig. 18.9 Reduction in width of the neutral zone after extraction of the natural teeth.

8 *Lower Anterior Teeth Placed Too Far Anteriorly*

The position of the lower anterior teeth is related to the muscle activity of the lower lip. In the older patient the mentalis muscle has encroached on the denture bearing area and the lower lip is lingually inclined. The lower anterior teeth must then be placed near the crest of the ridge. If they are positioned too far forward the lip displaces the denture backwards.

THE DENTURE BEARING AREAS

The examination includes a study of (1) the overall size and form of the residual alveolar ridges, (2) the ridge relations and (3) the covering mucosa and muco-periosteum. The examination is both visual and palpatory and may be supplemented by a radiographic assessment of the quality of the alveolar bone.

THE RESIDUAL ALVEOLAR RIDGES

Within limits, the larger the alveolar ridge, the greater is the potential for resistance of a denture to displacing forces. The limiting factor is when the ridges are so pronounced that there is insufficient space between them for dentures. The very large or bulbous ridge may require surgical reduction but presents a less frequent prosthetic problem than the grossly resorbed ridge.

The Arch Form

In the upper jaw it is usual to classify the arch form as being square, tapering, or ovoid. The lower arch form does not generally fit into these particular groups. Usually the vault of the palate in coronal section corresponds to the basic upper arch form.

The square and ovoid upper arch forms and palatal vaults are usually favourable for retention, whereas the tapering arch and palatal vault may be unfavourable because of the reduction of surface area that lies at right angles to any vertically or horizontally displacing force.

The cross section of the ridge form varies tremendously from patient to patient, between maxilla and mandible and in different areas in the same jaw. It may be parallel sided, undercut, V-shaped, narrow or broad. The most favourable ridge is one that is U-shaped with almost vertical walls, as this will provide the best resistance to both vertical and lateral displacement.

By palpation, the examiner must determine whether the form of the ridge is due to the bone contour or whether the latter has been modified by the covering soft tissue. The importance of this is evident in undercut areas. If the undercut is basically bony it may not be possible to adapt the denture closely to the tissue and some retention will be lost. A soft tissue undercut

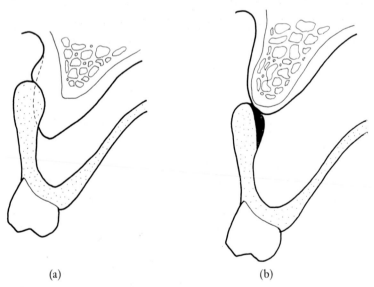

(a)   (b)

Fig. 18.10
(a) Soft tissue undercut which can be deformed on inserting the denture and used for denture retention;
(b) Hard tissue limiting the amount of undercut that can be used.

can be deformed temporarily on inserting the denture and the flange will then lie in contact with the tissue (Fig. 18.10).

The crests of the alveolar ridges should be palpated with the finger or with a ball-ended plastic instrument. An irregular crest is often found in the lower anterior region particularly in those cases with a history of extraction of lower anterior teeth due to chronic periodontitis. Radiographs may reveal the presence of sharp vertical spicules of bone (Fig. 18.11). If the mucoperiosteum is

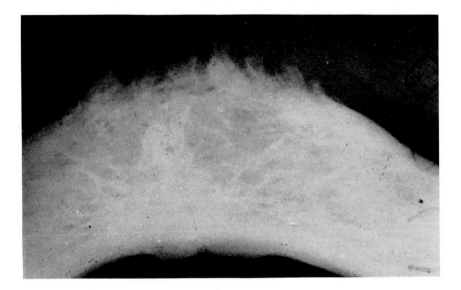

Fig. 18.11 Radiographic appearance of a lower anterior ridge showing sharp vertical spicules of bone.

reflected, the bony crest will be found to be very irregular and sharp to the touch. This type of ridge is commonly covered by a thin atrophic mucosa and it is not uncommon to obtain a painful response from the patient as a finger is passed lightly over the area. This clinical situation presents a real problem of tolerance to a denture for there is usually considerable pain on occlusal or incisal contact as the nerve endings in the submucosa are compressed between the bony spicules and the hard unyielding denture base.

In the mandible where gross resorption has occurred, the mylohyoid ridges and external oblique ridges are prominent and the genial tubercles often stand high. These bony prominences create problems of both denture extension and denture comfort. Palpation of the thin mucosa covering them usually elicits a marked response from the patient.

The Effect of Extreme Resorption on Denture Retention

A small ridge may present problems in denture wearing as it provides little resistance to lateral displacement and rotation of a denture. A slow resorption of bone over a period of years is less likely however to affect the ability of the regular denture wearer to control a prosthesis. The environmental musculature becomes the more important retention factor once adaptation to the form of the polished surfaces has been achieved. But when a patient is rendered edentulous late in life and where periodontal disease has destroyed much of the alveolar bone there may be difficulty in getting used to a first denture. The value of a well-formed ridge in this situation is that it provides mechanical resistance to displacement whilst the adjacent musculature is accommodating to the shape of the polished surfaces. When this has been achieved, the musculature plays the major part in retention and the ridge is not the vital factor it used to be.

Ridge Relations

Ideally, the upper alveolar ridge anteriorly should lie a little outside the lower and posteriorly be a little narrower than the lower. Then a normal horizontal overlap is possible anteriorly and the posterior teeth can be set up in normal relation. Unfortunately this is rarely seen due to the differing patterns of resorption in the two jaws. Although the precise vertical and horizontal relation of the ridges will be seen when the casts are mounted on the articulator, some idea of the relation can be obtained at this stage by separating the patient's lips when the mandible is in the postural position.

Note should be made of any gross malrelation of the jaws. If the patient is Class II or Class III then it is likely that a harmonious denture-tissue relation will be achieved only if the teeth on the dentures are set in a position similar to the teeth of the natural dentition. Many complete dentures fail because of an attempt by the clinician, or perhaps more frequently by the technician, to convert a marked Class II or Class III case into a Class I simply by setting the teeth on the dentures to that relation. The dentures fail because the teeth and the denture bases encroach beyond the confines of the neutral zone and interfere with the long-established patterns of movement of the adjacent musculature.

Radiography of the Denture Bearing Areas

The visual and digital examination of the alveolar ridges gives only a superficial concept of conditions and ideally the examination should be made complete by the use of radiographs. The radiographic examination has a twofold value; first, it discloses any pathological condition present in the jaws and secondly it enables the examiner to assess the quality of the bone of the denture bearing area and its possible reaction to masticatory stress. Three variations in bone structure have been described: dense, cancellous and non-cortical. The dense structure with a well-defined cortex reacts favourably to stress. The cancellous with a less well-defined cortex will tolerate stress provided it is not excessive; whereas the non-cortical type provides a very poor support for a denture and undergoes more rapid resorption. The last type is seen frequently in the lower incisor region.

A number of surveys of edentulous patients, where the alveolar ridges have been covered by a healthy-looking mucosa and where the patients were un-aware of any abnormality, have revealed that in as many as 30–40 per cent of cases there are retained roots, teeth and other abnormalities hidden beneath the mucosa.

THE COVERING MUCOSA

The soft tissues that cover the bony foundation of the denture bearing areas must be examined carefully. Like skin, the mucosa is protective in nature but differs from skin principally in that the stratum corneum is much thinner and may be absent in some areas. In the edentulous patient the mucosa has to support relatively inflexible dentures and is of consequence being used for a purpose for which it was not designed. It is not therefore surprising to find microscopic and macroscopic changes in the mucosa as a result of denture wearing.

Resilience of the Soft Tissues

So many inaccuracies, minor though they may be, creep in at the various technical stages that perfect fit of a denture is impossible. Therefore some resilience is desirable so that adaptation of the mucosa to the fitting surface of the denture can occur. A resilient mucosa also has a shock-absorbing effect on the stresses of mastication. Some of the force transmitted by the dentures to the tissues will be expended in the displacement of tissue fluids and there-fore less will be available to stimulate nerve endings lying in the mucosa.

If the mucosa is too thin the slightest inaccuracy in impression recording is likely to result in pain or inflammation of the mucosa. On the other hand, if the soft tissue is flabby and therefore mobile, the denture is likely to be unstable. Tissue which shows considerable variation in resilience may present problems in achieving even tissue loading by a denture.

Uneven thickness may result from irregular areas of bone resorption where the bone has been replaced by fibrous tissue. A common example is when a complete upper denture has been opposed by natural lower anterior teeth with no replacement of the missing lower posterior teeth. The constant overloading in the anterior region frequently results in considerable resorption of this portion of the upper alveolar crest. There is replacement of the lost bone by fibrous tissue and the production of the typical mobile flabby ridge.

The appearance of the mucosa and its histological structure may be affected at the climacteric, by age changes and as a result of denture wearing.

The Effect of the Climacteric on the Soft Tissues

At the climacteric it is not uncommon to find the mucosal surface reddened, swollen and glossy with bleeding a prominent feature. The epithelium strips easily from the underlying connective tissue leaving a raw sensitive surface. This is typical of the appearance of a gingivosis or chronic desquamative gingivitis. Microscopically the epithelium is thin and atrophic. The basement membrane may be absent and there is an inflammatory infiltration of the submucosa where the collagenous fibres may be atrophic or degenerated. Alternatively the mucosa may appear pale and parchment-like. With either the pale or reddened mucosa picture there may be an associated burning sensation and dryness of the mouth. The patient may also complain of joint and muscle pains (fibrositis, myositis).

Although such changes are found predominantly in women they may also be seen in males. Their predominance in women has suggested that the aetiology may be hormonal as the changes in the oral mucosa are similar to those found in the vaginal mucosa; the epithelium in both instances being reduced in thickness with decreased keratinization. The reduced oestrogen output associated with the climacteric and with increasing age results in the reduction in keratinization in both sites being in fact a correlated physiological atrophic phenomenon. The administration of oestrogen has a marked effect on vaginal epithelium with a rapid multiplication of the layers of stratified squamous epithelium. The effect of oestrogen on the oral mucosa is less marked but it has been used successfully in severe cases of gingivosis.

The adverse mucosal changes may also be related to malnutrition. It is not certain whether the vitamin deficiency that occurs is due primarily to dietary neglect or whether it is secondary to the low oestrogen level. Certainly it has been shown that a relationship exists between a vitamin B complex deficiency and a low oestrogen level. On the other hand, dietary neglect and peculiar dietary habits are often encountered during the climacteric and may result in malnutrition. For example the unpleasant taste sensations often experienced prevent the enjoyment of food and the result is that the patient forgoes regular meals and takes a poorly balanced diet. These symptoms are likely to be exaggerated if dentures are worn. In fact the patient frequently blames the dentures for the generalized discomfort and abnormal taste sensations that may exist. Even technically perfect dentures are likely to contribute to the patient's unhappiness by directing occlusal pressures onto supporting tissues which have a reduced resistance and poor response to loading.

The Effect of Age on the Soft Tissues

The picture is one of atrophy. The epithelial layers are less in number and the mucosa and submucosa show a decrease in thickness. This is particularly so in the lower jaw. It is generally agreed that the degree of keratinization of the epithelium is reduced with increasing age but in the edentulous patient the effect of the dentures on the epithelium is of importance and will be considered below.

The Effect of Denture Wearing on the Soft Tissues

It is recognized that well-designed and maintained dentures are likely to keep the supporting tissues in the best possible condition. There are, however, countless examples of patients who have worn ill-fitting dentures for many years in whom there are no clinical signs of trauma of the supporting tissues. In contrast, there are some patients in whom evidence of denture trauma is seen in spite of the most careful treatment planning and denture construction. There is perhaps a predisposition to earlier signs and symptoms of denture trauma when there are in addition manifestations of tissue change due to the climacteric or to the normal ageing processes. Although the changes in the mucosa as a result of denture wearing are not generally considered to be of a dangerous nature, it is obvious that the dentist should recognize that it is his responsibility to prevent chronic oral irritation particularly in an ageing patient and to take steps to ensure that the dentures are as atraumatic to the tissues as possible.

When a patient has neglected to attend for routine denture and tissue examination over the years, the dentures are frequently found to be ill-fitting and to have occlusal defects. Under such dentures are soft tissues which may appear deep red in colour, bruised and oedematous. The resulting inflammatory picture is commonly known as *denture stomatitis* (*denture sore mouth*), and is much more frequently seen under the upper denture than the lower. The clinical signs of denture stomatitis that may be present are:

1. Pinpoint inflammation

Small areas of inflammation in an otherwise normal tissue. These are usually found around the orifices of the ducts of the palatal mucous glands (Fig. 18.12).

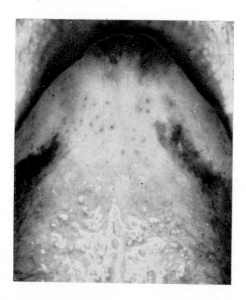

Fig. 18.12 Pinpoint inflammation of the palate.

2. *Localized inflammation*

Larger areas of inflammation in an otherwise normal tissue. Common sites are on the sides of the palate and the labial aspect of the denture bearing area.

3. *General inflammation*

A diffuse inflammation of the entire denture bearing area. The surface of the mucosa is smooth and may bleed easily. The area of redness is limited to the area covered by the denture (Fig. 18.13).

4. *Granular inflammation (Papillary Hyperplasia)*

The mucosa has a nodular hyperaemic surface which may be present over the entire denture bearing area but is more commonly restricted to the central area of the palate and is commonly found under relief areas of a denture (Fig. 18.14).

The principal causative factors suggested in the past have been heat build-up beneath the denture, poor oral hygiene with concomitant bacterial infection, chemotoxic effect of the denture base material, lowered tissue resistance due to systemic conditions (the anaemias, diabetes, vitamin and nutritional deficiencies, hormonal disturbances) and allergic reactions of the mucosa to constituents of the base material or to denture cleansing agents.

Whilst all these possibilities must be borne in mind by the examiner, careful

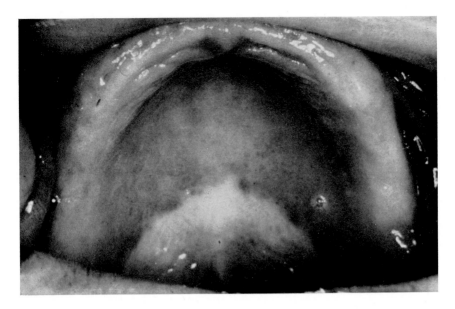

Fig. 18.13 Generalized inflammation of the palate.

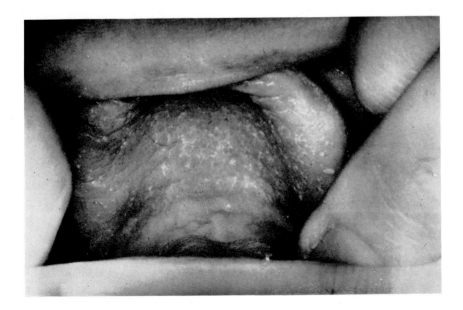

Fig. 18.14 Granular inflammation of the palate.

assessment of cases of denture stomatitis suggests that trauma and infection by *Candida albicans* are the most important etiological factors. Trauma may result from a rough denture fitting surface, inadequate adaptation to the tissues or premature contacts on occlusion or articulation. It is obvious that an ill-fitting denture with occlusal or articulatory faults will move considerably in function and is likely to cause local or general abrasion of the mucosa. Yet there remains the question whether some of the inflammatory conditions are due to primary infection by *C. albicans* or whether yeasts are secondary invaders of traumatized tissues. Studies have shown a 90 per cent positive yield of yeast-like fungi in patients with denture stomatitis, compared with 40 per cent in a control group of patients with dentures but not showing signs of denture stomatitis.

Yeast-like fungi are found particularly in the inflamed areas of the mucosa and there is a correlation between the degree of inflammation and the quantity of yeast colonies found on culture. The cases of generalized and granular inflammation seem to differ from cases showing localized inflammation in that yeast-like fungi are found in significantly greater quantities. Such cases are more likely to exhibit also symptoms of angular cheilitis and glossitis.

It seems probable that trauma of the oral mucosa predisposes to growth of *C. albicans*, although fungi may be isolated from inflamed mucosa beneath apparently non-traumatic dentures and also of course from non-inflamed mucosa. By removing trauma, inflamed areas often resolve and there is usually a concomitant reduction in candida growth. But there appears also to be a significant correlation between poor denture hygiene and candida growth. Organisms may be isolated from the fitting surface of a denture as well as from the soft tissues. The fitting surface of an acrylic denture may act as a highly satisfactory culture site for candidas. It is interesting to note that the provision of replacement non-infected dentures results in some reduction in inflammation. Later when the denture surface becomes heavily infected with *C. albicans* the signs of inflammation return.

Many cases of denture stomatitis are referred to hospital with a 'query allergy' diagnosis. The patients themselves often firmly believe they are allergic to plastic. But allergy to acrylic is rare. In contrast to denture stomatitis where the tissue reaction is confined to the denture bearing area, in cases of true allergy all tissues in contact with polished or fitting surfaces of the denture would be affected. Skin reaction tests can be performed on patients suspected of being allergic to denture base materials, but it must be noted that a negative skin result does not altogether exclude a positive reaction on mucosa.

A similarity has been noticed between the pinpoint inflammation type of denture stomatitis and the sweat retention syndrome often observed in persons reacting unfavourably to a hot climate. It has been suggested that the symptoms of this type of denture stomatitis may be due to lateral spread of saliva into the tissues following occlusion of the duct orifices of the palatal mucous glands. The four different and possibly successive stages of denture stomatitis may be analogous to the skin condition known as *miliaria rubra*. In the sweat retention syndrome, simple trauma has been shown to be capable of producing an allergic type of reaction and it has been suggested that the same mechanism may operate in the case of denture stomatitis. Here again though, the excitatory cause would be the occlusion of the glandular ducts as a result of trauma from a moving denture.

Clinical evidence of denture stomatitis is unfortunately fairly common, but as mentioned earlier, often goes unrecognized by both patient and dentist. The slow progress of the condition and the usual absence of pain are possible explanations. There is, however, no excuse for the dentist failing to observe evidence of denture injury to the tissues and thoughtlessly embarking on the construction of new dentures upon an inflamed mucosa.

The histological changes of the mucosa in denture stomatitis have been described by a number of workers. There seems to be general agreement that the connective tissue becomes oedematous and its papillae press towards the surface of the epithelium which may then show protuberances. The epithelium may be irregular in thickness in that cords of epithelium may be found deep in the submucosa, the surface of the denture bearing area may be denuded of epithelium which may result in occasional spontaneous haemorrhage. There is some disagreement regarding the effect of denture wearing on the stratum corneum. It may be that lack of agreement in the literature stems more from different definitions of *keratinization* than from differences observed in various biopsy sites, since many writers do not choose to define their criteria for keratinization. It is probable that the epithelium of individual denture wearers responds differently. Reduction in the degree of keratinization is perhaps usual under dentures. This can indicate one of two possibilities, either the layers of keratinized cells become less numerous, or the islands of keratinization become smaller in relation to the inter-island sea of parakeratosis. Female denture wearers in general tend to show less keratinization than male denture wearers. The clinical appearance of the soft tissues beneath dentures does not seem to be necessarily related to the presence or absence of keratinized cells.

In addition to gross signs of inflammation that may be present in a denture wearer, the examiner should be on the look-out for evidence of tissue deformation. When an ill-fitting denture has been worn for some time and where there is a fairly thick mucosal covering of the bone the movement of the denture in

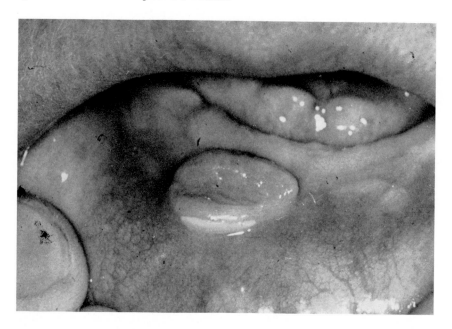

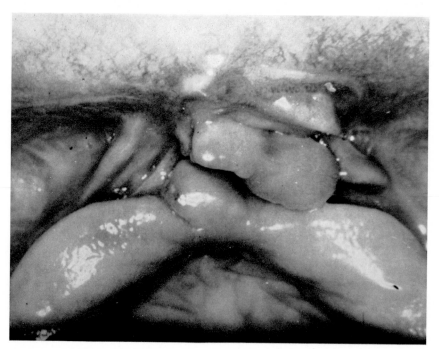

Fig. 18.15 Denture hyperplasia.

function is likely to lead to abuse and deformation. Again the first sign of accelerated resorption of the residual ridges under an ill-fitting denture is often the abused and deformed conditions of the soft tissues where there has been excessive pressure.

The flanges of dentures may be responsible for a tissue reaction known as denture hyperplasia (denture granuloma). This is a flap or roll of tissue commonly found at the mucosal reflection and related to the border of the denture. The flaps may be single or multiple (Fig. 18.15), and separated by clefts. The usual cause is sinkage of the denture due to alveolar resorption. Then the denture assumes an overextended relation to the sulcus.

Although digital examination was recommended for assessment of the resilience of the covering tissues the use of a ball–ended plastic instrument or blunt probe is suggested to pick out any trigger points that may be present in the mucosa overlying the crest of the ridge. These trigger points are usually about 2 mm in diameter and may be found in both jaws but more commonly in the lower and in the anterior region. They are believed to be caused by the abnormal distribution of nerve endings that may exist after tooth extraction.

A biopsy from a trigger point invariably shows the innervation to be locally more profuse. Large irregular nerve bundles are often seen in close proximity to the rough and sharp areas of the crest of bony spicules. Pressure on such tissue will give rise to a very painful response from the patient and is likely to make the wearing of a denture intolerable.

In his examination the dentist should pinpoint any trigger points for unless they are treated surgically or prosthetically, denture comfort will not be achieved.

SPECIAL INVESTIGATIONS

Various laboratory tests may be used to assist the clinician in his diagnosis and treatment planning. These include blood examination, bacterial cultures, patch testing, urine analysis. In dealing with a larger number of geriatric patients, more use may be made in the future of laboratory studies concerned with nutritional adequacy such as vitamin levels, gastric analysis and absorptive function tests.

It has not been the purpose of this chapter to describe all the lesions of the mucosa that may be present in the edentulous patient. For these the reader is referred to standard texts on oral pathology. It must be emphasized, however, that when examining an edentulous mouth prior to construction of complete dentures, the dentist must be alert for any pathology that may exist. The examination of the edentulous mouth prior to prosthetic treatment is frequently neglected and as a result painless yet potentially dangerous lesions may be missed. There is a moral and professional obligation to carry out the most careful examination before treatment of the edentulous case is commenced.

Chapter 19

Denture Copying

Whilst methods of copying existing dentures appear in the literature, unfortunately the techniques are by no means universally adopted, nor are they well known.

These techniques offer considerable advantages to both the patient and the operator in time, and in achieving a satisfactory conclusion to treatment, particularly of patients with denture problems. However, tradition in dentistry dies hard as it does in other fields, and many practitioners still persist in starting from the assumption that a patient presents with no valuable information from the existing prostheses but that the dentist's normal techniques can always produce 'better' dentures. It is only when this approach fails that he turns to look at the previous dentures to determine what has happened. It is much more sensible to start by using the information available from existing or previous dentures and to modify it as necessary.

When replacing dentures, any or all of the following features of the existing ones may need to be duplicated in the new prostheses:

1 Area and shape of fitting surface
2 Occlusal face height
3 Occlusal plane
4 Occlusal surface
5 Posterior tooth size and position
6 Anterior tooth size, position and arrangement
7 Shape of polished surfaces.

The first and most important stage is to decide what features of the existing dentures are acceptable and which require modification. The amount of actual 'duplication' undertaken depends on this decision. In some circumstances, the existing dentures may be duplicated in detail apart from a new fitting surface. On other occasions, both the fitting and occlusal surfaces may be changed whilst the anterior tooth position and relation and the general denture shape are all duplicated. When a large number of modifications are planned, there may be very little actual copying but the dimensions, shape and surfaces of the existing dentures may be utilized as guide lines to follow in the construction of the replacement dentures.

Techniques for duplicating dentures fall, therefore, into three main types:
1 Almost complete duplication of existing dentures
2 Modifications from the basic pattern of the existing dentures
3 Use of copies of the previous dentures as guides to assist in the setting up and shaping of the replacements.

CLINICAL STAGE COMMON TO ALL TECHNIQUES

The borders of the dentures may require modification, either by trimming where overextension exists or, more frequently, by the addition of compound or other materials where underextension is apparent. In some instances, the shape of the polished surfaces may be amended, for example, by trimming away a lingual overhang of the posterior teeth on the lower denture.

Any undercuts present on the fitting surfaces of the dentures are removed and the dentures then used as special trays for wash impressions in any suitable material. The removal of small undercuts does not affect the comfort with which the patient can wear the dentures after the new casts have been poured and the impression material removed. When large undercuts have been removed, the retention of the dentures may be seriously reduced. After the impression has been recorded, a temporary readaptation of the denture base may be achieved by placing a tissue conditioning material into the fitting surface.

Where the occlusal relation is to be modified in vertical or horizontal planes or both, a wax wafer is used to record the new occlusion. Appropriate facebow and other records are made according to the type of articulator to be used.

ALMOST COMPLETE DUPLICATION

When using almost complete duplication, one usually proceeds direct from the clinical stage to the finished denture without try-in or other clinical stage. The scope for modification of the denture, except the shape of the fitting surface, is very limited.

LABORATORY TECHNIQUE

A stone cast is poured to the impression recorded within the denture. Then the denture is invested in the first half of the flask by the inverted method. A layer of self-curing silicone elastomer is then applied to the teeth and the polished surfaces and allowed to polymerize. Flasking is completed by adding gypsum to fill the second half of the flask (Fig. 19.1).

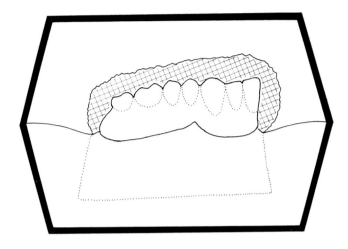

Fig. 19.1 Section of denture invested in combined silicone elastomer and gypsum mould.

On separating the hardened mould, the flexible silicone elastomer allows the denture to be withdrawn without fracturing the mould. The denture is removed from the cast and the impression material cleaned away. The denture can now be returned to the patient after checking the mould and shade of the teeth. If the teeth on the denture have not been modified from stock patterns, it is possible to insert duplicates of these into the impressions of the teeth in the silicone rubber and then to pack the mould either with self or heat-curing methyl methacrylate and so reproduce the denture. This technique is perhaps more suitable for duplication of a recently constructed denture rather than one in which the teeth have been abraded over a period of use.

Alternatively self-curing tooth-coloured polymer may be poured into the tooth impressions in the flask, allowed to polymerize, removed, trimmed and then replaced. The mould is packed with denture base as before and the denture completed. Whilst, with this technique, the teeth and denture base are duplicated with some precision, the aesthetics of the teeth moulded in the flask are not as good as those of stock teeth. Other methods involve pouring wax into the mould to form patterns from which teeth can be moulded separately. These are then replaced in the flask and the denture completed.

It is also possible to employ the silicone elastomer as the mould material for the fitting surface of the denture. Then large undercuts on the existing denture may be reproduced without fear of damaging the cast. For this purpose, the section of elastomer which forms the denture base mould should be stiffened and reinforced with wire mesh. Dimensional accuracy, however, may suffer a little unless care is taken when using this technique.

The denture may also be duplicated by making the upper half of the mould in a hydrocolloid material. Then by using a pour-technique self-curing base after the teeth have been made by any of the above methods, a duplicate denture can be prepared. Here dimensional accuracy is more doubtful and usually a reduction in occlusal face height occurs, together with other dimensional changes of the order of 1 to 2 mm.

PARTIAL DUPLICATION

In other duplicating techniques, one proceeds from impressions and occlusal adjustment to the stage of try-in. If a wax duplicate of the denture is first made, then this can act as the basis for the try-in. Teeth can be removed from the wax in a manner similar to that used for immediate dentures. The tooth position is maintained or slightly modified and there is controlled alteration of the shape of the polished surfaces if this is considered to be necessary. When an impression has not been recorded previously in the existing dentures, due to large undercuts, it may be necessary to incorporate a shellac base in the try-in to give a sufficiently stable structure in which an impression may be recorded.

LABORATORY TECHNIQUE

In the laboratory, casts are poured to the new impressions if these have been recorded. Where impressions have not been recorded due to the presence of large undercuts, it may be necessary to fit 'cores' of plaster to undercut areas. These are assembled after removal from the denture. Alternatively, the fitting surface may be covered with a layer of self-cure silicone rubber and the cast completed in gypsum.

The casts and dentures are placed in occlusion and mounted on the articulator.

The next stage is to duplicate each denture in wax. This is done by removing both the cast and the denture together from the articulator and recording an impression of both in alginate or other elastic material. To facilitate duplication, the cast is first soaked in water. A container, such as the deep half of a dental flask, is fitted with a metal gauze disc (approximately 3 mm mesh). Sufficient alginate material to fill the flask is mixed and is poured in. Then the denture and cast are dried superficially and pressed slowly tooth downwards into the alginate. There should be a sufficient amount of alginate in the flask and the latter must be deep enough to ensure that the alginate comes at least 10 mm up the side of the cast (Fig. 19.2).

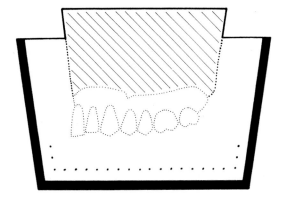

Fig. 19.2 Denture and cast placed in mix of alginate in a flask.

When the alginate has gelled, the mould is removed from the flask, the gauze giving the mould rigidity and reducing the amount of distortion which might occur on handling. The denture and cast are removed from the alginate mould. The denture is removed from the cast, cleaned, its shade recorded, weighed if necessary, and then returned to the patient. A tissue conditioner is applied if adaptation is poor. Both dentures are treated in the same way.

At the 'heels' of the lower mould and tuberosity regions of the upper,

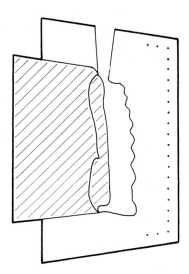

Fig. 19.3 After removal of the denture, the cast is replaced in the mould so that wax may be poured into the space previously occupied by the denture.

openings 6–10 mm diameter are cut through the alginate so that wax may be poured into the mould.

The casts are soaked in water and replaced in the alginate mould, being located by the impression of their outer surfaces (Fig. 19.3). An elastic band may be used to hold cast and mould together. Molten denture base wax, just above its melting point, is poured steadily in until the mould is full. When the wax is hard, the mould is removed, and the wax dentures on their respective casts can now be assembled on the articulator (Fig. 19.4). New teeth are selected and, by cutting off the wax teeth one at a time, the set-up may be completed without disturbing the shape of the polished surfaces.

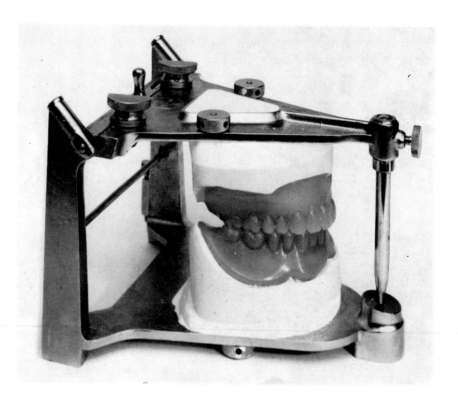

Fig. 19.4 Duplicate wax dentures on the articulator.

Wax contraction introduces some inaccuracies. However, contraction takes place mainly towards the wall of the mould and in practice, the accuracy achieved is good.

Where a shellac base is required, this is adapted to the cast before it is re-inserted into the alginate mould. As the wax is poured in, it becomes attached to the shellac base.

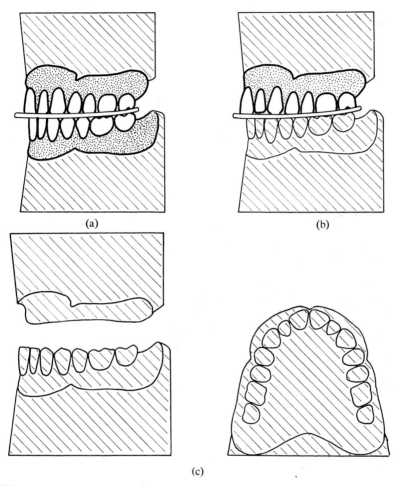

Fig. 19.5
(a) Dentures mounted on articulator using a wax record;
(b) Duplicate mounted in place of lower denture;
(c) Upper denture removed from cast. Ready for setting up to the lower duplicate using the upper duplicate for comparison.

Using Copies of Existing Dentures as Guides

In this technique, impressions are recorded of the polished and occlusal surfaces of the previous dentures. Gypsum casts are made from these and used as a basis for comparison with the new trial dentures. The clinical procedure is the same as that already described.

In the laboratory, after articulating the casts and dentures with a wax wafer, they are removed from the arms of the articulator. An impression is recorded of the shape of the previous dentures using a stock tray and alginate or impression compound and new casts made. The duplicate cast of one denture, usually the lower, is articulated in place of the previous cast using the same wax wafer. When mounting on the articulator the two casts are made removable so that they may be interchanged. The dentures are then returned to the patient. By setting up one trial denture to the stone cast of the opposing previous denture (Fig. 19.5) the occlusion and occlusal plane is maintained. Denture shape and tooth position are controlled by comparison with the duplicate of the previous denture and measurements made so that a similar shape of prosthesis is produced.

If an increase or reduction in occlusal height is contemplated in the new dentures, then provided that a facebow record has been taken, a small adjustment may be made on the articulator when setting up the trial dentures. In general, the increase or decrease in height should be shared between both dentures rather than added to, or subtracted from, one denture only.

With experience these techniques may be modified and improved upon but they form a useful guide to persons unfamiliar with them.

Chapter 20

Preparation of the Mouth

Thoughtful treatment planning and careful and meticulous surgery during the transition from the natural to the artificial dentition should result in the attainment of the ideal denture bearing area—that consisting of a U-shaped bony ridge covered by a mucosa that is relatively compressible but at the same time is tightly bound down to the underlying bone. There should be little need for preparation of the mouth prior to the construction of the first replacement dentures as all hard tissue abnormalities should have been treated before or at the time of insertion of the immediate dentures. Only when resorption has been less than was anticipated, is reshaping of the alveolar ridge necessary.

But not all patients presenting for complete dentures have had the benefits of a *well-planned* immediate denture service, nor may their dentures have been maintained at sufficiently frequent intervals. A number of patients have a 'denture history' extending over many years and there will be those who have been edentulous for some time but who have never had dentures.

Preparation of the mouth for complete dentures may therefore be necessary in the following groups of cases:

1 Where there is a history of denture failures and where examination reveals the presence of mouth abnormalities that have in fact precluded the possibility of successful prosthetic therapy
2 Where there has been considerable loss of alveolar bone and the attachments of the border tissues have become superficial
3 When anatomical abnormalities existed prior to the insertion of the immediate dentures, which were not dealt with adequately at the time of tooth extraction
4 Where soft tissue abnormalities have arisen during the wearing of previous dentures.

NON-SURGICAL PREPARATION

The need for careful examination of the soft tissues of the denture bearing areas in patients presenting for new dentures has been stressed. Before new dentures are constructed any abnormalities of the soft tissues must be recognized and treated.

Irritation from an overextended denture flange may have resulted in the formation of denture hyperplasia.

Ill-fitting dentures or those with defects in occlusion or articulation, may result in trauma of the soft tissues that varies from slight displacement to gross deformation, with or without denture stomatitis.

If the soft tissues, trapped between the denture base and the underlying bone, are displaced within normal physiological limits, they will return to normal contour if the denture is removed for a period. Where there has been severe trauma and there is clinical evidence of inflammation, structural changes in the tissues will have taken place and there will be a slower rate of recovery to normal.

Too often, in practice, the traumatic effect of dentures on the normal mucosa is ignored and impressions for the new dentures are taken of an already deformed foundation. The result is that pressure areas are perpetuated in the new dentures and pain and destruction of the underlying bone continues.

A convincing demonstration of the effect of rest on abused tissues can be seen if a patient is asked to remove the old dentures for 48 to 72 hours. When the dentures are replaced, gross errors in occlusion will often be evident and the dentures that originally seemed to be well-fitting now lack retention and stability. Carrying the demonstration further, if the dentures are now left to 'bed in' again, there will be a return to apparently good occlusal relations and adequate retention and stability, as the tissues are once more deformed to fit the dentures.

New dentures should be placed on healthy and non-traumatized basal tissues. It is therefore necessary for tissue recovery to take place before the major impressions are taken. As was noted above, this can be achieved by the patient leaving the dentures out of the mouth for a 48 to 72 hour period. Whereas a patient may cooperate in this way before the impression stage, he is unlikely to agree to do this before each succeeding clinical stage. Such a procedure will be necessary if there is a considerable delay between clinical stages, as it would be impossible to record the maxillo-mandibular relations, assess the trial dentures and insert the finished dentures on a deformed foundation when the major impressions were taken of the recovered tissues. In addition even if the patient is prepared to cooperate in this way, it is unlikely that the degree of tissue deformation and recovery will be identical between each clinical stage.

Therefore, in addition to obtaining tissue recovery before the major impressions are made, the soft tissue form must be controlled during the entire period of denture construction. Such control can be achieved by the use of 'tissue conditioning' materials. A conditioning material may be defined as a soft material which is applied temporarily to the fitting surface of a denture for the purpose of allowing a more equal distribution of load thus permitting the mucosal tissues to return to their normal position. The tissue conditioner should possess high elastic recovery with minimal flow properties and at the same time it should remain soft for a reasonable period. This means that the material will adapt to the soft tissues, partly by flow but mainly by elastic distortion produced by relatively small forces in the mouth. Products are usually supplied as a powder and a liquid but not all those available have the ideal properties required of a tissue conditioner. Where adequate elastic recovery has been achieved, softness may have been forfeited and tissue recovery be that much slower. The clinician must recognize that physical properties of the tissue conditioners vary and adjust his plan of treatment accordingly.

But mere placing of a tissue conditioner inside a denture will not allow adequate tissue recovery unless attention is paid to the defects in the old dentures that have caused the tissue deformation. These are:

1 Gross errors of adaptation of the denture base

2 Inadequate coverage of the denture bearing area

3 Insufficient freeway space

4 Errors in occlusion and articulation.

ACHIEVING TISSUE RECOVERY

Ideally the patient should be asked to leave the dentures out for a period of 12 hours before treatment is commenced so that some tissue recovery may take place. The fitting surfaces of the dentures are then covered with a pressure disclosing paste and any areas of heavy contact are relieved. Peripheral overextensions are reduced and underextensions built up with self-curing acrylic. If the freeway space is inadequate the occlusal surfaces of the teeth are reduced. Errors in occlusion and articulation must be modified as much as possible by providing a relatively flat, non-interfering occlusal surface. Time will then be available for an incorrect closure pattern to be eliminated and a return to the previous muscular position to occur. Alternatively, it is helpful to build up the occlusal surface of one denture with self-cure acrylic and to record a new relation whilst this is at the dough stage. These alterations both help to simplify the recording of the jaw relations at the appropriate clinical stage.

The fitting surface of the denture is now ground out to a depth of 1 to 2 mm to provide room for the treatment material. The instructions of the manufacturer must be followed carefully with regard to the mixing of the tissue conditioner, the viscosity at the time of insertion in the mouth and the time of removal from the mouth. When the denture is removed, excess material round the border is removed with a warm knife or a pair of scissors. Pressure points and overextended borders which show as areas denuded of material are reduced with a stone. Repair of such areas can then be achieved by (1) patching in the defect, (2) adding a complete second layer, or (3) removing the original layer and replacing it.

When the impression is complete the patient is dismissed for 2 days with instructions to adopt a fairly soft diet and to massage the soft tissues of the denture bearing area with a soft mouth brush.

On return, the lining is inspected; any newly developed pressure points are indicated by exposure of the denture base. These areas are stoned, the soft material removed and a new lining inserted. The occlusion and articulation should be checked and adjusted if necessary.

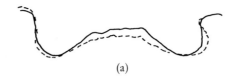

(a)

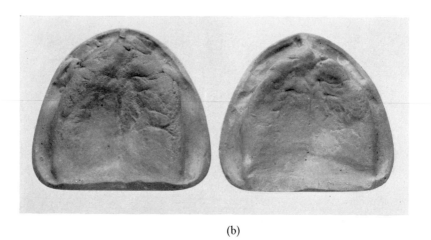

(b)

Fig. 20.1 Tissue recovery after conditioning:
(a) contour record (dotted line—before treatment);
(b) study casts—before and after treatment.

A number of such treatments may be necessary before the clinician is satisfied that complete tissue recovery, shown by a change to normal contour and colour, has taken place. It will be useful to take progress impressions in order to assess the degree of tissue recovery (Fig. 20.1).

It is sometimes possible to use the treatment lining in a denture as the major impression. Stone is poured into it and the resultant cast used for denture construction. The denture with its lining intact is returned to the patient for wear until the new denture is ready. After taking such care in conditioning the tissue, the new dentures should obviously be constructed in the shortest possible time.

Since *C. albicans* or other yeasts may play an important part in the pathology of denture stomatitis, antifungal treament may be instituted during the period of tissue conditioning.

By carrying out tissue conditioning where it is indicated, the clinician is providing a real health service to his patient. If the need for the treatment is explained to the patient and the tissue response demonstrated, he will begin to appreciate that the construction of satisfactory dentures is not just a simple mechanical procedure. The patient is also more likely to return regularly for inspection of dentures and the supporting tissues.

SURGICAL PREPARATION

Surgical preparation may involve both hard and soft tissues. It is not proposed to discuss the surgical procedures in detail but rather to indicate the types of preparative treatment that may be necessary if successful dentures are to be made. For detailed description of the surgical procedures the reader is referred to standard texts on oral surgery.

SURGERY OF THE SOFT TISSUES

Surgery of the soft tissues may be necessary in cases where previous dentures have caused severe irritation. This may have resulted from gross errors in denture construction, or have been caused by dentures that have become ill-fitting due to bone resorption which has not been compensated by correction of the fitting surface of the denture.

FLABBY RIDGES

These pendulous 'ridges' lack alveolar bone support; they arise from excessive incisal or occlusal trauma which has caused resorption of the underlying bone.

Commonly they are found in the anterior part of the upper denture bearing area, although they may be present in other areas where there has been abnormal denture pressure. A mobile ridge does not form a good foundation for a denture, but where there is very little alveolar bone remaining beneath, a mobile ridge is a better foundation than no ridge at all. There is evidence, however, that resorption of alveolar bone proceeds more rapidly beneath a flabby ridge than beneath normal mucosa. Therefore in the interests of bone preservation, surgical removal of surplus tissue has been recommended.

The decision to retain or resect a mass of hyperplastic tissue overlying the bony ridge will depend on the patient's age, state of health, and the amount of bone loss. If some alveolar bone remains and the patient is able to withstand surgery, then most of the excess tissue should be removed. Total resection will result in a mucoperiosteum that is tightly bound down to the underlying bone, but partial resection will have the effect of 'stiffening' the original pendulous ridge and may be preferred where little or no alveolar bone remains. If, however, it is decided to retain a mobile ridge, the clinician must be aware of the need for varying his standard impression technique as it is essential to register the mobile tissue in the position in which it will suffer least damage and provide the best support for the denture.

DENTURE HYPERPLASIA

New dentures should never be made to cover areas of denture hyperplasia, but it is seldom necessary to remove them surgically particularly if they are small. In all cases the denture should be eased well away from the area. Usually, in a remarkably short period of time, shrinkage of the hyperplastic tissue occurs. This non-surgical approach is always recommended; it avoids the scarred groove in the sulcus which often follows surgical treatment and which is such a poor supporting tissue for the border of the new denture.

When the denture hyperplasia is large and fibrous and does not resolve after removal of the irritation, surgical removal is indicated. Because chronic irritation is a known etiological factor in oral malignancy, it is always advisable to have a histological examination of all resected hyperplastic tissue.

GRANULAR INFLAMMATION

This condition, which is considered by some to be precancerous, is usually, although not always, associated with the wearing of dentures. In denture wearers, the multiple small elevations of tissue may be found to coincide with the site where a relief chamber is present on the palate of the denture (Fig. 20.2). This condition is one of the stages of denture stomatitis. It is the only stage that warrants surgical intervention.

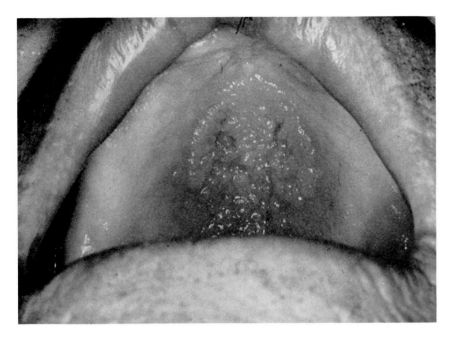

Fig. 20.2 Localized area of granular inflammation coinciding with position of relief chamber.

In cases of extensive granular inflammation and where there is any doubt that the lesion might become malignant, radical excision of the entire affected area should be carried out. In less severe cases removal may be achieved by the use of electrosurgery, cryosurgery, or rotary abrasives by which the elevations can be 'shaved off'. If surgery is not warranted, the fitting surface of the denture that covers the granular mucosal surface should be smooth. This may be achieved either by the use of a swaged metal base or by tinfoiling the cast before acrylic polymer is processed against it.

FIBROUS ENLARGEMENT OF THE TUBEROSITY

Where a large mass of avascular and dense connective tissue covers the tuberosity, there may be interference with correct denture extension and tooth positioning. In such cases the surplus fibrous tissue should be removed.

TRIGGER POINTS IN THE MUCOSA

Trigger points in the mucosa should be marked by tattooing with sterile

Indian ink when they are first discovered. Then they may be excised individually or at the same time as alveoloplasty or smoothing of the bony ridge beneath them is undertaken.

INCREASING THE SIZE OF THE DENTURE BEARING AREA

Although the environmental musculature acting on correctly shaped denture flanges plays a vital part in denture retention, there is no doubt that a well-formed alveolar ridge is *initially* the major factor. Consequently, as the height of the alveolar ridge decreases and the attachments of the soft tissues become comparatively more superficial, problems of retention increase. In cases of extreme resorption the whole of the alveolar process may be lost and atrophy may involve basal bone in both mandible and maxilla. In many atrophic mandibles an alveolar groove exists rather than an alveolar ridge.

Because of the problems of denture retention associated with ridge resorption, many techniques have been developed to increase the size of the denture bearing area. Such techniques are directed at either building up the ridge by implanting substitutes for lost alveolar bone, or deepening the sulcus by repositioning the soft tissue attachments. The aim is the same in both instances —to achieve larger vertical retaining flanges on the dentures.

SUBSTITUTES FOR LOST ALVEOLAR BONE

Various materials may be implanted to act as substitutes for lost alveolar bone.

Bone and Cartilage

Although experimental work continues on the use of graft material from other sources, at present the best type of graft material is autogenous in origin. Whilst large pieces of autogenous cartilage may be used in facial reconstructions (i.e. nose, zygoma), they are not generally used in alveolar ridge reconstruction and autogenous bone is preferred by most oral surgeons. The bone may be taken from a rib or from the ileac crest and cut to the desired form and shape. Recent research has suggested a different bone regeneration technique using a cobalt-chromium mesh tray containing haematopoietic marrow encased in a cellulose acetate filter. The filter material appears to enhance bone regeneration at the surgical site by excluding connective tissue from the area in which bone formation is required. The metal implant which had been constructed to conform to the desired increase in height of the alveolar ridge is removed some 2 to 3 months after the insertion of the marrow graft.

However, although autogenous bone and cartilage grafts are generally well tolerated by the tissues, it must be said that attempts to reconstruct the alveolar ridge by grafting have not in the past met with outstanding success. The major problem is always to obtain sufficient soft tissue covering for the implanted material without tension and without sacrificing sulcus depth. This is particularly so in the mandible where the covering mucoperiosteum is frequently thin and lacking in resilience. This, together with the generalized reduction in surface area of the oral mucosa with increasing age, means that considerable pressure may be exerted on the implanted material. This in turn results in the rapid resorption of the new 'ridge'. It does seem that in those patients where there has been extreme alveolar atrophy the process of rapid resorption also affects the newly implanted tissue. Chances of success are probably best in the maxilla where there is usually a sufficient amount of soft tissue to provide coverage of the implant without tension. It is unfortunate that the chances of success are least where the need is greatest—that is in the mandible.

Metals and Polymers

Metal implants have been used extensively in many branches of surgery and it is natural that their use in the oral cavity should be considered. Although stainless steel, vitallium and tantalum, because of their biological inertness, may be implanted with safety, the results in building up an alveolar ridge have not been encouraging. The problem again has been of finding enough soft tissue to cover the implant particularly when it is placed under functional stress, by a denture. The same problem has occurred with acrylic and other polymeric implants, including polyvinyl sponge. There is a further problem associated with polymer implants, namely that of the eventual tissue reaction to the materials concerned.

TREATMENT OF THE THIN UNDERCUT RIDGE

If the undercut of this type of ridge is reduced, the resultant denture bearing area, although smoother, is too narrow. It is therefore worth considering the possibility of filling in the undercut. Such undercuts are often found lingually in the lower premolar region and labially in the lower anterior region (Fig. 20.3). Several workers have reported success with building out these lateral undercuts by the subperiosteal implantation of various materials. It is essential that the subperiosteal incision for all these implants extends right up to the sharp edges of the bone, thus protecting them. Otherwise discomfort will persist on pressure from the denture.

Tantalum gauze has been implanted successfully in these areas, where it becomes covered with fibrous tissue. Drugs have also been implanted to stimulate the formation of fibrous tissue and so fill up the undercut.

The injection of a self-cure silicone rubber has been recommended for minor ridge reconstruction in undercut areas and to supply a protective layer

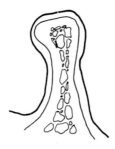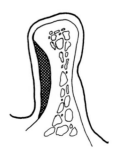

Fig. 20.3 Reduction of labial undercut by subperiosteal implantation rather than surgical removal of the overhanging bone.

over irregular ridge crests and other prominences such as the mylohyoid ridges and the genial tubercles. It has been suggested that the resilience of the rubber is sufficient to absorb the stresses of mastication. Histological studies in animals show good tissue tolerance but there is a tendency for a condensation of connective tissue to occur around the implanted rubber. There may be some resorption of bone if the implant is under compression from the surrounding soft tissues.

This condensation around a non-absorbable and solid material has caused concern in the past. Implantation of such materials as dacron, nylon, polyethylene, polymethylmethacrylate or polyvinyl chloride has sometimes led to tumour formation in animals. It has been suggested that the mechanism of tumour formation is related to an interference in the normal exchange of metabolites, nutrients and oxygen in the dense avascular tissue surrounding the implant, in addition to the obvious possibility of the irritant nature of some of the chemical constituents of these materials.

As an alternative to the injection of a solid silicone rubber, silicone foam rubber has been suggested. A possible advantage in the use of silicone foam is that fibrous tissue infiltrates into the pores of the rubber and a solid connective tissue barrier is not formed around the implant.

SULCUS EXTENSION

The operation of sulcus extension or deepening is only feasible if some alveolar bone remains or if the basal bone has sufficient height (Fig. 20.4). Whilst sulcus deepening is often possible in the maxilla, improvement of lower denture retention is usually of greater necessity. Unfortunately the mandible is often very thin and gives no opportunity for deepening the sulcus. The shape of the basal bone is also of importance in determining whether sulcus deepening is possible. Not uncommonly, in the anterior region, the mandible presents a flat surface extending from the mental protuberance to the superior genial tubercles, the latter being prominent. The amount of sulcus extension possible also depends on the amount of mucous membrane available and in the case of the lower jaw the position of the mental nerves.

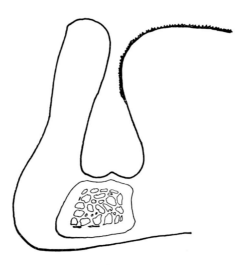

Fig. 20.4 Insufficient basal bone to allow sulcus deepening.

Epithelial Inlays

A variety of techniques have been devised for achieving sulcus extension. Of these the most successful have been those using epithelial inlays. The inlay consists of a Thiersch graft from another part of the body, usually the inner aspect of the arm. The raw surfaces of the incised and deepened sulcus are lined with the epithelial graft. This has the effect of reducing the amount of fibrous tissue formation in the surgical area and prevents the obliteration of the newly created sulcus by contracting fibrous tissue. The shape of the new sulcus is largely determined by the shape of the mould which fits into the epithelial inlay cavity and therefore care should be taken in its design. It should always be made in a retentive shape, so that pressure from the epithelial inlay does not displace the denture. Despite the epithelial lining, there is still a tendency for the new sulcus to become shallower and therefore for a period of 3 months, the denture should not be left out of the cavity for more than a few minutes. Later the contractile phase passes and the denture can be left out for longer periods.

The grafted epithelium survives well in its new environment, but it never completely assumes the characteristics of the surrounding mucosal surface. It has the advantage of covering a large area without tension and this is to be preferred to techniques which have to rely on epithelialization of a denuded area.

Although success may be obtained with many types of ridge extension operations when some ridge remains, they are not so successful when the need is desperate—that is when all alveolar bone has been resorbed. Too frequently the initial results are good only to be followed by some obliteration of the sulcus from the bottom upwards. This loss of depth of the newly created sulcus is invariably observed after all methods of sulcus extension and regardless of the type of soft tissue fixation that has been used. Often, after surgery, the newly created sulcus is scarred and narrow at its deepest point where the border of the denture is to lie and scar tissue is not the best foundation for a denture.

Other Methods of Sulcus Extension

Apart from the complex procedures designed to deepen the sulcus, simpler and more successful procedures for increasing the size of the denture bearing area, are the removal of frena and of the hard bony ridges to which muscles are attached. In this way the sulcus is deepened locally. Perhaps the greatest improvement is attained by such procedures on the lingual side of the mandible, for the ability to have well-extended denture flanges in the anterolingual and distolingual areas contributes much to the retention of a lower denture and, in particular, to its resistance to lateral displacement.

Resection of the mylohyoid ridge and the portion of muscle attached to it has a twofold advantage. Not only is a sharp bony prominence removed but the lingual sulcus is considerably deepened as the mylohyoid muscle is allowed to fall into the submandibular space (Fig. 20.5). Reattachment of the muscle to the mandible may then occur at a lower level.

In the anterior lingual region the greatest problem is related to the superior genial tubercles. They are invariably covered by a thin incompressible mucosa. Many prosthodontists wish to extend the flange of the lower denture to the sublingual folds and use the elastic recoil of the soft tissues here to develop a positive seal. Large superior genial tubercles or a short lingual frenum may not only make it exceedingly difficult or impossible to achieve such extension, but may make the siting of the periphery of the denture a most difficult

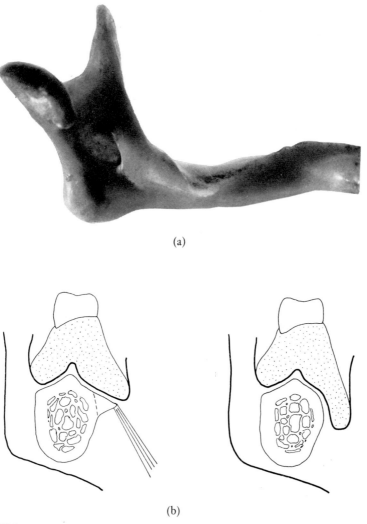

(a)

(b)

Fig. 20.5
(a) Prominent mylohyoid ridge;
(b) resection of mylohyoid ridge. The mylohyoid muscle may subsequently reattach
at a lower level.

procedure. The surgical elimination of these structures is therefore sometimes indicated.

Local sulcus extension labially and buccally in either jaw can be achieved by resection of the appropriate labial and buccal frena. Resection of a frenum

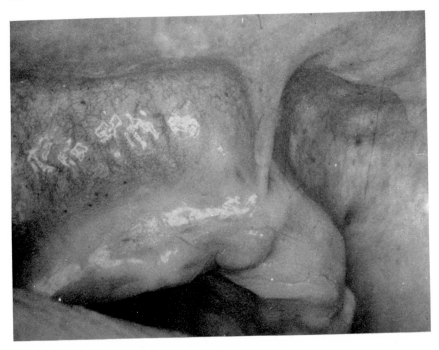

Fig. 20.6 Prominent labial frenum extending to the crest of the alveolar ridge.

is recommended when it extends to the crest of the ridge and is likely to be a displacing factor on the denture, particularly in the lower jaw. Resection of the labial frenum in the upper jaw (Fig. 20.6) allows complete flange extension and the attaining of maximal border seal in the anterior region—a retentive factor which is often adversely affected by too enthusiastic relieving of the denture flange for the reception of the labial frenum. But perhaps of greater significance is that removal of the frenum obviates the need for the labial notch. Midline fracture of an upper denture usually begins at the base of this notch. Hence, removal of the frenum reduces the risk of recurrent fracture of a denture which is heavily stressed during mastication. Therefore in patients with a history of repeated midline fracture, resection of the labial frenum should always be considered before prescribing a metal palate. The operation is simple although there is a danger of subsequent contraction and shallowing of the sulcus in the surgical area. The frena do not usually contain muscle fibres, although they are commonly called 'muscle attachments', but consist of strands of connective tissue stretching from the soft tissues of the cheek or lip to the alveolar process.

In order to retain the sulcus depth, it is preferable that a denture is inserted immediately after resection of the frenum. In the construction of this denture, the frenum is trimmed from the cast and the border shaped to that required after surgery. Otherwise after resection of the frenum, the required depth of the sulcus must be maintained by an anchor suture joining the mucosal edges to the periosteum at the highest point. When a denture is available, simple resection of the frenum from the alveolar process is all that is required.

SURGERY OF THE HARD TISSUES

ALVEOLOPLASTY

Alveoloplasty or shaping of the alveolar ridge is necessary to remedy the mutilation associated with careless forceps extraction or accidental removal of bone attached to a tooth during extraction. The irregularities of the ridge produce difficulties for the dentist and often pain to the patient when dentures are worn (Fig. 20.7).

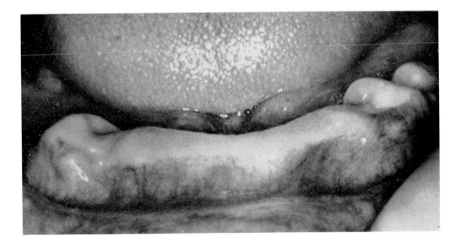

Fig. 20.7 Irregular lower alveolar ridge.

A bur or chisel is used to remove the spurs, exostoses or excess bone. At all times, however, the operator should be conservative in his approach.

In the anterior region of either jaw, undercut areas may hinder the provision of a complete labial flange. If a complete flange is considered necessary for reasons of retention and if the undercut areas may not be engaged by a flange despite analysis of a variety of paths of insertion of the denture, then surgical reduction of the undercut is necessary.

The irregular alveolar crest is a constant source of trouble. It is seen particularly in the anterior regions of both jaws, in cases where the dental history is of extraction of the teeth in that area after long-standing periodontal involvement. When the alveolar crest is exposed by reflecting the mucoperiosteum, the appearance of the bone can be likened to a sawblade. The production of a smooth surface to the ridge is essential if the patient is to have comfort.

LACK OF INTERMAXILLARY SPACE

Removal of bone locally may be necessary in the tuberosity region of the upper jaw (Fig. 20.8). A dental history of extraction of lower third molars and

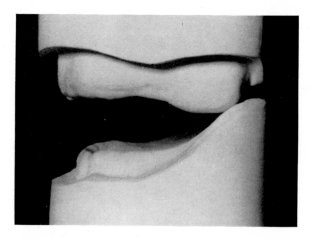

Fig. 20.8 Prominent tuberosity in contact with the retromolar pad and requiring surgical reduction.

retention of the uppers often leads to over-eruption of the upper teeth. After extraction of the upper molars the tuberosity is so close to the retromolar pad that coverage of both by the denture bases is impossible. Prominent tuberosities may also occur in cases of fibrous dysplasia. Radiographs should be taken so that the operator knows the relation of the maxillary sinus to the ridge. It must be realized, however, that close proximity of the sinus to the crest of the ridge does not necessarily preclude surgery. It is also advisable to record impressions and the occlusion so that the amount of bone to be removed may be estimated with some degree of accuracy.

A general reduction of ridge height may be necessary to provide room for two denture bases and their attached teeth (Fig. 20.9). If surgery is avoided where the ridges are closely approximated there is a real danger of the new dentures encroaching on the freeway space.

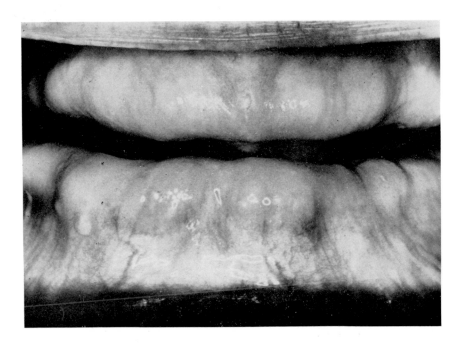

Fig. 20.9 Lack of interalveolar space between massive ridges with the mandible in the postural position.

OPPOSING BONY UNDERCUTS

Bilateral or opposing bony undercuts occurring on the labial and buccal surfaces present problems in the insertion of correctly extended denture flanges. Where they are not substantial, blocking out of one or both on the major cast before processing the denture may suffice. But where the undercuts are very pronounced, surgical reduction on one or both sides may be necessary.

EXOSTOSES

The removal of small bony protuberances is often necessary because the undercuts formed by them may prevent correct extension of denture flanges. Apart from those occurring on the labial and buccal surfaces one that creates particular difficulty is the torus mandibularis (Fig. 20.10). This is usually bilateral and is situated on the lingual side of the lower ridge in the premolar regions. When large, these swellings should be removed. In the upper jaw the torus palatinus (Fig. 20.11), should be removed when:

1 It is excessively lobulated or irregular
2 It is sufficiently large to cause some displacement of the tongue when covered by a denture base
3 When the mucosa covering it is very thin and will not tolerate the minor irritations inevitable when covered by a denture.

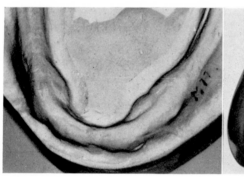 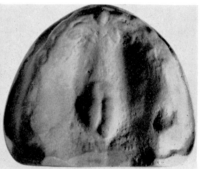

Fig. 20.10 Torus mandibularis—bilateral.   **Fig.20.11** Torus palatinus.

AESTHETICALLY UNFAVOURABLE BONE FORMATIONS

To a limited extent, the appearance of a Class II or Class III jaw relation can be reduced by removal of some alveolar bone. The best effect is likely to be achieved in pseudo Class II cases where the basal bones are in fact in a Class I relation but where the upper alveolar bone has been deformed labially as a result of labial tooth migration in periodontal disease, or by a thumb sucking habit when the natural teeth were present. Here the clinician is able to position the anterior teeth more normally in relation to the adjacent musculature. But where the skeletal bases are Class II, reduction of the premaxillae in an attempt to convert the cases into Class I must only be performed after the most careful thought and consideration for the eventual aesthetic effect and the effect of the changed tooth relation on the environmental musculature.

In gross Class II and Class III cases where aesthetic and functional improvement is necessary, the necessary improvement will only be achieved by osteotomy or bone grafting or a combination of both.

RETAINED ELEMENTS

Between 30 and 40 per cent of apparently normal edentulous alveolar ridges have been shown by radiographic examination to contain retained roots, foreign bodies, residual cysts, unerupted teeth and other pathological processes. Routine radiographic examination of edentulous ridges is therefore recommended. This is not to say that all retained elements should be removed. Each item will require individual consideration and when the surgical cure is likely to result in much trauma and postoperative discomfort, then it is not justified.

Residual cysts, active pathological processes and any that might have a possible systemic effect should obviously be eradicated, although age and the general physical condition of the patient have to be considered.

The difficult decisions are those relating to retained tooth fragments and to unerupted teeth. The clinician should ask two questions:

1 Are the retained elements having any effect on the patient's general health?
2 Are the retained elements likely to interfere with the fitting and wearing of a satisfactory denture?

If the answer to either question is 'Yes' surgical removal is indicated. If the answers are both 'No' then the retained elements may be left *provided* the patient is aware of their presence and of the possible need for their removal at a later date if they cause symptoms. There must be regular follow-up clinical and radiographic examination.

Where the erupted teeth or retained roots are close to the surface of the alveolar ridge there are of course grounds for removing them in the younger patient even though they are asymptomatic. First, such surgical procedures are easier in younger patients than in the elderly. Secondly, if roots or unerupted teeth are close to the surface, the normal process of alveolar resorption that occurs under denture pressure, is more likely to uncover them and lead to pain. It may result in infection later when they penetrate the oral mucosa.

Before the clinician can state that a retained element can be left he must be absolutely sure of its position. Therefore the most careful diagnostic radiographs must be taken involving both lateral and occlusal views. Likewise if removal is contemplated, correct location is necessary to avoid unnecessary removal of precious alveolar bone in an attempt to find an elusive root.

At surgery, every attempt should be made to preserve the height of the alveolar ridge; any depressions in the side of the ridge resulting from bone removal may be filled in with one of the absorbable cellulose products. By thus providing a framework for future bone formation, depressions in the ridge can be prevented.

AIDS TO RETENTION

When complete dentures of conventional design have failed to be tolerated by the patient, the operator may consider the use of various aids to retention. Those which require surgical preparation are:

Subperiosteal implants

Endosseous implants.

SUBPERIOSTEAL IMPLANTS

These consist of a cobalt-chromium alloy framework which is placed beneath the periosteum. Vertical posts project from the framework through the covering mucoperiosteum. These posts support a denture of normal appearance which is retained either by the frictional resistance of the vertical sides of the posts or by clasping devices which have positive retention onto the posts (Fig. 20.12).

The advantage of the subperiosteal implant is that it ensures maximum retention and stability of the denture and that pressure onto the mucosa is relieved and placed more directly on the bone via the implant substructure.

The main indications for a subperiosteal implant are in the lower jaw where there has been complete loss of the alveolar ridge. Other indications are where the muscle attachments are lying on the upper surface of the ridge remnants, in certain mutilated mouth conditions and in patients who for psychological

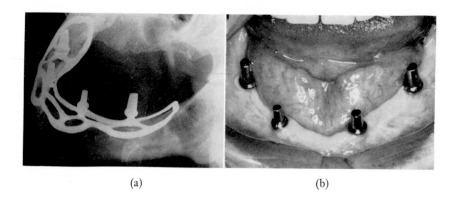

(a)   (b)

Fig. 20.12 Subperiosteal implant:
(a) radiograph;
(b) the intraoral appearance of the implant 1 year after fitting.

reasons cannot tolerate a denture of conventional design.

Reconstruction of the alveolar ridge by grafting or sulcus extension by epithelial inlays requires surgical procedures that are quite traumatic and not certain of success. In cases of extreme atrophy of the mandible, therefore, subperiosteal implants are to be preferred to some of the complex surgical reconstruction procedures aimed at increasing the size of the denture bearing area.

Implant dentures are not substitutes for well-planned and well-made conventional dentures and they should only be constructed for those patients in whom all other procedures have failed. It should be emphasized that just as much care must be given to the design of the superstructure or denture as is given to the design and surgical technique involved in positioning of the sub-periosteal framework. The rules of flange contour, position of teeth, occlusion and articulation are just as important with implant dentures as with conventional dentures.

The major criticism of the implant denture has been the possibility of infection of the underlying bone because the continuity of the epithelium is broken by the protruding posts. Histological examination of implants in monkeys has shown that there is a downgrowth of epithelium at the sites of penetration of the mucosa by the posts and that this eventually surrounds the implant framework. It has been suggested that this 'exteriorization' of the implant may be the reason why bone infection does not usually occur. Another factor in preventing infection may be the production of a seal around the posts by tight adaptation of the mucosa. After healing, there appears to be a normal gingival crevice and attempts to inject dye between the metal posts and the surrounding tissue have demonstrated that the attachment is relatively impenetrable.

A very slow process of rejection of the implant by tissue downgrowth can perhaps be regarded more as a physiological than a pathological process. It seems justifiable to use subperiosteal implants where normal prosthodontic treatment is impracticable provided that the known metallurgical, surgical and technical procedures are followed.

Implant failures may be attributed to poor diagnosis, inadequate impressions, lack of bone coverage by the framework and errors in occlusion and articulation of the dentures. The choice of patient is of the greatest importance for success is unlikely without cooperation and an understanding of the problems involved and the maintenance of meticulous oral hygiene.

SURGICAL TECHNIQUE

At operation the soft tissues are retracted to expose not only the alveolar ridge or what remains of it but also a considerable amount of surrounding skeletal bone. The early implants were usually positioned over the alveolar ridge and failure occurred because of further bone resorption beneath the framework. Success is more likely if the implant lies on those areas of the mandible that are resistant to resorption. The soft tissues should therefore be retracted to expose in the lower jaw, the external oblique ridge, the mental protuberance, the genial tubercles and the mylohyoid ridges.

Before taking the impression any bony spicules or sharp ridges are removed and the surface of the bone washed clean of blood clots with normal saline.

The impression of the bone surface is taken in composition or rubber base using an acrylic tray which was constructed on a cast obtained from a muco-compressive impression of the denture bearing area before surgery.

Later, the implant is inserted beneath the mucoperiosteum. This may be 3 to 4 weeks or only a few hours after the first surgical stage. Placing the implant after only a few hours avoids the necessity of surgery near to recently healed wounds. If a delay of 3 to 4 weeks is decided upon, the second incisions follow exactly the first ones to avoid subsequent sloughing of small areas of tissue between two separate cuts and subsequent exposure of parts of the implant framework.

Some 6 weeks after the second surgical stage final impressions are taken and the superstructure and conventional upper denture completed.

ENDOSSEOUS IMPLANTS

Endosseous implants lie *within* the bone. Various materials have been investigated as potential endosseous implant materials—metals (in the form of pure metals and alloys), polymers such as polymethylmethacrylate, and ceramics (sintered alumina and vitreous carbon). The basic problems have always been those of producing an implant in a material which has the necessary physical and chemical properties to withstand the oral and tissue environments, and which is compatible with the living tissues, so that it becomes permanently incorporated in the jaw, and prevents the ingress of microorganisms and epithelium from the mouth into the deeper tissues.

Metallic implants in the form of screws, pins and blades and made of vitallium, titanium and stainless steel have been used with some apparent success. Research has however shown that all such implants either become exteriorized by epithelial downgrowth or are surrounded by a fibrous tissue capsule or areas of inflammation.

Of the other potential endosseous implant materials, vitreous carbon and sintered alumina are the only ones which have been shown to remain *in situ* directly adjacent to the normal tissues of the region. This suggests a high degree of compatibility with the host tissues, and when considered with their physical properties suggests that they might find a use as endosseous implants.

Chapter 21

Impression Procedures for Complete Dentures

A large number of techniques are recommended for recording impressions of the edentulous denture bearing areas. Almost every dental surgeon favours a particular technique because the results obtained with it are satisfactory. There are, therefore, many theories upon which the various techniques are based. In this chapter, precise techniques will not be given. An understanding of the principles involved and how they apply in practice is considered to be more important in enabling the dentist to use an impression method suited to the clinical conditions which are present.

The authors recommend a two-stage impression procedure for replacement complete dentures. As indicated in Chapter 12 when considering impressions for immediate dentures, the casts obtained from the primary impressions are used for the construction of special or individual trays which will enable the operator to determine the denture extension with some precision and to record a more accurate final impression than would be achieved using a stock tray. Primary impressions may be recorded in alginate or compound. Compound is particularly indicated in the lower jaw when there has been considerable alveolar resorption and where the environmental tissues have encroached into the potential denture space.

When providing an immediate denture, slight inaccuracies in recording the shape of the ridge tissues may pass unnoticed. Dimensional changes in the soft and hard tissues after extraction cannot be forecast with precision. An immediate denture, therefore, is not adapted precisely to the tissues on insertion. Oedema during the first few hours after surgery improves the adaptation, whilst resorption after a few weeks of wear often causes some loss of fit. It is important, however, to define the sulcus extension with accuracy if discomfort and pain for the patient is to be avoided.

On the other hand, replacement dentures are constructed after the major post-extraction changes have occurred and a precise fit of denture to tissue is essential to ensure maximum retention.

THEORIES OF IMPRESSION TECHNIQUES

A denture may be divided into three main surfaces. First the fitting surface, secondly the polished surface, including the sulcus, and thirdly, the occlusal surface of the teeth.

At one time the impression recorded was of the fitting surface only and the sulcus and polished surfaces were shaped arbitrarily by the dentist and his technician (Fig. 21.1). At this period theories considered mainly the effects of pressure upon the soft tissues of the ridges and the palate, both during impression recording and during denture function. Following this, techniques evolved which were concerned with the accurate determination of the sulcus shape so

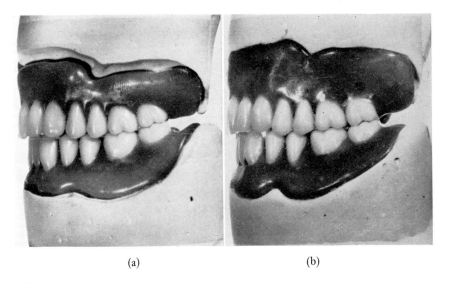

(a)　　　　　　　　　　　　　　(b)

Fig. 21.1
(a) Arbitrary trimming of the border and polished denture surfaces—the borders are underextended.
(b) Correct border extension.

that an impression of the volume and the shape of the denture at its border was prescribed with precision and not left to freehand carving of the wax trial denture, nor to filing and trimming of the finished dentures. The impression area recorded then extended past the sulcus and joined with the polished surface, which was, however, still carved in an arbitrary manner. Not unnaturally, the concept of recording the polished surface shape also, now gains ground.

Thus instead of an impression recording only a surface, the volume and the bulk of the denture may be determined with some degree of accuracy. Such an impression also indicates the width and general position of the artificial teeth, leaving only the occlusal shape of the posterior teeth and the detailed position of the anteriors to be determined. The shape of the denture is then defined by recording the space available for it within the soft and hard tissues forming its environment.

PRESSURE ON THE RIDGES AND PALATE

The denture bearing areas are not covered evenly by soft tissues but vary in the depth and quality of covering from one area to another. Some theories of impression technique are related mainly to compensation for these differences.

MUCOCOMPRESSION

It is argued that if a denture under no occlusal load touches the surface of the epithelium over its entire area, then, on occlusion of the teeth, the denture will apply a large force to the harder areas (Fig. 21.2). Areas in which the submucosa is present will therefore move away slightly under load whilst those with only a thin covering of tissue, i.e. without submucosa, will bear most of the applied load. This may cause 'rocking' of an upper denture in the midline, particularly after slight ridge resorption has taken place. When a torus palatinus is present,

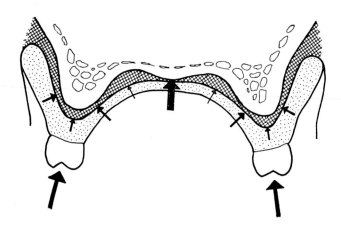

Fig. 21.2 Theoretical effects of pressure from an upper denture on areas of basal tissue of different degrees of softness.

this effect may be marked. This prominent area of bone in the centre of the palate has only a thin tissue covering and therefore may become traumatized by a denture after only slight ridge resorption has occurred. It has often been suggested that flexure of the denture about this pivot may result in midline fracture. It is more likely, however, that such fractures result from a general weakness of the denture base.

Mucocompressive techniques, therefore, have been suggested to avoid the difficulties due to the differences in the depth of soft tissue covering. Such impressions are recorded under a force similar to that used in occlusion and on mastication, so that the softer areas are compressed by the impression. A denture made to a cast from such an impression touches the soft tissues only at rest; a small space full of saliva is present over the harder areas. On occlusion, however, all the tissues are loaded evenly as the softer areas are compressed and the saliva expelled over the hard areas. A similar but somewhat arbitrary 'relief' of hard areas can be achieved by modifying the cast before constructing the denture. Tinfoil is placed over the hard areas marked out on the cast and produces a space or 'relief chamber' between the denture and tissues.

Compression of soft tissues occurs in two ways. In the centre of the palate and over the edentulous ridges within the limits of the mucoperiosteum, a reduction in tissue volume can be achieved only by displacement of a fluid. This may be tissue fluid from the middle and deeper layers of the epithelium, or blood or lymph from within the vessels of the lamina propria. More laterally in the palate, some displacement of the submucous layer backwards is possible, together with displacement of fluids from within this layer.

MUCOSTASIS

Arguments against mucocompression point out the inadvisability of removing essential tissue fluids and also that for the greater part of its life a denture is not under either occlusal or masticatory stress. Whilst agreeing that the greatest retention is necessary during mastication, only a transient force and not a continuous one is applied. In addition, any small space between a denture and the tissues is rapidly filled by hyperplasia of the mucosa. This tends, of course, to make the covering more even, increasing it where it was previously too thin.

Practical difficulties exist in recording an impression under a pressure similar to that which will be used in practice as masticatory loads are not necessarily related to static occlusal loads nor to the pressure applied by the hands of the operator. Advocates of a non-pressure or mucostatic theory, advise careful recording of minute surface detail to ensure an even loading over the entire fitting surface. They argue that the mucosa and saliva act as an hydraulic fluid and so balance up the pressures applied to the tissues by the denture.

It is probable that the small inaccuracies which inevitably accompany our present techniques of denture construction produce a change in denture shape greater than the difference between a mucocompressive and a mucostatic impression. For example, an upper denture constructed of heat-cure acrylic base is more retentive initially than one made of self-cure material. Thermal shrinkage of a heat-cure base after processing produces a slightly smaller upper denture and this creates slight border compression, thus improving the retention. Only where there is a marked difference between hard and soft areas of the ridge and palate do the differences between a mucocompressive and a mucostatic impression have any practical significance.

When trying to describe an impression technique the subtle tactile sense of the operator cannot be put into words. This causes a difference between two impressions recorded by apparently identical techniques.

It must be realized also that the shape of the denture bearing area itself is not static. The volume of the soft tissue alters slightly with changes in peripheral blood volume; e.g. in the early morning or after a meal a slight loss of retention of a denture may be noticed. These difficulties of controlling all the factors which affect the shape of the fitting surface of a denture lead to confusion and a multiplicity of impression techniques in the literature.

PRESSURE IN THE SULCUS

At the sulcus, a slight compressive displacement of the mucosa is possible due to the presence of a submucous layer and the absence of a bony support beneath. Only where the periphery of the denture is in close relation to bone, e.g. at the root of the zygoma, is there insufficient tissue to provide some possibility of compression. Slight pressure of the denture periphery extends the sulcus depth fractionally. The slight elasticity of the submucous layer then maintains a good air seal at the border of the denture. Provided that the pressure is not excessive, no inflammation is seen. Where the sulcus mucosa joins the alveolar process, its attachment is at first loose and here an additional light pressure inwards towards the underlying bone is also possible. Besides making the denture physically a little tighter, this also enhances the valve seal. Care must be exercised in controlling the degree of lateral pressure as heavy loading only produces bone resorption followed rapidly by loss of the initially good retention.

THE DENTURE SPACE

The denture base and teeth should occupy the neutral zone where pressure from the lips, cheeks and tongue are in relative equilibrium. The contours of the denture surface should be such that the pressures from these structures do not result in denture displacement and instability. Whilst an approximation to the correct denture shape can be achieved by carving the record block and subsequently the trial denture, an impression of the space available may be recorded.

When replacing a denture which has been worn for a long time, the functional denture space is that occupied by the existing denture. Copying the shape of the existing denture enables one to maintain the same general denture shape and to prescribe this in detail for the technician. This is a more accurate procedure than the recording of measurements from a previous denture and applying these in the construction of a new prosthesis.

GENERAL PRINCIPLES OF
IMPRESSION RECORDING

When recording an impression the following points should be borne in mind:

1 Record an impression of the mucoperiosteum, compressing soft areas where a marked difference exists between them and the harder areas. Alternatively, modify the cast by placing reliefs over the hard areas.

2 Record an impression of the volume of the sulcus similar to the space to be occupied by the denture. Create slight pressure against the sulcus mucosa, so obtaining a border seal.

3 Avoid tissue distortion over the edentulous ridges. Whilst a normal mucoperiosteum can be pushed sideways only by a very heavy pressure, an excess of fibrous tissue (flabby ridge) is more readily distorted. Such tissue must not be pushed aside on recording the impression, otherwise denture instability leading to further resorption will result.

4 Define the denture space by recording the denture shape and position of the teeth by an impression of the space available. Alternatively, this may be defined by carving the record block and the trial denture base, or by copying the existing satisfactory denture shape. The latter may be done either by a copying technique, or by taking measurements.

RECORDING THE IMPRESSION

An impression may be considered in two parts. First the support (tray) and secondly the impression material.

Support of impression material is necessary on two counts. By using a well-fitting support, the bulk of impression material, and therefore the patient's discomfort, is reduced. Support is necessary to carry the impression material into the lingual areas of the lower jaw and the labial and buccal sulcus areas of both jaws. Sideways displacement of the related soft tissues enables the potential denture space to be recorded. For example in the lower lingual area the tongue often lies in contact with the inner side of the alveolar ridge. The firmness of this contact increases when the tongue is protruded in order to develop the correct lingual sulcus shape. Only by interposing a support between tongue and impression material can a satisfactory impression of this area be recorded.

A more fluid material requires a more precisely shaped support than a more viscous one. An unsupported material of low viscosity is squeezed out of the sulcus during any tension or movement of lips and cheeks, leaving a sharp edge to the impression. Whilst this sharp edge may be correctly extended, trimming and polishing of a denture made to the cast usually reduces it to an underextended position (Fig. 21.3).

Conversely a large mass of viscous material presses strongly against the soft tissues of the sulcus and produces an overextended impression. A similar effect is achieved by an overextended support. A viscous material does not flow readily in thin sections unless time is allowed. Some materials flow very slowly and an impression may be developed in hours or even days. Other materials

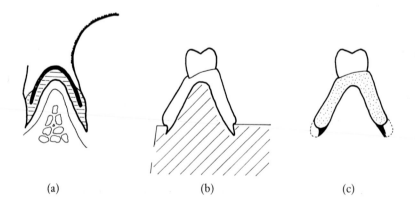

(a)   (b)   (c)

Fig. 21.3 The effect of an underextended impression tray on the subsequent cast and denture extension:
(a) knife-edged impression periphery;
(b) sharp edge on the waxed-up denture;
(c) trimming and polishing the sharp edge of the border results in underextension of
    the denture.

flow only for a limited period of time, during which recording of the complete impression must take place.

The surface of an impression may be subdivided into mucoperiosteal (including the palate) and sulcus areas.

MUCOPERIOSTEAL AND PALATAL AREAS

As already described, the impression of these areas may be either mucocompressive or mucostatic. To achieve tissue compression a thin layer or 'wash' of impression material is used inside a close fitting tray or baseplate. Little or no compression can be produced with a thicker layer of impression material unless it has a high viscosity; for example, impression compound. Even this material, however, is used with the surface softened to a higher temperature than the material beneath to get better flow of the superficial layer. In providing a close fitting support for a mucocompressive or mucostatic impression, a preliminary impression is necessary. This records the general shape of the tissue surface of the denture bearing area and gives reasonably accurate adaptation of the tray for the second impression. In some cases the first impression itself may be used as a support for a further layer of another impression material. This is often referred to as a '*wash impression*'.

Where a layer of 1 to 2 mm of impression material is used, any slight discrepancies in the fit of the special tray or baseplate pass unnoticed, but on using a very thin layer of approximately 0.6 mm, more accurate adaptation of the support is necessary to prevent irregular pressure from the tray itself. When following such a technique, the accuracy of adaptation of the tray may be seen by making it out of clear acrylic base. This is placed against the tissues and checked for contact, particularly over the harder areas. The surface of the tray is then adjusted until pressure is seen to be correct over both hard and soft areas.

Thus, an impression of the mucoperiosteum proceeds by a series of approximations towards accuracy. The first impression is usually moderately accurate and the second, by control of thickness, can eliminate irregular pressure and distortion of soft tissues. It can also produce selective pressure over different areas of the mucoperiosteum.

The post dam area is one which is often selected for greater pressure. By adding compound (tracing stick) or wax to the fitting surface of the impression tray extra pressure can be brought to bear in this area. Similarly an avoidance of pressure over the sphenopalatine foramen and the mental foramen, if within the denture bearing area, can also be arranged, by leaving a larger space between the support and the tissues.

Mucostatic impression techniques use a layer of impression material of low viscosity some 3 to 5 mm thick so that pressure on the soft tissues is largely avoided. A spaced impression tray is loaded with a suitable volume of impression material and placed in correct relation to the tissues. 'Stops' or localizing registers may be necessary to ensure correct location of the tray (Fig. 21.4).

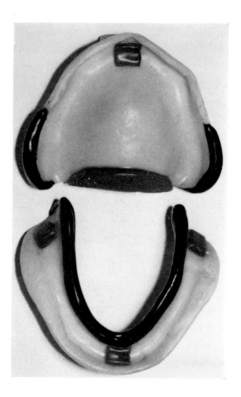

Fig. 21.4 'Stops' or localizing registers on spaced upper and lower trays.

These are placed in the upper tray along the post dam and just behind the incisive papilla. In the lower jaw three stops, two over the pear-shaped pads and one centrally are used. These may be moulded in the mouth or alternatively the position of the tray may be prearranged by making suitable stops adapted to the cast from the preliminary impression. For preference, stops should be of a relatively soft material to avoid local areas of high pressure. Soft carding wax is most suitable, but a harder wax or impression compound is frequently used.

Flabby Tissue

When an excessive amount of mobile tissue covers the crest of the bony alveolar ridge and when it is considered inadvisable to remove it, care should be taken, when recording the impression, not to distort or bend this mobile tissue. The 'flabby' ridge should be recorded in its resting position. If distortion occurs on recording the first impression, a tray or support may well continue this tissue distortion unless its fitting surface is modified. An impression taken in a loose-fitting tray using a material of low viscosity such as an alginate or plaster is less likely to cause distortion than a mass of viscous material pressed against the crest of a flabby ridge (Fig. 21.5).

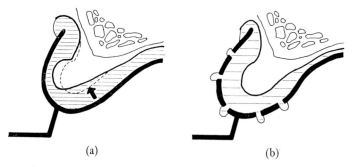

(a)   (b)

Fig. 21.5 Recording the impression of a 'flabby' ridge:
(a) viscous material causes tissue displacement;
(b) a more fluid material in a perforated tray records the resting shape of the displaceable tissue.

SULCUS AREAS

Stock impression trays are usually inaccurate in their adaptation to the sulcus. As a result two things can happen. Either the tray impinges on the sulcus and distorts it, or alternatively, it is short and the impression material must fill the gap. If a large mass of viscous impression material is used, this distorts the sulcus giving overextension. Less material, particularly if it is of a more fluid nature, does not fill the space completely and an underextended impression is produced. Usually with a stock tray some lateral distortion of the alveolar mucosa occurs due to outward pressure of the tray on the cheeks and lips. A denture constructed to such an impression does not fit closely at the periphery and is lacking in retention.

We have, therefore, two main possibilities of support to record a functional sulcus shape with slight elastic compression of the mucosa. First a support some 2 to 3 mm away from the sulcus (Fig.21.6a). By using an impression material of moderate viscosity and not in too great a bulk, a compressed sulcus shape is recorded. Such a technique requires some means of location of the support the correct distance away from the sulcus, or it may rely on tactile or visual appreciation of the position of the tray by the operator.

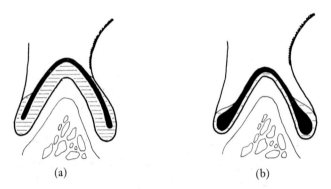

(a)   (b)

Fig. 21.6
(a) A spaced tray (3 mm) for use with a moderately viscous impression material;
(b) a closely adapted tray (0.6 mm) for use with a more fluid impression material (note the borders of the tray have been extended to the functional sulcus depth and width).

Secondly a more precise sulcus support may be used. This implies the use of a rigid acrylic tray which is close fitting and particularly designed for use with a thin layer of impression material such as zinc oxide–eugenol paste. The correct extent and shape of the border of the impression tray is obtained by the addition of a mouldable material which is functionally trimmed by the sulcus tissues (Fig. 21.6b). Before the material is added to the tray, the border should be reduced so that it is 2 mm short of the sulcus. Various border trimming materials may be used including tracing stick and specially formulated polymers. The shape of the sulcus in the labial and buccal areas of both jaws is developed either by manipulating the lips and cheeks or by asking the patient to contract and then dilate the circumoral musculature. The lower lingual border is obtained by asking the patient to swallow first and then to protrude the tongue just beyond the lips. Where considerable resorption of the lower ridge has occurred, the amount of tongue protrusion must be controlled, otherwise folds of mylohyoid muscle and the sublingual salivary glands may be forced between the tray and the ridge. Care must also be taken when placing the lower tray, to avoid trapping folds of buccinator muscle (Fig.21.7). As the tray is seated the cheeks are moved upwards and outwards by light finger pressure, thus releasing these folds. The border trimming with the upper tray should include the post dam area. The extent of the tray should be trimmed to coincide with the axis of rotation of the soft palate, for it is here in most cases that the posterior border of the complete upper denture will lie. The border trimming material of choice is now added to the fitting surface of the tray which is returned to the mouth and held in position with finger pressure. Selective displacement of tissue will occur and is a means of functionally

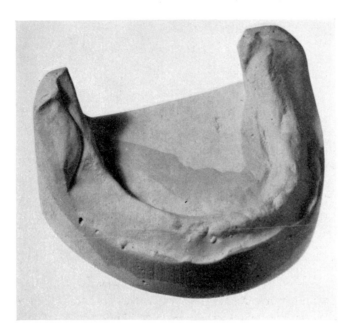

Fig. 21.7 A fold of buccinator muscle that has been trapped between the impression material and the alveolar ridge.

recording the post dam. On removal, excess material that has flowed beyond the posterior border of the tray is removed. Close-fitting trays whose borders have been moulded with tracing stick are shown in Fig. 21.8.

The impression of the mucoperiosteal areas is easily obtained by using an impression material that will flow readily over the tissues, loading it in the support or impression tray and holding it in contact with the tissues until it is ready for removal. In the sulcus, however, the correct compressed sulcus shape must be recorded with accuracy in the impression material before it sets. If a special tray is used where the border of the tray is short of the sulcus

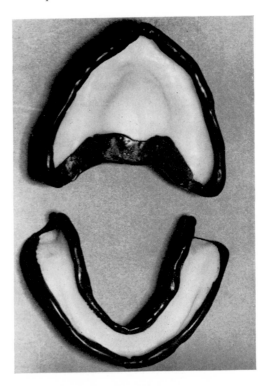

Fig. 21.8 Close-fitting trays with border moulding.

by 2 to 3 mm the operator, having loaded the tray with an impression material of moderate viscosity and inserted in the mouth, must ensure that the impression material is moulded by the sulcus tissues to the correct shape (Fig. 21.9). He will achieve this by manipulating the lips and cheeks for labial and buccal areas. The lingual border shape will be recorded by asking the patient first to swallow which will mould the distolingual aspect of the impression. The other areas of the lingual border will be moulded by asking the patient to move the tongue from side to side and then to protrude it just beyond the lips. As mentioned earlier the amount of tongue protrusion must be controlled.

If a closely adapted tray is used, the border of which has been trimmed with a suitable material, trimming of the impression material when the tray is in place in the mouth should be unnecessary as there should only be a very thin layer of impression material covering the tray border. The operator's main aim is to ensure that the tray is properly seated. However, it is usually advisable to go through the routine of lip and cheek manipulation and ask the patient to make the appropriate tongue movements to make doubly sure

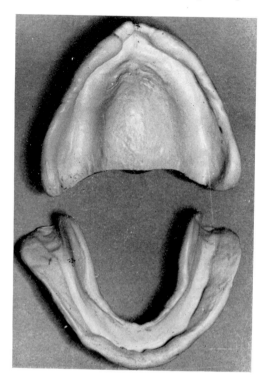

Fig. 21.9 Completed impressions.

that the borders of the impression faithfully reproduce the shape of the sulcus.

OPEN AND CLOSED MOUTH TECHNIQUES

Whenever the operator's fingers hold a tray or other support in the mouth, the patient's mouth must be open to a certain extent. It is inadvisable to ask the patient to open the mouth widely as this changes the sulcus shape. The facial musculature is stretched and this reduces the sulcus width besides making it more difficult to insert the impression tray. On partial opening of the mouth there is only a small change in sulcus shape. However, even with a partly open mouth technique limitations are imposed upon the development of a correct sulcus shape in the anterior region if there is a handle on the tray gripped by the operator's fingers. Whilst this source of inaccuracy can be reduced by suitable positioning of the handle, a closed mouth technique obviates this difficulty. The support of the impression is in the form of a record block which is held in place by the patient in light occlusion.

Whilst the labial and buccal sulcus can be well developed in a closed mouth technique by asking the patient to grimace and to pout the lips, the lingual sulcus is less readily defined. The bulk of the record block may limit the amount of tongue movement and thus produce an overextended lingual sulcus. By thrusting the tongue against the record block and by swallowing, the lingual shape can be developed. Alternatively, the tongue may be protruded to establish the lingual sulcus shape before asking the patient to occlude.

In older patients who have worn the same dentures for many years it is often advisable to use the existing denture base as an impression tray, or alternatively, to duplicate its tissue surface and construct a tray or baseplate of the same shape. Often an old denture (particularly for the lower jaw) touches only at its periphery and not over the crest of the ridge. This pattern of pressure distribution is often the only one which the patient can tolerate. Occasionally any attempt to apply load to the ridge crest produces pain. Then the original 'fitting' surface should be retained.

RECORDING THE DENTURE VOLUME

Techniques have been described by which the denture shape including the position of the teeth may be recorded. Such techniques are of value in the case of the lower denture for an elderly patient where a denture copying technique is not indicated or where a denture has not been worn previously. A suitable baseplate is used to record the denture bearing area and to this is added a rim to support the remainder of the impression (Fig. 21.10). To

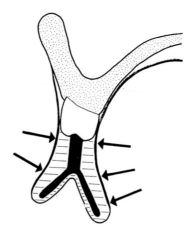

Fig. 21.10 A baseplate impression tray for recording the denture space. The alginate (cross lines) is moulded by the environmental musculature.

develop an impression under functional stresses, the patient should be asked
to practise the sucking and tongue-thrusting movements usually employed to
shape the impression. Then the support is covered with a thin layer of impression material, is inserted into the mouth and moulded by the patient using
similar movements (Fig. 21.11). Whilst it is preferable to record the area and
volume available for one denture at a time, it is possible to record both at once.
If the patient's dentures are approximately satisfactory for bulk, they may be
employed as a support in a similar manner.

(a)

(b)

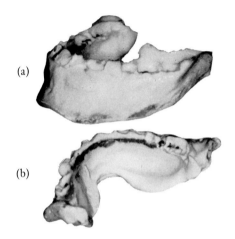

Fig. 21.11
(a) The buccal surface of the impression;
(b) the lingual surface.

IMPRESSION MATERIALS

A material which ceases to flow in a few minutes allows only a short period
of time to mould the material in the sulcus to the correct shape. If the correct
conditions are created, i.e. position of the support or tray, viscosity of impression material, amount of material, and degree of moulding by the related
muscles, an accurate impression will be recorded.

The materials commonly used for edentulous impressions are: zinc oxide
paste; synthetic elastomer; alginate; plaster; impression compound; impression waxes; tissue conditioners. Flow, speed of setting, palatability, dimensional
stability, reproduction of detail, together with elasticity or brittleness on removal from undercut areas are important properties of all impression materials.

ZINC OXIDE PASTE (*recommended tray : acrylic, spacer 0.6 mm*)

This material is usually provided in two differently coloured pastes which set when mixed together, particularly when subjected to warmth and humidity. Impression pastes vary widely in their initial consistency. Some of low viscosity require a very precise support particularly at the borders. Others have a higher viscosity and will compensate for errors of up to 2 to 3 mm in the accuracy of extension of the tray, baseplate, or denture. Little variation in either viscosity or setting time is practicable and a paste should be selected which is suitable to the technique to be used. Additions to paste impressions can readily be made if, after removal, the impression is found to be deficient in any areas.

Some patients find that the eugenol content of these pastes produces a burning sensation when applied to the mucosa. Others find the material to have a marked, but not unpleasant taste. One advantage of a mild stimulus from an impression material is that the patient's attention is diverted to this and away from the normal stimulus of having the impression recorded. Rarely a patient's mucosa may become sensitized to eugenol and produce an allergic reaction when the material is used again. Other essential oils are used in some brands of pastes in order to avoid the marked flavour of eugenol. Alternative non-eugenol materials with similar properties are based on the reaction between zinc oxide and a carboxylic acid, such as ortho-ethoxybenzoic acid to form an insoluble soap.

Dimensional stability of zinc oxide pastes is good at cool room temperatures. Some materials will flow in a warm room, particularly if the impression surface is placed downwards against the bench. Accuracy of these impressions is probably related more to the stability of the support. Stress relief of a shellac baseplate or tray on storage in a warm atmosphere, causes distortion. Inaccuracy of zinc oxide impressions may be due to uneven pressure on recording the impression or elastic distortion of the tray, denture or baseplate. These pastes gradually increase in viscosity. If pressure is applied initially to one side of the tray and then later to the other, the first side moves out of contact with the tissues and results in an inaccurate impression. Heavy biting pressure by the patient upon an occlusal rim or upper denture may cause an elastic distortion of the support which springs back on removal from the mouth.

Reproduction of tissue detail is excellent, due to the moderate and sustained pressure usually necessary to seat an impression particularly in the upper jaw.

Zinc oxide pastes are frequently used when rebasing existing dentures or when using old dentures as the support for impressions. Since the dentures may be well adapted in areas which have undergone but little resorption, a rebase impression is often very thin in places indicating excess pressure and overdisplacement of tissue. This is difficult to avoid but can be rectified by cutting away a portion of the denture surface in these areas and then adding a further thin layer of impression paste.

Difficulties occur when trying to remove the paste impression from the mouth due to its adhesion to the tissue. This presents only minor problems when a tray with a handle is used, but causes difficulty in a closed mouth or rebase technique when no handle is available. It is essential, therefore, to dry the support before recording the impression as otherwise the paste will adhere more strongly to the tissue than to the support.

SYNTHETIC ELASTOMERS (*recommended tray : acrylic, spacer 1.5 mm*)

The main advantage of polysulphide and silicone impression materials is their high degree of elasticity on setting. However, this degree of elasticity is usually not essential for edentulous impressions. These materials are usually employed in thin sections of 1 to 2 mm. Whilst the viscosity of the material varies between different brands, the consistency of any one brand cannot readily be changed. Both materials produce a relatively smooth surface to the cast without sharp irregularities as neither is miscible with saliva or mucin. The polysulphides have the advantage in general of a longer working time and if this is coupled with a moderately high viscosity, give a longer time for the operator to develop the correct border extension of the impression. Both materials are readily tolerated by the patient and since they are used in small bulk, seldom cause nausea.

ALGINATES (*recommended tray : shellac or acrylic, spacer 3 mm*)

Flow of alginate materials varies between different brands and also with the powder/water ratio used. Variations in the consistency of mix from any one material occur mainly due to errors in proportioning powder by scoopfuls. Weighed portions of powder eliminate this source of variation. The powder/water ratio of most alginates can be varied to suit any impression technique for *edentulous* patients as the loss in elastic properties which often results is unimportant for most edentulous impressions. Some alginates maintain a fairly constant viscosity until they gel suddenly. Others gradually thicken and have an imprecise gel point spread over some 20 to 30 seconds. The former type have some advantages as with them there is less danger of trying to mould an already partly elastic material. Also, the time of insertion of the tray and manipulation of lips and cheeks to mould the sulcus area is not critical, provided that it is done before gelation. The speed of setting can be controlled by the temperature of the mix.

Alginates can be used in a thin film for mucocompressive techniques but find a more frequent use in thicker sections for mucostatic impressions. In thin sections, alginates may peel or tear away from the supporting tray or baseplate. It is usual, therefore, to record alginate impressions in a tray which leaves a space of 2 to 4 mm between it and the tissues. For such an impression a moderate to low viscosity is required. A smooth shiny mix which will not flow out of the tray on inverting it is usually satisfactory. Where much fibrous tissue is present over the ridge, a more fluid mix in a well-spaced tray ensures the minimum of distortion of the flabby tissue on recording the impression. Alginates flow well but require good support from a correctly extended tray. Prepacking of difficult areas, e.g. the tuberosities, centre of palate and lower posterolingual areas is often necessary to reduce the volume of air which may be trapped there.

Alginates are generally acceptable by the patient, although their bulk may cause stimulation to the dorsum of the tongue and so cause nausea. They are more than sufficiently elastic to record edentulous undercuts into which a denture can be placed. An alginate impression is accurate only if it is well supported and also attached to the support, preferably by means of an adhesive. Slow removal, particularly of an upper impression, may tear the impression material away from the tray and produce distortion. If facilities for pouring the cast immediately are not available, the impression can be wrapped in damp napkins and stored in a closed container, or alternatively placed in liquid paraffin. With some materials the change in dimension due to storage for several hours, under good conditions, does not appear to have any clinical significance in the edentulous case. Alginates reproduce good detail but record the surface of any mucin lying on the tissues, rather than the tissues themselves. This is seen at the hard and soft palate junction particularly if a vomiting reflex is stimulated during impression recording. A denture made to such an impression is not well adapted in this area and is therefore lacking in retention. An astringent mouthwash used prior to impression recording assists in the removal of a thick mucin film, as does wiping the area with cotton wool or a dental napkin.

Alginate impressions pull cleanly away from the surface of a cast poured in a suitable dental stone, and therefore all the detail of the impression is reproduced in the cast.

Alginate finds a general use for edentulous impressions. It is subject to inaccuracies from several sources, however, and care in its manipulation is necessary to ensure good results.

PLASTER (*recommended tray: shellac or acrylic, spacer 3 mm*)

At one time plaster was the most frequently used impression material. Suitably modified with chemicals to control its setting time and expansion, reduce its strength and to give it colour, it has several good properties. It absorbs mucin and saliva, thus reproducing the tissue surface instead of the superficial surface of any mucin film. Unfortunately, in the lower jaw it mixes readily with saliva. This weakens the impression sufficiently for the plaster to break up, losing correct sulcus extension. It is not pleasant to taste. Plaster is brittle on removal, it cannot therefore be distorted on removal from an undercut, but the resulting jigsaw puzzle may present difficulties in accurate reassembly.

Plaster can be mixed to a consistency suitable for either a mucostatic (3 to 4 mm) layer or a thin wash of 1 mm or less within a modified compound impression. At any particular consistency its setting time may be controlled by the temperature of the added water. Plaster passes quickly from a plastic state to a consistency which can no longer be moulded. Whilst it is at first rather friable on setting, it quickly becomes sufficiently strong to enable the operator to remove the impression. Although plaster records good detail of a dry surface all the detail of the mucosa is not necessarily reproduced on the cast. Plaster which enters small depressions in the mucosa may be so weak that these portions are left behind in the mouth after removal of the impression. Also after making the cast, on removing the impression small prominences of its surface are again seen embedded in the surface of the cast, thus reducing again the amount of sharp detail which is recorded.

Because plaster is brittle the accuracy of an impression is readily seen on examination. Plaster is not as palatable to the patient, but is capable of wide variations in consistency and speed of setting and this makes it suitable for various impression techniques. It adheres well to impression trays, baseplates, etc., without an adhesive. There are no problems in storing a plaster impression before it is cast.

IMPRESSION COMPOUND (*recommended tray : metal or acrylic, spacer 3 mm*)

The viscosity of impression compound varies with temperature. As one is limited to a maximum of 60 to 65° C for oral use, impression compounds vary in their fusing points and therefore in the range of usable viscosities. Some low fusing materials are quite fluid at 60 to 65° C whilst others are still highly viscous. Impression compound cools slowly at mouth temperature. If used in thick sections it is not an accurate material, as the time necessary for it to cool down becomes inordinately long. Therefore the material is usually removed whilst still plastic thus creating good conditions for distortion to take place. Compound is a very suitable material for recording a good support over which a wash impression may be taken. High-fusing tray compounds are generally used for this purpose. The compound impression may be modified to create suitable space for a thin wash of another impression material. Alternatively, the compound impression may be chilled, the surface resoftened by heating and the thin layer of softened material used for recording the impression over a firm base of harder compound.

Because of its viscosity, compound can be used to produce pressure in selected areas. For example, peripheral pressure from a close-fitting support or tray can be produced by adding a thin layer of compound to the edge of the support. Similar additions over the post dam or pear-shaped pad areas can be made.

One of the main advantages of compound is that one may trim the impression or add further material, or resoften local areas and then reshape them until the impression is satisfactory. The compound impression can be reinserted and tested for accuracy as many times as are necessary.

Reproduction of detail is not high with compound. It is completely bland to the patient, however, and the impression can be stored before being cast.

Due to the setting or hardening time of all the materials presently discussed, impressions recorded with them tend to be 'snapshots'. A longer time may, however, be necessary to allow for a balance to be achieved between the flow of the impression material and the slight mobility of the soft tissues covering the ridge and palate. After gross resorption of the mandibular ridge the tissue covering it may move slightly with the sulcus tissues. Then it is important to record the tissue surface when the sulcus is filled with a bulk similar to that to be used in the final denture. For this purpose, an impression material must have the property of being able to flow for a long time at mouth temperature in order to give selective and physiological compression of tissue and allow excess material to escape to the periphery. In addition, it should reproduce surface detail and be capable of being added to as the impression is made. Such a material can be found amongst the impression waxes and tissue conditioning materials.

IMPRESSION WAXES *(recommended tray : acrylic, spacer 0.6 mm)*

Waxes are available with different softening temperatures and therefore different flow rates at or slightly above mouth temperature. These materials are added to a close-fitting acrylic tray or other rigid support such as a denture, either by a series of local applications or in a thin sheet over the entire impression area. Wax impressions can be moulded during function under existing or new dentures.

Four grades of wax may be described:

1 Extra hard—recommended to extend borders prior to covering with one of the softer waxes

2 Hard—recommended in rebasing as a hard foundation for softer waxes when extensive resorption necessitates a bulk of material

3 Soft—recommended for minor tray corrections and as an initial lining to stabilize the tray

4 Extra soft—recommended to secure a completely adapted impression under normal occlusal load. It registers fine tissue detail.

An extra soft wax is recommended as a final impression material. Used in thin sections it is said to produce a selectively compressive impression of the edentulous area. Having no setting phase the wax will flow continuously at mouth temperature. This flow can take place under a physiological occlusal load and therefore it is logical to assume that a physiological compression of the mucosa can be achieved.

Impression wax is prepared for use in a container within a thermostatically controlled water bath. The fitting surface of the support (whether it be a tray or an existing denture) is thoroughly cleansed and dried with compressed air. A camel hair brush is used to coat the fitting surface with wax. The support is immersed in warm water for a few moments, in order to temper the wax, after which it is inserted in the mouth. If a denture is used as the support the patient is asked to close into light occlusal contact for a minute. If a tray is used, the operator maintains light finger pressure on the tray for the same period. The impression is then removed and inspected. All areas of the wax on the fitting surface that are in a bearing contact with the tissues will have a glossy surface. If any of the support material shows through the wax, relief is made with a bur or stone to avoid overdisplacement and the area resurfaced with wax; any dull spots or imperfections are coated with molten wax. The impression is immersed in warm water as before and reinserted in the mouth. On removal, if the entire surface has a glossy appearance and all the borders show a definite roll, the impression is said to be in correct bearing adaptation to the basal tissues.

Wax impression materials are suitable therefore for a wide range of techniques. They produce a smooth surface which is reproduced on the cast. These materials are well tolerated by patients. Addition and trimming of the wax to build up a perfect impression can be done, but the materials are a little laborious to use and require careful handling to produce accurate results.

TISSUE CONDITIONING MATERIALS

Circumstances also arise where the soft tissues have been traumatized by an ill-fitting denture. Before a new impression is recorded it is essential to 'condition' the ridge tissues and allow them to return to a normal shape.

To allow tissues to recover from trauma and the impression surface to be developed gradually, impression recording may take place over several hours or even days.

In general, recent impressions recorded with tissue conditioners produce a well detailed yet smoothly contoured impression surface, similar to that recorded by the impression waxes.

REMOVAL OF IMPRESSIONS

Impressions recorded by closed mouth techniques may use a denture, record block or close fitting tray without a handle. In the upper jaw difficulties sometimes occur in the removal of the impression, particularly one of plaster or zinc oxide paste. The introduction of air or water between the impression and the tissues will usually enable it to be removed without distortion. If the patient is asked to close the lips and to inflate the cheeks, air and saliva are forced in. Alternatively a small amount of water from a syringe applied to the border of the impression may assist in removal. To enable air to enter the space created between tissues and impression on the removal of the latter, the patient should be asked to relax the lips which are then displaced laterally by the operator's fingers so moving them away from the border of the impression. The operator should avoid heavy pressure on the impression border, particularly when the material is still capable of flow, e.g. zinc oxide paste and waxes.

ASSESSMENT OF AN IMPRESSION

It is not always possible to produce a perfect impression due to a variety of reasons. Small surface imperfections due to the trapping of air occur on occasions. Where the prognosis for denture retention is good, these small defects can be filled in with wax and smoothed off, particularly if they are at the border (Fig. 21·12). Similarly, *slight* underextension in the posterolingual pouch, or anteriorly in the upper jaw, due to inadequate support, may be tolerated if retention over the rest of the denture bearing area is good. Where difficulties of denture support exist, due to resorption, nothing other than an accurate record of the mucoperiosteum and sulcus is satisfactory and it may be necessary to go through two or more impression stages each one improving in accuracy.

One of the commonest causes of an inaccurate impression is to load the tray with a large amount of impression material in the hope of improving the

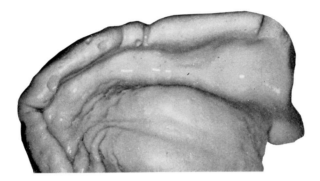

Fig. 21.12 Small defects in the border of an impression that may be filled in with wax.

chances of recording the entire area. In fact, the use of an excessive volume of material reduces the possibility of seating the support or tray correctly, or even of being aware of its correct position in the mouth. The tray becomes

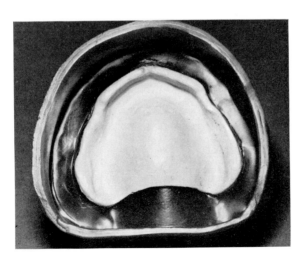

Fig. 21.13 A boxed upper impression.

lost in a mass of impression material. Also, excess material in the sulcus traps air, besides distorting the sulcus laterally.

Having carefully produced an accurate record of the sulcus shape, boxing of the impression is recommended to ensure that this sulcus shape is reproduced in the cast and in the completed denture (Fig. 21.13).

Chapter 22

Jaw Relations in the Edentulous Patient

The recording of jaw relations of an edentulous patient, so that new dentures may be constructed, will occur in three different circumstances:

1 When replacing dentures which have been successful, i.e. immediate restoration or previous non-immediate dentures
2 When replacing unsatisfactory dentures
3 When constructing dentures for an edentulous person who has not previously had dentures.

REPLACEMENT OF DENTURES WHICH HAVE BEEN SUCCESSFUL

A patient may attend requiring replacement of immediate dentures a year or more after the extractions, or replacement of non-immediate dentures after a much longer period. The vertical and horizontal relations of the jaws should have been maintained by the rebasing procedures and the patient will have become familiar with the shape of the polished and occlusal surfaces of the dentures. He will appreciate the nature and timing of tooth contact; control of the dentures, which may have presented initial problems, will now be reflex in nature.

If the replacement dentures are not a fairly accurate copy of the immediate or previous dentures, the patient will be conscious not only of the differences that exist but may also find difficulty in learning new patterns of movement of the oral musculature in order to control and use the dentures. The younger the patient the shorter will be the time necessary to accommodate to the shape and dimensions of the new dentures. But in the elderly patient new reflex actions are learnt with difficulty and a period of discomfort, unhappiness and possibly intolerance to the new dentures may ensue. In these circumstances the patient may revert to the previous dentures and continue to use them even though they are ill-fitting and traumatic to the tissues.

When replacement dentures are prescribed, every effort should be made to reproduce the shape and dimensions of the previous dentures. Despite the obvious advantages to be gained by so doing, it is more usual to find that little attempt is made to use the information available. Sometimes impressions are taken of the old dentures. However, the casts obtained from these do not provide the essential information—that of the spatial relation of the teeth on the denture to the alveolar ridge. The result is that when the replacement dentures are compared with the previous ones the arch form may be seen to have been misplaced with the teeth usually placed too far lingually and the plane of occlusion altered in height or inclination or both.

The authors recommend that when successful dentures need to be replaced, a denture copying technique be used as described in Chapter 19.

REPLACEMENT OF UNSUCCESSFUL DENTURES AND THE PROVISION OF DENTURES FOR THE ALREADY EDENTULOUS PATIENT

A copying technique is not advocated when the existing dentures that may have proved satisfactory to the patient, incorporate a gross malocclusion or errors in tooth form, position and arrangement. The technique is also inadvisable when the *patient* has been unhappy with previous dentures. In these cases the conventional method of recording jaw relation must be used, relating the area, bulk and occlusal surface of the new dentures to those factors which are acceptable in the previous dentures, and amending elsewhere. The existing dentures have some value in giving an indication of the jaw relation and tooth positions. Whilst these will not all be correct, some valuable evidence is always available and may be used as a guide when decisions are made regarding the construction of new dentures. The previous dentures should be examined carefully to ensure that those errors which have caused the dissatisfaction or failure are not repeated in the new ones.

Every effort should be made to reduce the guesswork that is so often a prominent feature of jaw registration. The only instance when total guesswork should be necessary is when an edentulous patient attends who has never had dentures and of whom there are no pre-extraction records of any description. Such patients are in diminishing numbers as the profession and the public appreciate the advantages of immediate denture therapy.

After the major impressions have been recorded, record blocks are made. These will be shaped by the dentist as the prescription for the technician and the success or failure of the new dentures is frequently related to the care which is taken at the clinical stage of registering jaw relations. The record blocks should be constructed carefully. So often the base of the cord block is made haphazardly and yet its adaptation to the tissues and its rigidity have a vital bearing on the accuracy of the registrations recorded in the mouth. Bases may be temporary or permanent.

TEMPORARY BASES

These are preferably made of shellac or self-cure acrylic. Wax is sometimes used but is considered unsatisfactory since if it is left in the mouth for more than a few minutes, the base softens and distorts.

PERMANENT BASES

These are made of heat-cure acrylic and are prepared on the master cast. This usually results in the destruction of the cast during deflasking. Such bases form the fitting surface of the finished denture and the teeth are attached to them with a self-cure acrylic material.

Many clinicians believe that it is only by the use of permanent bases that accurate intra-oral records can be obtained and this accuracy maintained on transfer to the articulator. The advantages claimed for the permanent type of base are:
1 The base feels like the permanent denture
2 Errors in extent and adaptation of the base, due to a faulty impression, can be detected and corrected before the denture is completed
3 Because of the superior retention and stability of the base the patient's mandibular movements are more likely to be normal and this will result in easier recording of the horizontal relation of mandible to maxilla. This is particularly so with the nervous patient. If he is able to retain the trial denture base for speaking, swallowing and normal oral functions, he is more likely to cooperate in the recording procedures.

The disadvantages of the permanent type of base are:
1 The difficulty of setting teeth on the relatively thick base where there is little inter-ridge space
2 The need for the use of self-cure acrylic material to attach the teeth to the base in order to avoid the dimensional changes in the base which might take place if heat-cure acrylic was used.

THE OCCLUSAL RIMS

These are made of wax and contoured by the dentist as a prescription to the technician, to give him information regarding the arch form, the arch position in relation to the underlying ridge and the position of the occlusal plane. The upper and lower occlusal rims related to each other indicate the correct vertical and horizontal relations of the jaws. The importance of careful contouring of the occlusal rims cannot be overemphasized. Only by receiving such information will the technician be able to set teeth on the trial bases so that they are in a harmonious relation with the adjacent oral tissues.

Before attempting to contour the record blocks they must be examined carefully both in and out of the mouth.

Where the bases are temporary and made of shellac or self-cure acrylic their adaptation to the casts is checked. The opportunity is taken also to examine the casts to confirm that they have not been damaged. In the mouth the blocks are examined for retention and fit. Although blocks with temporary bases will not exhibit the same positive retention as those with permanent bases, no movement should be apparent when the mouth is half open or when limited oral movements are performed. Displacement of the blocks indicates either overextension of the border or positioning of the wax rim so that the neutral zone is exceeded. In each case the tissues displace the blocks. Minor overextension of the border, in the area of the frena or the sulcus is corrected by suitable reduction of the base. But where overextension is considerable a new major impression must be recorded. Displacement of the block by encroachment of the wax rim beyond the confines of the neutral zone may be corrected by trimming of its labial, buccal or lingual surfaces.

If the bases are permanent, the retention of the blocks will be superior to those with temporary bases and will give some indication of that to be expected with the finished dentures. If displacement occurs during mouth opening and mandibular movements, the cause must be found and the necessary corrections made *before* the jaw relation records are obtained.

Too frequently an operator labours with record blocks that are too bulky and have to be held in place either with adhesive or by the operator's fingers. It is true to say that the retention of a finished lower denture will not be significantly greater than the retention of the lower record block. Retention is achieved largely by shaping the rim to avoid the field of actively moving musculature—adjacent to the periphery or the polished surfaces of the denture. If the block 'floats' when the mouth is partly open, something must be done or the denture also will be poorly retained.

TRIMMING THE UPPER RECORD BLOCK

THE LABIAL SURFACE

The upper anterior teeth will be set up to the labial surface of the upper block and therefore when this surface is trimmed consideration must be given both to appearance and to function. The labial surface should be sufficiently prominent to give support to the upper lip, in particular to its lower border. A correctly supported upper lip is slightly concave, revealing the vermilion border, and showing a depression at the philtrum. The retentive potential of the upper denture must be assessed. Where this is good then the labial surface may be brought forward of the ridge to give good support to the lip and the best cosmetic result; where the retentive potential is poor then some appearance must be sacrificed in favour of better retention and stability, and the rim positioned closer to the crest of the ridge. When previous dentures are available, the relation of the upper anterior teeth to the ridge on the denture is compared with the labial surface of the record block, and used as a guide in assessing the labial contour for the new denture.

THE INCISAL LEVEL

By trimming the height of the rim in the upper anterior region, the position of the incisal edges of the upper anterior teeth is determined. Part of the rim should show below the level of the correctly supported, resting lip, usually to the extent of 1 to 2 mm. Variations occur and are related to the length of the upper lip. With a long pendulous lip the level of the rim may be so trimmed that no wax shows; with a short bow-shaped and possibly incompetent lip 4 to 6 mm of the incisors may be revealed below the lip at rest. Comparison with previous dentures may modify the incisal level to be selected, as changes of more than 3 to 4 mm are generally unacceptable to the patient for appearance and for ease of speech.

THE OCCLUSAL PLANE

Having established the shape and height of the anterior part of the rim, the plane of occlusion is now determined. Anteriorly this should be horizontal and a useful guide is to make it parallel with an imaginary line passing between the pupils of the patient's eyes. Posteriorly it should be similar to the plane of occlusion of the natural teeth. An approximation to this plane is given by the ala-tragus line. To confirm parallelism, an occlusal plane guide may be used (Fig. 22.1).

Whilst the plane of the incisor teeth in the natural dentition may not be horizontal within the face, it is usual to set the artificial teeth to a plane that is horizontal. What is accepted in the natural dentition may be the cause of critical comment on careful examination of a denture. In addition, the use of a horizontal plane makes the arrangement of the posterior teeth simpler.

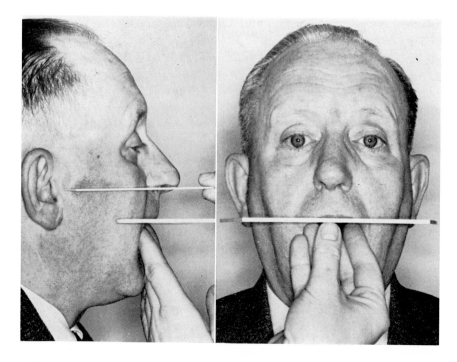

Fig. 22.1 Use of an occlusal plane guide to check parallelism of the upper record block rim with the ala-tragus line and the interpupillary line.

TRIMMING THE LOWER RECORD BLOCK

In trimming the lower occlusal rim, the aim is to achieve even contact with the upper rim at the correct occlusal face height with the mandible in the muscular horizontal relation to the maxilla. The clinician should think of these three factors simultaneously. Whilst achieving even contact of the rims, he will be considering the occlusal face height and will automatically be guiding the mandible into the muscular position each time the rims are brought into contact. The less experienced clinician, however, is advised to consider the requirement of lower block trimming in the sequence—even contact with the upper, vertical relation, horizontal relation. He must also bear in mind the relation of the labial, buccal and lingual surfaces of the rim to the adjacent musculature.

EVEN CONTACT

This is of vital importance if the denture bearing areas are to be loaded evenly. Indiscriminate softening of the occlusal surface of the lower rim followed by a 'squashbite' closure controls neither the occlusal height nor the muscular position.

The operator ensures that the blocks are firmly seated and asks the patient to close very slowly. Any premature contacts of the rims should be detected and a correction made. If the patient closes too quickly, or if the blocks are not maintained firmly on the basal tissues an initial contact may be obscured by a tilting of the block and a simulation of apparently even contact.

THE OCCLUSAL FACE HEIGHT (VERTICAL DIMENSION)

This is the vertical separation of the upper and lower jaws when the occlusal surfaces of the rims (and subsequently the teeth) are in contact. When this is recorded correctly there will be an adequate freeway space when the mandible is in the postural position. If the vertical separation of the jaws is too great or too small the freeway space is reduced or increased. The freeway space is said to vary between 2 and 4 mm in the *average* patient. The clinician should not consider every patient to be average; each case must be carefully assessed. There is probably some degree of latitude in the recording of the occlusal face height but one should err on the side of caution and aim at a slightly reduced height rather than impinge upon or even eliminate the freeway space. Various methods of assessing the correct occlusal face height are employed, though clinical experience and mature judgment are of prime importance in ensuring satisfactory results.

The most valuable methods of assessing the correct occlusal face height are a combination of measurements of the freeway space and an examination of the facial appearance with the record blocks in place, together with a comparison with any previous dentures.

Freeway Space Determination

The success of the dentures is conditional on there being an adequate freeway space. It is obvious that the assessment of this should be the most important way of recording the correct vertical jaw separation.

A measurement between some external facial reference points is made with the mandible in the postural position. From this measurement is subtracted the amount of freeway space required and the occlusal height adjusted to this reduced figure when the upper and lower rims are in contact. There are three problems—first that of obtaining the true postural position of the mandible, secondly that of deciding how much freeway space the patient needs and thirdly making accurate measurements.

The postural position changes with the contents of the mouth. Consequently if previous dentures are available they should be inserted before recording this position. Only when the occlusal face height of the existing dentures is too great should one denture be removed before taking the measurements. When no dentures are available it is preferable to record the postural position with the record blocks in the mouth. Otherwise the mandible moves closer to the maxilla in order to reduce the amount of intra-oral space. On the other hand, if the mouth is overfilled with bulky record blocks, the mandible moves away from the maxilla. Therefore the rims must be trimmed to a minimum bulk, similar to that of the completed dentures.

To achieve the postural position, the patient should be seated upright in the chair without any tension of the throat or head muscles and must be relaxed. The arms should hang limply by the sides of the chair, the legs should be uncrossed and the lips should be moistened by the patient to ensure that they do not tend to stick together. The lips may or may not be in contact when the mandible is in the postural position. Patients with short upper lips (often previously associated with proclined natural upper anterior teeth) may have their lips separated.

Several methods have been described for measuring between reference points on the face. Either a Willis gauge or a pair of calipers may be used (Fig. 22.2). Either is satisfactory provided the operator uses them in the same way for making each measurement. Neither is a precise method, however, as slight movement or compression of the face tissues brings about a change in the measurement similar in size to that of the average freeway space. Measurements made by different people show a variation and a record by one person is not applicable to another. Lateral skull cephalographs are perhaps the nearest to an accurate form of measurement but cannot of course be used for every patient.

Having taken a measurement with the mandible in the postural position, the second problem arises—that of deciding how much freeway space is required. An indication is given by any existing dentures. If a large freeway space has existed for some time then a larger than average one should be continued. When treating an old patient an increase in occlusal face height of 3 to 4 mm is usually the maximum that can be tolerated. In young patients a greater correction of overclosure can be made and changes of 4 to 6 mm made. It must be appreciated, however, that not many young edentulous patients with existing dentures will have become overclosed by such an amount.

The skeletal relation of the jaws has some effect on the freeway space to be used in complete dentures. Skeletal Class I patients usually have an average freeway space of between 2 and 4 mm. In Class II cases, particularly, and sometimes in Class III, the freeway space may be in excess of 4 mm. In Class II and III patients, the operator should analyse with care the patient's postural

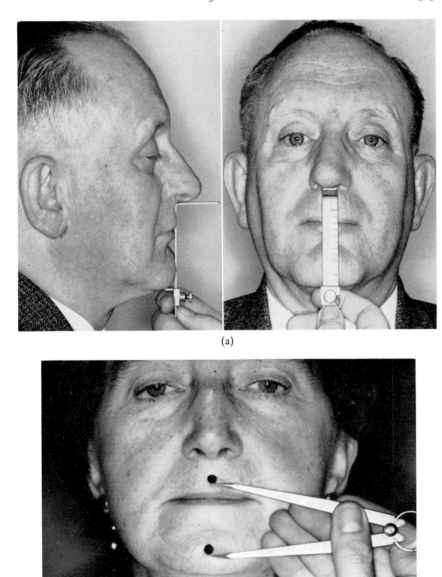

(a)

(b)

Fig. 22.2 Determination of the freeway space by external measurement, using
(a) the Willis gauge;
(b) dividers.

position. It may well have been that in the natural dentition an 'habitual' postural position was used in order to effect an anterior oral seal in speech and other activities requiring lip contact.

If there is a history of tooth clenching or discomfort under one or both dentures, the freeway space should be made greater than the average in order to reduce the possibility of heavy occlusal pressure being applied to the ridges.

One must not ignore the obvious method of observing the relation of the occlusal rims when the mandible is in the postural position. The patient should be asked to relax and the lips should be gently parted by the operator and the presence of a suitable freeway space confirmed.

The use of speech sounds is a useful aid only if there is good retention of the record blocks and if they have been correctly contoured, particularly in respect of arch width. Therefore if the permanent type of base has been used the evidence of phonetics may be helpful. The patient is asked to make the 'Th' sound. When this is produced the tongue is protruded between the occlusal rims. If there is insufficient freeway space this will not be possible and a hissing sound will be heard.

Many dentists with a considerable amount of clinical experience are able to tell simply by looking at the profile of the patient whether the occlusal face height is too great or too small. Here they are using the evidence of the appearance of the facial tissues.

The Labiomental Angle

This angle or depression found between the lower lip and the chin is always present, but varies in degree from patient to patient. The amount of jaw separation by the record blocks in the mouth affects this angle. If the separation is too great the angle is flattened as the patient strains the lower lip to make contact with the upper (Fig. 22.3). On the other hand if the separation is not enough the lower lip bulges forward as it contacts the upper, causing a deepening of the labiomental groove.

A deep labiomental depression is not always indicative of a reduced occlusal face height and the operator should be aware that the angle is often very pronounced in skeletal Class II cases when the vertical jaw separation is perfectly normal.

The Lips

At the correct degree of jaw separation the lips should be able to come into a relaxed and easy contact. If the separation is too great the patient will have difficulty in making the lips touch. If the upper lip is short, bow-shaped and

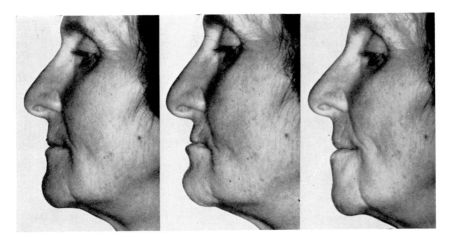

Fig. 22.3 The effect of variations in the occlusal face height on the lip relation and the labiomental angle:
(a) normal occlusal face height;
(b) overclosed;
(c) overopen.

incompetent there would not have been contact when the natural teeth were in occlusion. This should be repeated with the artificial dentition and the operator should therefore examine very carefully the shape and size of the upper lip.

If the separation is insufficient the lower lip becomes everted with the normally hidden, inner aspect, which is moist and shiny, becoming visible. This latter picture is seen where there has been minimal atrophy of the lip tissues and when the alveolar ridge is still well formed (Fig. 22.4). But where the alveolar ridge has undergone much resorption and atrophy of soft tissue has occured, the lips may be inverted with insufficient jaw separation and with only a narrow line of vermilion border of the lips visible (Fig. 22.5).

The Angles of the Mouth

Often, too much reliance is placed on the appearance of angular folds at the corners of the mouth. These creases naturally become deeper as the patient grows older and are not eliminated by increasing the occlusal face height. The really deep folds which are liable to become macerated and infected—a condition known as angular cheilitis—can usually be eliminated more effectively by correct positioning of the anterior teeth and by providing sufficient support for the angles of the mouth by the denture flanges.

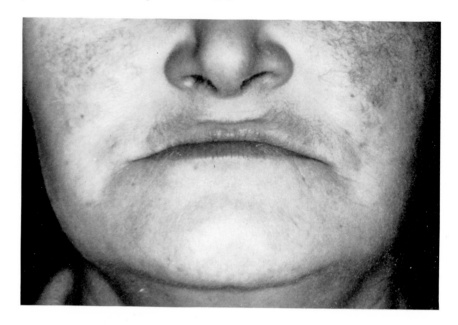

Fig. 22.4 Eversion of lower lip with overclosure in a young patient.

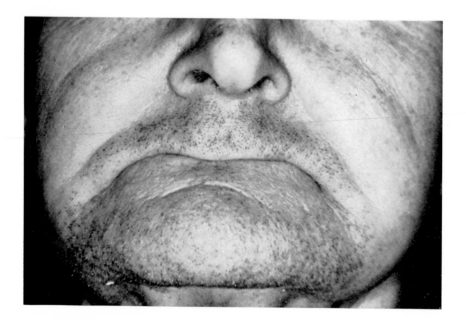

Fig. 22.5 Inversion of lower lip with overclosure in an older patient.

The dentist should be wary of the hypercritical middle aged female who is anxious to have the multiple fine lines radiating from the corners of the mouth and the vertical lines in the lips eliminated by an increase in occlusal face height (Fig. 22.6). Such patients must be advised that denture comfort and the aesthetics of youth become more incompatible with increasing age; the use of cosmetics should be suggested.

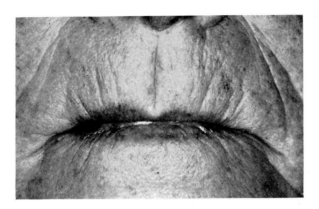

Fig. 22.6 Fine radiating lines on the lips caused by normal tissue ageing and which cannot be eliminated by flange contouring.

Other methods involve assistance from the patient in assessing the most comfortable vertical relation. By means of a screw mechanism between the record blocks, the vertical relation is gradually changed. It is considered that the patient can recognize the correct jaw relationship. It is also thought that the correct occlusal face height is some 2 to 3 mm below the height at which the maximum force can be applied to the record blocks by the patient.

None of the methods or aids mentioned above are critical or may be used by themselves as the sole basis for determining the vertical dimension; used in combination they provide a guide for the assessment of the most suitable occlusal face height and freeway space for the patient. In the final analysis it is the experience of the operator that is perhaps of greatest use. This is probably not much consolation for the struggling student but he must be encouraged to make occlusal height and freeway space assessments on as many patients as possible, whatever the state of their dentition. By gaining proficiency in obtaining a postural mandibular position, by measuring freeway spaces and by relating these to skeletal jaw relations and age, he will become rich in experience and a more competent clinician.

THE HORIZONTAL JAW RELATION

Whenever possible the muscular horizontal jaw relation should be recorded. This is usually easier to achieve when adopting the denture copying technique mentioned earlier in this chapter. Difficulties may arise when the horizontal relation is registered with conventional record blocks but they are minimized if the operator has a clear understanding of the factors that influence the various mandibular positions in relation to the maxilla.

Much depends on the previous dental history of the natural dentition and of any artificial dentition. When the natural teeth were present, the proprioceptors in their periodontal membranes were an important source of afferent signals which influenced muscle movements. After removal of all occluding teeth, the movements of the mandible are controlled mainly by proprioceptors in the muscles and in the joints. When record blocks or complete dentures are inserted, the mechanoreceptors of pressure and touch of the oral cavity and particularly of the denture bearing areas, take the place of the periodontal receptors. Provided that the consciousness of a different shape or bulk in the

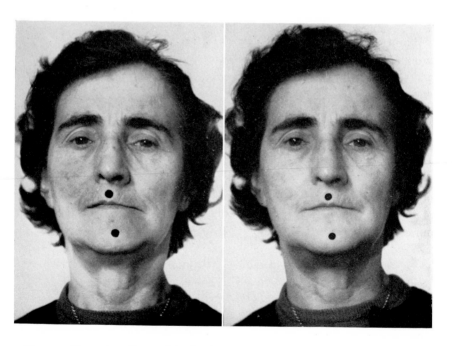

Fig. 22.7 Correction of a previous denture malocclusion with new dentures:
(a) marked left lateral deviation;
(b) corrected horizontal jaw relation.

mouth does not influence the previous movement pattern, the patient will usually close into the muscular horizontal position. The operator can assist the patient by eliminating any oral discomfort and thus any conscious control of jaw movements.

Some patients presenting for the provision of complete dentures have a bad occlusal record, in that over the years, a number of different horizontal relationships may have been learnt. A non-coincidence of intercuspal and muscular positions in existing dentures may have occurred because of errors at a previous registration stage or may have been acquired because of wear of denture teeth or as a consequence of alveolar resorption. Such malocclusions must be recognized and if at all possible corrected in the new dentures (Fig. 22.7).

Longstanding occlusal disharmonies establish new movement patterns. To begin with the patient is *conscious* of the need to posture the mandible to get maximum tooth contact but soon the movements become reflex and a situation develops where intercuspal and muscular positions do not coincide. The longer the incorrect movement patterns have been established the more difficult it will be to record the mandible in its original and natural muscular relation to the maxilla. Unless care is taken the mandible will again be related in a protrusive or lateral relation.

There may of course be indications for accepting a malocclusion and reproducing it in the new dentures. This is particularly applicable in old patients and also when the malocclusion has been established for many years. But in most cases an attempt should be made to record the muscular horizontal relation. In common with all the movements controlled by muscles, jaw movements become less precise with increasing age. Some old patients do not have a clearly defined muscular position and it may be necessary to accept an *area* of reproducible contact rather than a definitive position.

Difficulties of recording the muscular position can be reduced if the malocclusion of previous dentures is adjusted at earlier visits. A gradual correction of the occlusion by selective grinding will often return the patient to the muscular position and thus simplify the recording of the occlusion. Alternatively, the stimulus from the incorrect occlusal pattern can be masked by covering the posterior teeth of the lower denture with a thin film of self-cure acrylic which presents a flat surface to the upper teeth.

Recording the Muscular Position

There are many methods by which the mandible can be 'persuaded' to go into the muscular horizontal relation to the maxilla. Sedation may on occasion be indicated when dealing with a very nervous, tense patient. Temporary exhaustion of the muscles which protrude the mandible can be achieved by asking the patient to open and close or to protrude the mandible repeatedly. The attachment of the genioglossus muscle to the mandible may also be used. If the tongue is curled upward and backward to touch the posterior palatal border of the record block base this will restrain mandibular protrusion. A small blob of wax placed here will help the patient to position the tongue more readily.

Forced retrusion, either by tongue positioning or by pressure on the mandible by the operator may, however, push the mandible behind the muscular position and into the ligamentous position. Forced retrusion is to be avoided but occasionally is the only possible method to prevent protrusion or lateral movement of the mandible on closure.

In the majority of cases the mandible will go into the muscular position if no foreign objects other than properly contoured and adequately retained record blocks are in the mouth.

A prerequisite of accurate recording is that the patient must be able to relax the muscles controlling jaw protrusion.

To induce a complete state of relaxation in a patient in a dental chair is difficult and is only achieved after considerable practice and experience. The operator must aim virtually at inducing a state of light hypnosis in his patient. Any excitement or apprehension on the operator's behalf will be transferred to the patient. If the attempt to obtain the muscular position is prolonged, the possibility of success diminishes rapidly. Sometimes a more relaxed patient can be achieved by placing the patient in the prone position, the operator sitting comfortably by the patient's head. By talking quietly and calmly to the patient, a state of relaxation can be induced during which the mandible can be gently positioned.

The operator should explain to the patient what is required and he should then *guide* the mandible into the correct position. Slow closure should take place from the postural position. If rapid closure is allowed from a wide open position, displacement of the condyles may take place and an incorrect relation be recorded. Whereas if closure occurs from the postural position, there is only rotation of the condyles and a more accurate record is likely.

There are many methods by which the mandible may be guided into the correct position. One method is to hold the lower block in place with the fingers of one hand. The thumb is placed on the symphysis. The other hand may be used to support the upper block where necessary. The patient is asked to close from the postural position (Fig. 22.8). The thumb does not exert any backward pressure on the mandible—it is simply used as an indicator of any tendency for the patient to protrude the mandible. The hand supporting the lower block now guides the mandible into place. Usually a backward movement can be felt as the condyles move into the correct position in the glenoid fossae. The patient is asked to close into occlusal contact. Another method is illustrated in Fig. 22.9.

The ability to guide the mandible into the muscular position is a clinical skill that can only be achieved with practice and experience.

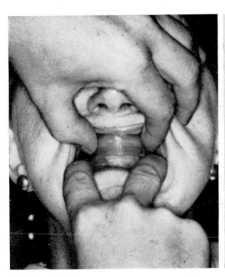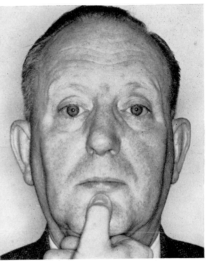

Fig. 22.8 Finger control of record blocks when recording the muscular horizontal position. The thumb of the right hand (hidden) is placed on the symphysis and senses any protrusion of the mandible.

Fig. 22.9 Another method of controlling the path of closure of the mandible. The thumb again senses any attempt at protrusion.

The operator must check the accuracy and reproducibility of the relation he has obtained. For this purpose guide lines are marked on the blocks. A minimum of three are required; they must cross the occlusal plane and be well defined. One of the cuts is the centre line and the two lateral cuts are in the canine or premolar regions. Then the patient is asked to open and close from the postural position a number of times. If the three lines coincide on each occasion the reproducible muscular relation has been recorded.

It is important to check the labial and buccal contours of the lower rim. The labial contour indicates the amount of horizontal overlap between upper and lower teeth. There may be little or no horizontal overlap in skeletal Class III cases, or a very large overlap in Class II. Modification of the contour of the lower to decrease the overlap can only be carried out in relation to the form and function of the lower lip. With the mouth in the half-open position, the lower block should remain in place on the basal tissues. If the labial and buccal surfaces are too prominent the labial and buccal musculature may cause a backwards and upwards displacement of the block. This is particularly likely when the lower alveolar ridge is poorly formed.

The blocks are now sealed together, having ensured that the occlusal surfaces of the rims are in even contact at the correct vertical separation. Staples may be used or alternatively, notches may be cut in the premolar regions of one rim and small pieces of soft wax moulded into them when the patient occludes. A recommended alternative is to place a thin layer of zinc oxide paste, plaster or specially compounded registration paste on the occlusal surface of one rim (usually the upper). With the other record block in place, the patient is asked to close into occlusion until the interposed material has set.

Many operators prefer to record the horizontal jaw relation by asking the patient to close into soft wax—either carding wax or softened baseplate wax. The disadvantage of carding wax is the danger of the relation between the blocks being altered in the laboratory prior to or during mounting on the articulator as a small force distorts the carding wax. A further disadvantage of using soft wax is that in closing, the vertical relation will not be maintained unless great care is taken. However, with considerable experience, it is possible to record both the vertical and horizontal jaw relations at the same time by letting the patient close slowly into a mass of *well softened wax*. In this technique, the lower record block should consist of a base carrying two very narrow pointed rims just in the premolar and molar regions. The lower record block can be stabilized with the finger and thumb placed in the incisor region and control over the patient's closing movements achieved. The use of a very narrow lower rim reduces to the minimum the force which the patient applies in closing into the soft wax and leaves good control in the hands of the operator.

If the record blocks are also used to record impressions, then the rims should be located but not sealed together. This enables the technician to pour each cast separately and then relocate the record blocks. When satisfactory impressions have been recorded previously, then the record blocks are sealed together, and are replaced carefully on the upper and lower casts. The heels of the casts must not touch each other or the blocks will be incorrectly seated. Any excess stone should be trimmed away from the casts but care taken not to damage the retromolar pad of the lower and the tuberosity and hamular regions of the upper.

INDICATIONS FOR RECORDING THE LIGAMENTOUS POSITION

Although in the majority of cases the muscular position can be recorded, there are indications for recording the most retruded position of the mandible in relation to the maxilla, that is, the ligamentous position. This may be achieved by forceful manual retrusion of the mandible, by recording a Gothic arch tracing or by using the hinge-axis facebow.

Recording the ligamentous position is indicated particularly for those patients in whom it is difficult or impossible to obtain a reproducible muscular position and in whom it is considered undesirable to reproduce the malocclusion in the replacement dentures. Similarly in edentulous patients who have not had dentures previously it may not be easy to record the muscular position. In both instances unless the ligamentous position is recorded, a horizontal relation is likely to be observed at the trial denture stage which varies from that recorded at the registration stage. A number of try-ins may be necessary before a reproducible result is obtained.

In most natural dentitions there is a clear difference between the occlusal contacts in the ligamentous position and the maximal intercuspation that occurs in the muscular position. It has therefore been suggested that the teeth on complete dentures should be routinely set up to the ligamentous position and subsequently ground to give balanced contact in the muscular position.

This procedure should be adopted in those patients in whom it is not possible to record a reproducible muscular position.

Gothic Arch Tracing

On lateral excursion of the mandible, the condyle on the side toward which the mandible moves, rotates about a vertical axis with only a slight backward and sideways (Bennett) movement, limited by the jaw ligaments. Hence, the path of the other condyle is along a curve. Lateral excursion of the mandible to the other side produces a similar curve. If the patient does not make a pure lateral movement but protrudes the rotating condyle, then an irregular curve is produced instead of a smooth one since the protrusion of the condyle is not usually carried out in a smooth manner. By attaching a tracing stylus to the maxilla, a pointed shape can be produced (Fig. 22.10). If each line is the tracing of a pure lateral jaw movement, then each indicates the path of movement of one condyle down the eminentia articularis whilst the other condyle rotates on the lower surface of the articular disc. We may assume that the rotating condyle does not move far away from its ligamentous position. Hence, where the two lines meet, both condyles should be in the ligamentous position.

There is doubt however, as to whether the condyles always move into the ligamentous position. They may be held in the muscular position. Then the apex of the gothic arch tracing indicates the muscular position and not the ligamentous position.

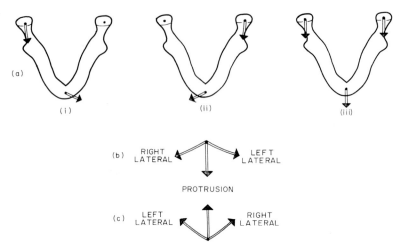

Fig. 22.10

(a) The movement of the condyles and symphysis in
- (i)   left lateral excursion;
- (ii) right lateral excursion;
- (iii) protrusion.

(b) The movement of the mandible in relation to the maxilla;

(c) Gothic arch tracing produced by attaching a stylus to the upper record block. This is the reverse of (b).

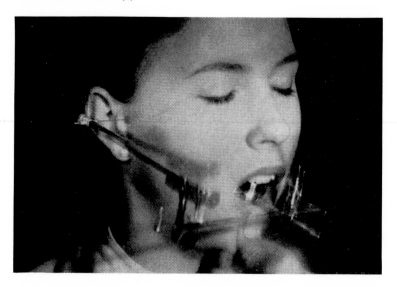

Fig. 22.11 Hinge axis locator *in situ*. Exposure during hinge opening. Notice the stationary condyle pins rotating, whereas other parts of the appliance and the chin are indistinct due to movement.

Unfortunately, many patients do not produce a good gothic arch tracing and some are able to produce one despite the fact that the condyle which should only rotate is also being brought forward. Hence the recording is not entirely reliable.

Hinge-axis Determination

The movement of the mandible from the postural position to occlusal contact in the muscular position, is generally about an axis passing through the two condyles. For this small movement, a hinge-like movement is used and the axis is appropriately called the hinge-axis. A greater hinge movement of between 20 and 25 mm, measured at the incisors, can take place but with both condyles in the ligamentous position. The amount of hinge movement possible depends upon the control of the posterior fibres of the temporalis muscles in preventing forward displacement of the condyles. On wider opening, a translation or forward movement occurs. The hinge movement is seen best at the end of closing rather than at the beginning of an opening movement. It is therefore called the terminal hinge movement. A suitable facebow may be attached to the mandible with adjustable extensions which can be positioned near the condyles. On asking the patient to open and close the jaw, a position of these styli will be found where the jaw rotates about an axis (Fig. 20.11). If this movement is between the postural position and correct occlusal face height, it terminates at the muscular position. If the larger hinge movement is recorded, it terminates at the ligamentous position. On inserting the record blocks, the patient should make the same movement with the styli rotating about the same point. Any protrusion or lateral movement is noted by the change in position of the styli.

Neither of these methods is satisfactory unless the base of the record block is firmly seated and well retained. Indeed, when using the facebow method a clamp under the chin is usually employed to ensure stability of the lower record block against the displacing effect of the facebow.

MARKINGS RECORDED ON THE WAX RIMS

These lines are made as a guide to the selection of the upper anterior teeth.

The Centre Line

This is marked with reference to the centre of the face. It is not necessarily in line with the philtrum or the labial frenum. The operator should stand in front of the patient when assessing the midline of the face. The centre line on the wax rim indicates where the mesial surfaces of the two central incisors contact.

The Canine Line

Bilateral canine lines may be scribed on the wax rims. They follow an imaginary line joining the inner canthus of the eye and the ala of the nose. The point where the canine line crosses the occlusal plane represents approximately the position of the tip of the canine. An indication of the width of the anterior teeth can be obtained by measuring the distance between the canine lines. With a flexible ruler, the intercanine distance is measured and the width of a set of teeth selected accordingly. Naturally the width of tooth selected is related also to any spacing or crowding which may be necessary in the arrangement.

The High Lip Line

This is the smile line and marks the extreme functional position of the upper lip. Some operators make use of this in determining the length of the anterior teeth. This was of greater value when vulcanite was used as the denture base material. Today, however, with the good aesthetic properties of acrylic polymers, and the possibilities of tinting and contouring the labial flange to simulate normal mucosa, the high lip line is probably of limited use in selecting teeth.

FUNCTIONAL LIP ACTIVITY

Apart from a consideration of the need for support of the resting lip, it must be realized that the type of lip activity peculiar to any individual patient has an important influence on the satisfactory positioning of both the upper and lower anterior teeth. Observation of functional activity of the lips is difficult and even the most careful shaping of the labial surface of the wax rim may not result in the teeth being positioned in a harmonious relation with the functioning lip musculature.

The difficulties are perhaps greatest in skeletal Class II and III cases. An added problem exists in the skeletal Class II case where the natural upper anteriors may have been either proclined or retroclined. It is difficult, if not impossible, to determine just how the natural teeth were positioned in relation to the lips if pre-extraction records are not available. Just as the available denture space may be measured by an impression, it is possible to record the amount and direction of lip pressure and thus indicate tooth position. If the lips act on a mouldable material on the labial surfaces of the record blocks, this will be shaped according to the pressures exerted.

After the vertical and horizontal jaw relations have been recorded, the wax rims are removed from the anterior part of the upper and lower blocks extending as far back as the first premolar area. Soft wax or alginate impression material is put into the space and, using a denture adhesive, the blocks firmly positioned on the tissues. The patient is asked to open and close on to the occlusal rims and to swallow several times. The pattern of lip activity will be

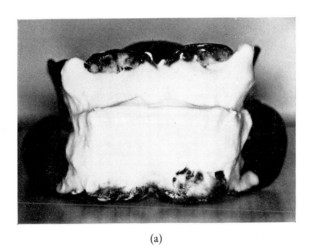

(a)

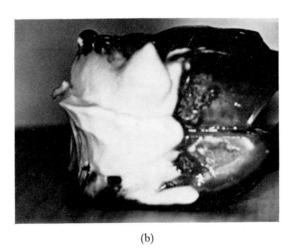

(b)

Fig. 22.12 The pattern of lip activity of a Class III case recorded in alginate placed on the anterior surfaces of the record blocks.

recorded. (Fig. 22.12.) The value of asking the patient to swallow is that in skeletal Class II cases a tongue thrust may be present during swallowing. Obviously if the anterior teeth are inadvertently set too far lingually such tongue thrusting may well cause displacement of the finished dentures or soreness of the tongue.

When the record blocks have been mounted on the articulator, plaster may be poured against the alginate to form an index which then prescribes the position of the teeth for the technician.

THE CHOICE OF ARTICULATOR

A survey of the literature indicates the controversy that exists with regard to the reproduction of jaw movements. Each designer of an articulator considers that his instrument reproduces mandibular movement more closely than others. In fact this simply means that the instrument is conforming to that person's concept of mandibular movement.

The closer the instrument imitates mandibular movement the more efficiently will the technician be able to set up the teeth to a balanced occlusion and articulation. But the precise mandibular movement pattern which will be employed by the patient is very difficult, if not impossible, to define. It is therefore inadvisable to spend unnecessary hours of clinical and laboratory time on mounting casts and setting up teeth on a very complex articulator when just as satisfactory an articulation can be produced on a simpler type of instrument.

Articulators may be classified as 1 plane-line or simple hinge, 2 average value, and 3 fully adjustable.

The writers' preference is for an articulator of the average value type with a fixed condyle path and either a fixed or adjustable incisal path. Such an articulator is capable of reproducing average lateral and protrusive movements.

THE USE OF THE FACEBOW

A simple facebow may be used with the fixed condyle path type of articulator. It provides a transfer record that relates the casts to the hinge-axis of the articulator. Since the mandible rotates about a hinge-axis between occlusion and the postural position, *small* changes in vertical relation of the jaws can be made by adjusting the articulator. Without a hinge-axis record *any* change in vertical relation necessitates the recording of a new occlusal position.

PRESCRIPTION

At this stage, the prescription to the technician should cover the following points:

Information given by the record blocks
1 Vertical and horizontal jaw relations
2 General positions of the upper and lower anterior teeth
3 Denture outline
4 Neutral zone.

Further information.
1 Type of articulator to be used
2 Shade, mould and material of anterior teeth. (Chapter 23)
3 Anterior tooth arrangement
4 Material, cusp formation, width of posterior teeth. (Chapter 10)

Try-in: Aesthetics

The try-in stage enables the accuracy of previous records to be checked, further details to be considered and the necessary adjustments to be made before the dentures are finished.

ACCURACY OF THE CASTS

It is advisable to ensure perfect adaptation of the trial bases to the casts and to confirm that a similar degree of 'fit' is present in the mouth. Good adaptation of the bases is essential before one can try the occlusion or check the aesthetic appearance of the denture. If the trial dentures are non-retentive, difficulties in checking the occlusion are created. Also, the patient can hardly form an opinion of the aesthetics of mobile dentures. Whilst a denture adhesive may occasionally be necessary to provide adequate retention, complete lack of retention of a try-in indicates an error in construction which must be rectified before the dentures are completed.

It is inadvisable to leave a wax try-in in the mouth for more than a few minutes at a time, particularly in warm weather. Distortion of the softened wax, and tooth movement soon take place. On removal from the mouth the trial dentures should be chilled and replaced on the casts.

It is preferable to insert the trial dentures one at a time and to test their adaptation to the ridges and palate and their peripheral extension. Finger pressure applied to the molar teeth alternately, or to a canine on one side and the last molar on the opposite side will elucidate any distortion of the impression and consequent inaccuracy of the cast.

EXTENSION OF BASES

Peripheral underextension is readily seen on direct examination in the labial and buccal sulcus by moving the lips aside slightly and examining the relation of the denture to the sulcus. Elsewhere underextension of the base is more difficult to discover and reliance is placed more upon the earlier assessment of the impression and complete coverage of the recorded area on the cast by the try-in. If doubts exist as to adequate extension, a temporary wax addition is made and the area tested for extension in the mouth. If this addition is tolerated then a new impression must be recorded to include this area.

Peripheral overextension is indicated by the denture moving away from the basal tissues. In the upper jaw the denture falls down whilst in the lower jaw it jumps up again after it has been placed in position. When trying-in a denture with good retentive possibility, however, a lesser degree of over-extension may not be so obvious. Lack of freedom of movement of the frena can be seen by direct examination in the labial sulcus. Overtrimming of these areas should, however, be avoided as otherwise they will allow ingress of air between the denture and the tissues. To test for overextension during oral function, a finger is placed lightly on the occlusal surface of the posterior teeth and with the other hand the cheeks and lips are pulled slightly outwards and over the denture to simulate the amount of movement used during speech, chewing, etc. Too vigorous manipulation of these soft tissues must be avoided as it brings about a reduction in sulcus depth that is much greater than that encountered during normal function.

Lingual extension is tested by asking the patient to move the tongue. Denture displacement when the tongue is protruded just beyond the lips reveals overextension onto the genioglossus muscles or in posterolingual areas. Care must be taken, however, to differentiate between upward pressure from the muscles in the sulcus and the direct pressure of the tongue itself on the lingual aspect of the denture. Hence the degree of tongue protrusion should be limited to that described. Lateral movement of the tongue into the cheeks reveals any overextension at the mylohyoid muscle and sublingual gland areas of the opposite side, whilst swallowing brings forward the palatoglossal arch and reveals distolingual overextension.

The posterior border of the palate is checked with the 'ah' or vibrating line and the area is palpated to ensure that post dam pressure is applied to slightly yielding tissues and not to a hard bony area.

OCCLUSION

When both dentures are properly extended and are stable, the patient is asked to close the teeth gently together. If everything is correct then the same inter-digitation of teeth is seen in the mouth as exists on the articulator. An even posterior tooth contact, however, does not necessarily mean that a correct occlusion has been recorded.

Space Between Posterior Teeth

On occasions the lower denture may rise away from the ridge so that it occludes with the upper teeth but a space exists between the denture and the basal tissues. This error occurs more commonly in the lower posterior region. By attempting to insert the blade of a spatula or wax-knife between the posterior teeth, the denture will be displaced out of occlusion and back onto the basal tissues if a space exists. Care must be taken, however, to limit to a minimum the amount of force applied in trying to separate the teeth and also to ensure that the patient maintains the 'apparent' occlusal contact whilst the test is being made. If much force is used the patient experiences pain and quickly separates the jaws slightly in order to relieve the pressure. If there is much displaceable tissue over the alveolar ridge crest, excessive force will result in depression of the denture into the tissues, suggesting an error in occlusion that does not in fact exist.

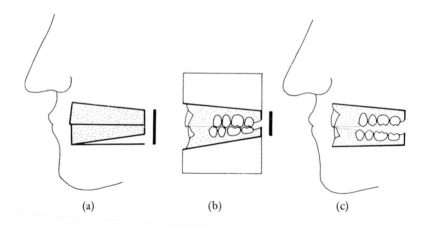

(a)   (b)   (c)

Fig. 23.1
(a) Record blocks in the mouth. The lower block has moved away from the basal tissues;
(b) dentures set up to this incorrect vertical relation;
(c) trial dentures in contact with the basal tissues with a space between the occlusal surfaces.

This lack of occlusion of the posterior teeth arises from a similar movement of the record block when recording the occlusion. Unless slight pressure is applied bilaterally in the premolar region, the base of the block may not be touching the tissues. Then the distance recorded between the ridges by the occlusal rims is smaller than it should be (Fig. 23.1). Thus whilst the posterior teeth meet on the articulator, they are apart in the mouth. This type of error is of clinical origin. To rectify it, wedges of softened wax of suitable thickness are placed on either side and the correct inter-ridge distance is recorded. No teeth need be removed nor should any attempt be made to raise the posterior teeth into occlusion by resetting them in the mouth. This is a time-consuming and inaccurate method. Having recorded the correct occlusion, the technician will then remount the casts and set the lower teeth to occlude with the uppers, as usually with this type of error, the upper record block has been fitting correctly and the upper occlusal plane is therefore correct.

On occasions, lack of contact of posterior teeth is also caused by an increase in the distance separating the casts anteriorly. This may occur when mounting the casts on the articulator but it is not a common error.

Anterior 'Open Bite'

The second common occlusal error is indicated by reduction or elimination of the vertical incisal overlap present on the articulator, or the presence of a definite space between the anterior teeth. Here the occlusal height is increased and the patient is unable to approximate the lips comfortably. To produce this type of error, the distance between the casts posteriorly must be greater than that which separates the same areas in the mouth.

Clinically, a small degree of increase posteriorly can be produced by compression of the soft tissues covering the ridges. Heavy pressure when the occlusal rims are in contact, increases the space between the ridges by 1 to 2 mm depending upon the amount of soft tissue which can be displaced. No change of the surface contour of the stone casts can take place. Therefore, they remain too far apart in this region and the posterior teeth meet first when the patient occludes. This type of occlusal error also arises unilaterally. If hard wax is placed on one side of the jaw and soft wax on the other, the tissues beneath the hard wax are compressed and a greater height of occlusal rim is accommodated on this side. A similar degree of error arises from stress relief of a large mass of partially softened wax. If the occlusion has been registered by a 'squashbite' technique, and the wax left in a warm atmosphere for a day or two, distortion by relief of stresses set up within the wax increases the height of the rims and the distance between the casts. This may occur at the occlusion stage or when correcting an error of a previous try-in.

The error which produces premature contact of the molar teeth can also be due to a technical error in the laboratory. Contact of the cast behind the denture bearing area on either upper, lower or both casts, does not allow them to fit accurately into the base of the record block but increases the distance between the ridges.

Alternatively, lack of good adaptation of the record block to the cast may cause a similar error by not allowing the base to fit back accurately on to the cast. This type of error recurs where there is an inaccuracy of the cast. A wax trial base will accommodate itself partly to the shape of the mouth and then is a poor fit when replaced on the inaccurate cast. As a result the distance between the ridges will continue to be too great unless the true source of error is realized.

To rectify the occlusion, the position of the upper teeth is checked. If satisfactory, the lower posterior teeth are removed and replaced by a rim of wax of similar height. If wax is added until it just touches the upper teeth, then after softening the surface the correct occlusal height can readily be recorded.

Incorrect Occlusal Relation

An error of occlusion may also present itself as a lack of interdigitation of the posterior tooth cusps. If the occlusal relation is seen to be forward of that in which the teeth were set up, then the patient is usually protruding the mandible or moving it into a lateral position. Relaxation of the patient and a further occlusal contact may then confirm the correct, previously registered muscular position.

Sometimes, however, the occlusal relation is behind that to which the teeth have been set. Then it must be determined whether the new position is the ligamentous or the true muscular position. As the difference between these two positions is in most patients only 1 mm this type of occlusal error invariably results from an incorrect recording of the muscular position. The posterior teeth of one denture are removed to prevent guiding the mandible into the incorrect tooth position of the set-up. These teeth are replaced by softened wax of the same height and a light indentation of the opposing teeth in the correct muscular position is recorded.

Recording of the correct relation changes the amount of horizontal incisal overlap and a decision will then be necessary as to if, and how, this should be decreased in amount.

Where a lateral position of the mandible in relation to the maxilla was previously recorded, the centre line of the upper denture no longer coincides with that of the lower, and the posterior teeth of one side do not interdigitate. Removal of these teeth and replacement with wax, combined with the placing of a small amount of soft wax on the teeth of the other side of the jaw enables the correct muscular position to be recorded.

OCCLUSAL FACE HEIGHT

Changes in occlusal face height of the try-in may be necessary due either to an original error or to a new assessment of the occlusal problem on seeing it for a second time. A more accurate comparison between previous dentures and the trial bases can be made at this time. If only small changes in occlusion have been decided upon, the trial dentures may be checked one at a time against the previous dentures thus revealing any marked changes in occlusion which have become incorporated in the try-in.

An increase in height is readily made by placing wax between the teeth. To reduce the occlusal height, however, all the teeth should be removed from the lower denture and a wax rim formed just out of occlusion with the upper teeth so that new jaw relations may be recorded. If the lower anterior teeth remain in position they may restrict closure into the correct position since the mandible comes forward as the occlusal height is reduced. When a moderate vertical incisal overlap exists, however, or when the degree of closure required is only small, there is an advantage in leaving the incisors in position as from their relation with the upper incisors the amount of reduction of height can be readily gauged.

POSTERIOR TOOTH POSITION AND WIDTH

Stability of the lower denture is affected by pressure from the cheek and tongue and the posterior teeth should be of such a size and position that they lie in the zone of neutral pressure between these two structures. Encroachment on tongue space is indicated by the tongue covering a large amount of the occlusal surfaces of the posterior teeth. Normally only about 1 to 2 mm of the lingual aspect of these teeth should be covered. It may be necessary where coverage is greater than this either to move the teeth to a more buccal position or to reduce their width by grinding the lingual surfaces. Alternatively of course one may select a narrower mould of tooth. A line is drawn on the surface of the teeth to indicate the adjustment which is necessary, together with a suitable prescription for the technician.

The occlusal plane of the lower posterior teeth should be related to normal tongue and cheek function. For stability the tongue should lie just above the occlusal surfaces of the lower posterior teeth, thus applying a little downward pressure onto the denture. If the posterior teeth stand up above the tongue, the denture is less stable on tongue movement. When lower denture retention is poor it may be necessary to lower the occlusal plane in order to improve denture control by the tongue.

AESTHETICS

Where large errors of occlusal relations or of accuracy of the casts have been discovered and new records taken, a decision must be made as to whether a further try-in is necessary. Usually, after correcting large errors or when considerable difficulties exist in recording the occlusion a further try-in is preferable. In these circumstances only the general tooth position is assessed at the first try-in and the detailed examination left until the next visit. Naturally any obvious errors of centre line or incisal level are modified at this stage and indicated to the technician by the movement of one or two anterior teeth.

When, however, the accuracy of the casts and of the occlusal record is confirmed, the appearance of the anterior teeth must be critically assessed.

Awareness of the Natural Dentition

Few patients have any precise knowledge of the shape, size and arrangement of their natural dentition. This can be realized very readily if the reader pauses for a minute to try and visualize the details of his own anterior teeth and draw, from memory, their main characteristics of shape and position. One usually has only a hazy impression of general tooth position and is aware only of marked irregularities of the dentition. Prominence of all the teeth, large spaces, gross overcrowding, large fillings, particularly in gold—these are distinguishing features that remain in the patient's mind.

It is only when we concentrate the patient's attention on dentures that a critical assessment of tooth position begins. Unlike the natural teeth which are accepted as they erupt, new dentures are examined carefully. They also can be removed and inspected for colour, shape and arrangement of the teeth—a facility not available with one's natural teeth. Consequently, some patients criticize the arrangement of teeth on their dentures as being unlike their natural ones. The patients know that the teeth on their dentures do not appear to be the same, but they can offer only destructive criticism and cannot describe their actual desires on the arrangement of the teeth with any precision. This is particularly so after an extended period of edentulousness when memory of natural tooth detail becomes very hazy. The patient becomes confused and frustrated at not being able to achieve a restoration of their dimly remembered appearance with natural teeth. The dental practitioner must then give some guidance on tooth arrangement and position and be able to support his opinion in discussion with the patient. Hence the development of various theories of tooth position and arrangement related to the residual ridge structures.

INCISAL LEVEL

The amount of tooth displayed beneath the resting upper lip depends upon the relation between the ridge and the lip. Generally, the canine teeth are barely visible, whilst a varying amount of the incisor teeth is shown. When a patient has a short upper lip, it rises in a cupid's bow from the canine and reveals more of the crowns of the central and lateral incisors. (Fig. 23.2). In addition when there is protrusion of the upper teeth and a moderate overjet, little wear of the incisal edges of the natural teeth takes place. Conversely, when the lip is relatively straight, very little of the crowns of the incisors is shown after attrition has reduced their length. This is usually found in the older patient. (Fig. 23.3). Thus the incisal level should be taken more from the sides than from the centre of the lip.

The amount of tooth shown depends not only on the incisal level selected, but also on the anteroposterior tooth position. The more forward the teeth are set, the greater will be the amount of tooth exposed on movement of the lips.

SIZE OF TEETH

In general, artificial teeth are smaller than their natural predecessors. If a patient has been edentulous for some time and has not had the benefits of immediate dentures, the sudden insertion of teeth of a size similar to the natural ones usually causes the patient to comment on their large size. This arises from various factors. Natural teeth prior to extraction usually have restorations which break up their area whilst many artificial teeth resemble perfect natural teeth. Artificial teeth are cleaner than many natural ones particularly when the dentures are first inserted and they therefore appear to be rather large. Their labial surface is often rather flat and less rounded, so that the apparent form of the tooth appears to be larger than if a tooth with a more convex surface was used. One has a less precise appreciation of the dimensions of a well-rounded object than of a flat surface. If, in addition, the surface of the artificial tooth is not broken up by horizontal imbrication lines or vertical developmental grooves, the flatter surface reflects a broad patch of light. Such a tooth appears to be larger than one which has a broken reflecting surface.

The wishes of the patient on tooth size should always be considered, but if a patient requests very small teeth, the unsatisfactory appearance of these should be pointed out; a tooth size *slightly* smaller than one would normally use, should be selected. Outside the mouth, teeth look considerably larger than when they are partly covered by lips and less well illuminated within the oral cavity. Consequently, it is not advisable to place the articulated try-in on the

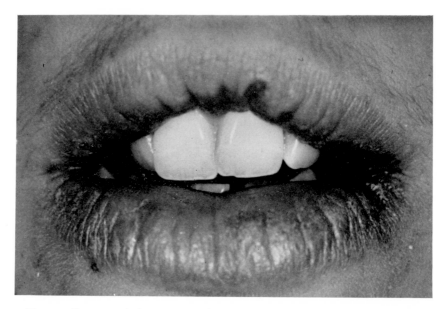

Fig. 23.2 Exposure of a large amount of the upper incisor teeth in a young person. The lip is bow shaped.

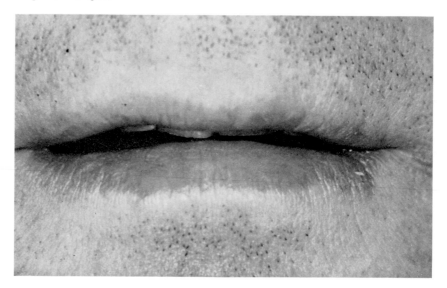

Fig. 23.3 Exposure of little of the crowns of the upper incisor teeth in an older person. The lip is relatively straight.

bracket table in front of the patient; this is particularly important when the patient is requesting somewhat smaller teeth than one would normally advise.

With modern denture base materials there is little reason for extending the teeth up to the high lip or smile line. Tinting of acrylic resins and suitable gingival carving produces a more pleasing result than the use of disproportionately long teeth, which as a result appear to be very narrow.

If the anterior teeth are to be arranged with only a small vertical overlap, it may be necessary on occasions to modify the incisal level of the upper teeth in order to allow the use of slightly longer lower teeth. Otherwise the patient may show but little of the lower teeth. This difficulty arises particularly when the natural incisors had a large vertical but little horizontal overlap (Class II, div 2). If it is essential to achieve balanced articulation, some loss of lower tooth appearance must be accepted.

SHAPE OR FORM OF TEETH

Over half a century ago, a method of selecting anterior teeth was suggested by Leon Williams. He divided face shapes into square, ovoid and tapering and considered that tooth shapes should be similar. In nature such a correlation only appears in about one third of the population as there is no genetic relationship between tooth shape and skull development.

The Williams classification therefore has little scientific background and, in addition, it is virtually impossible to describe either a tooth or a facial shape as belonging to one of the three categories. Where no other information is available, however, harmony of tooth and face shape is a safer starting point than disharmony. Complementary shapes seldom conflict but, on the other hand, it should not be forgotten that a pleasing effect may also be achieved by the use of teeth dissimilar in shape from that of the patient's face.

Other methods of tooth selection suggest that the tooth shape, convexity, surface detail and gum contouring should portray the personality, sex and age of the patient. A vigorous male personality should be provided with broad, convex-surfaced teeth with marked surface irregularities. The incisal edges should show signs of attrition due to the vigorous masticatory function which such a person would have employed. The gum contour should also be shaped to expose the necks of the teeth (Fig. 23.4). Conversely, for a delicately featured female person, slender, relatively flat-surfaced teeth with rounded incisal edges should be used, and the interdental papillae shaped as in a younger person. Between these two, a wide range of 'tooth' personalities may be achieved to reflect the personality of the patient.

One should consider the teeth purchased more as raw material rather than a finished product whose shape cannot be altered. Porcelain teeth lend themselves less to modification than acrylic teeth which can be readily ground and polished. The teeth of most people with a normal jaw relation have become

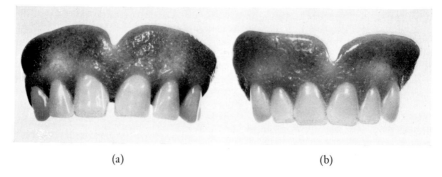

(a)   (b)

Fig. 23.4 Variations in incisal grinding, tooth shape, position and gingival contouring to produce:
(a) a vigorous;
(b) a delicate appearance.

worn by attrition by the time dentures are required, yet most manufactured teeth have unworn incisal edges. The effect of incisal grinding of teeth is shown in Fig. 23.5. The placing of restorations in artificial teeth or the use of 'characterized' teeth helps to break up the appearance of newness of artificial teeth. In females, the lateral incisors are proportionately smaller than in the male yet in many artificial teeth the lateral is a relatively broad tooth and requires modification before being set up.

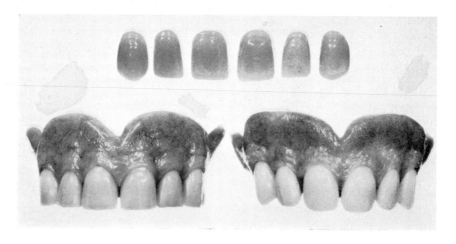

Fig. 23.5 The effect of incisal grinding on the appearance of the same mould of anterior teeth.

DETAILED TOOTH ARRANGEMENT

If teeth are set so that their labial surfaces each reflect an equal amount of light, then despite their differences in size and shape, they will appear to be similar. Differences in *angulation* between the various teeth alter the area from which light is reflected and emphasize their different shapes. Whilst a large patch of light should preferably be reflected from the centrals, only the tips of the laterals should reflect light. Prominence of the neck of the canines causes light reflection from these areas and emphasizes the breadth of the tooth arrangement when the patient smiles.

Irregularity of teeth occurs in certain fairly well-defined patterns related to the times of eruption of teeth and the jaw relation (Fig. 23.6). When tooth size

(a)

(b)   (c)

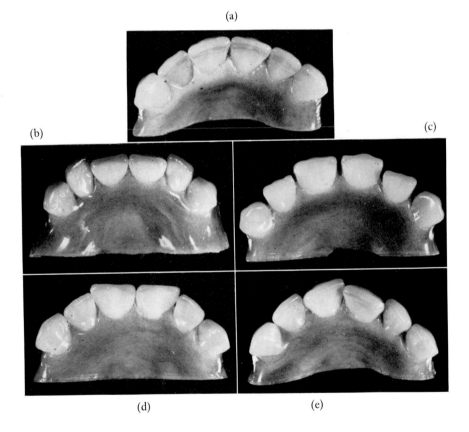

(d)   (e)

Fig. 23.6
(a) Classical setting of the anterior teeth;
(b)–(e) some common irregularities of the anterior teeth.

is small compared with the jaw size, an even spacing of teeth results and this is usually associated with attrition of the incisal edges. Overcrowding causes overlapping of the centrals and laterals and the canines usually slope forward as they erupt last into the small space available. Alternatively, the centrals may be arranged with their distal edges rotated outwards and the laterals tucked in behind them. Class II div 2 cases show a classical retroclination of the centrals with protrusion of the tips of the laterals and prominence of the canine necks.

If one compiles a representative sample from casts of patients with natural dentitions, these may be used as the basis of a prescription for the technician. Alternatively samples of tooth arrangements mounted in acrylic base may be kept both in the surgery and in the laboratory so that a prescription for tooth arrangement may be made. It should be realized that many dentists and their technicians favour a particular type of tooth irregularity. This may be related subconsciously to the arrangement of their own natural teeth.

When there is little assistance from the patient towards tooth selection and arrangement the dentist must have something positive to say, hence the various theories of denture aesthetics. It is largely, however, a matter of artistic prefer-ence to be arranged between the patient and the dentist rather than something which follows rules and principles. The variations in tooth shape and arrange-ment of the natural dentition are so numerous that it is only when we make a marked error in tooth position that a totally unsatisfactory appearance is created.

There are some patients, however, with perfectionist tendencies who are apparently determined to ensure the precisely correct arrangement of each tooth. Some time must be spent in seeking the 'perfect arrangement' but it is preferable not to spend too long. The patient should be advised when the result appears to be satisfactory. Otherwise 'plus ça change, plus c'est la même chose'. An experienced chairside assistant is invaluable when dealing with the dental appearance of ladies. By leaving the patient to talk with another female, one can frequently get agreement of tooth position if the assistant confirms the opinion expressed by the dentist.

SHADE OF TEETH

The colour of teeth is derived from internal reflection from the dentine and enamel structure and from surface staining of the teeth due to smoking, stand-ard of oral hygiene, etc. The hues or shades of teeth appear also to be related to general facial skin colour and the colour of the hair and the eyes. A swarthy person usually has teeth of a darker shade than a fair-skinned, naturally blonde person. There is usually some balance or harmony between skin colour and tooth shade. The teeth of a darker person may appear to be very white, but, in fact, it is only by contrast with the skin colour that they do so. With age, the teeth darken and appear to be more grey, due to a greater degree of mineralization of their structure. This greying is probably due to less light being reflected from the layers of tooth near the surface and more entering deeper into the tooth and being lost sideways. In the young patient, the teeth are of a creamier or yellower hue.

Suitable teeth are often described as being of yellow or red hue rather than blue or green-yellow. Warmth and light are given by the hues yellow and red, whilst teeth with a blue-grey tinge do not resemble the natural teeth to the same extent. The precise mechanism of 'colour' or hue in natural teeth is unknown and the tooth manufacturer is therefore presented with a problem in matching artificial and natural tooth shades. In addition, colour of the surroundings, lighting and visual fatigue all affect the appearance of the teeth.

When recording tooth shade, a comparison should be made by holding a tooth against the skin and then, after moistening it with the patient's saliva, it should be placed in position partly hidden by the upper lip. It will then be in a similar colour environment to the teeth on the denture.

As with tooth size, the shade of tooth should be examined by the patient when the trial dentures are in the mouth. Freqently a comparison is made of the teeth set up in wax against the white cast or articulating plaster. Comparison with this white surface makes the teeth appear too dark in shade to the critical patient.

GINGIVAL CONTOUR

The waxing up of the denture has a marked effect upon the appearance of the teeth. Too often craftsmanship or expediency in finishing and polishing the denture result in a gingival contour unlike that of the natural dentition. Healthy, natural gingival tissues are only moderately contoured and their surface resembles 'orange peel' rather than a smooth, polished surface. A heavily contoured denture is simply difficult to clean whilst large, smooth interdental papillae spoil the appearance of the artificial teeth.

Changes occur in the gingival tissue contour with age, and waxing up, suitable for a patient in the 30 to 40 year age group, is different from that required in an older patient. Loss of interdental papillae and exposure of cement at the necks of the teeth are normal features in the older patient. These changes in gingival contour can be prescribed by the dentist if a standard is set for use both in the surgery and by the technician. Only two or three types of contouring need be defined, related to the age of the patient (Fig. 23.7). On occasion, however, with a patient who does not keep the denture clean, it is advisable to provide an uncontoured denture with a highly polished surface

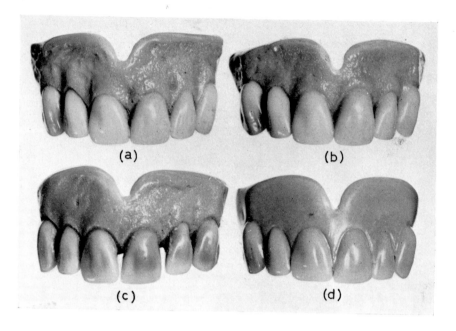

Fig. 23.7 Variations in gingival contour:
(a) up to 40 years;
(b) 40 to 60 years;
(c) over 60 years;
(d) smooth surface for a patient with poor oral hygiene.

and with moderate papillae filling the interdental spaces, so preventing the accumulation of debris or stain in these areas.

In patients with a very short upper lip who will expose the gumwork of the denture, this should not only be contoured, but should also be coloured to resemble natural gum tissue. One may use different shades of veined denture base materials to simulate the difference between the lighter gingivae and the more deeply coloured reflected mucosa. Alternatively, a veneer of acrylic resin may be made which forms the labial flange of the denture. This veneer is painted on its inner aspect to the required colour and is then joined to the remainder of the denture base.

TRY-IN COMPLETION

The dentist, having come to his own assessment of the appearance of the dentures, then consults the patient for his or her comments. The patient should be given a hand mirror or may stand in front of a wall mirror and so examine their appearance in normal room lighting away from the dental chair. Then by discussion and comment, aided particularly in the case of a female patient by the dental surgery assistant, the patient's comments can usually be obtained and alterations made within the limits imposed by denture function. Again the trial dentures should not remain in the mouth for too long a time as softening of the wax and movement or displacement of the teeth may occur.

The amount of lip support afforded by the denture bases may have to be changed. Frequently, additions to the base on the canine and premolar regions, particularly of the upper denture, are necessary in order to reduce the nasolabial folds.

Modifications to the Casts

Routine relief of certain areas, e.g. the centre of the palate, is not advocated. Reduction of pressure from the denture is, however, necessary over hard bony nodules with a thin mucosal covering, over trigger points or over a very prominent torus palatinus. Areas of pressure from the impression tray should also be relieved and these should already be shown in outline on the cast.

Whilst the edge of any relief area must eventually be chamfered, the outline of the area to be relieved is marked on the cast. The thickness of tinfoil is then prescribed. Usually gauge 4 (0.25 mm) tinfoil is used for normal relief and gauge 7 (0·50 mm) where it is necessary to create a large space. With the thicker tinfoil some hyperplasia of mucosa into the space will take place after a few months' wear.

Tissue undercuts should be assessed for their effect in preventing the insertion

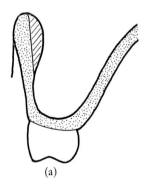   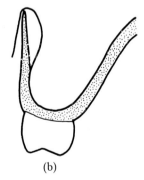

(a)   (b)

Fig. 23.8 Treatment of undercuts:
(a) the flange is thickened and the hatched part trimmed away subsequently at the chairside allowing insertion of the denture;
(b) the effect of trimming the fitting surface of a flange of normal thickness is to leave an unfavourable knife-edged border.

of the denture. Palpation reveals whether the undercut is bony or fibrous and the depth of undercut can be assessed on the cast. Unilateral undercuts present little difficulty, but where undercuts oppose each other, one or both must be modified. In the upper jaw undercuts in the canine region may oppose a tuberosity undercut on the other side. A general undercut in the anterior region of the lower jaw extending buccally, labially and lingually to the premolar regions also causes difficulties. The casts should be surveyed to determine the most suitable path of insertion.

Since the denture should extend fully into the sulcus even if not sideways into the undercut, it is advisable to modify the cast where a large undercut exists. Fibrous tissue undercuts of 3 to 4 mm can be accepted whereas a bony undercut must be reduced until only 1 to 2 mm remains.

Two methods are used. Either the undercut is partly filled in on the cast leaving slightly more than one thinks will be tolerated; usually plaster is applied to the undercut area reaching into the sulcus. Alternatively, the technician is asked to thicken the periphery of the denture over the undercut and so allow for trimming on the fitting surface of the denture before inserting it (Fig. 23.8). If only a small amount of adjustment is necessary on inserting the denture, the extra bulk on the polished surface can quickly be removed.

If the impression procedure did not incorporate selective tissue displacement at the post dam area, this area is palpated and a suitable amount is scraped from the cast. The post dam should extend laterally to the hamular notches. More pressure should be created on either side of the midline where a greater thickness of submucosa exists.

In cases where the surface of the palatal mucosa is nodular, it is advisable to prescribe that the entire surface of the cast be covered by a very thin tinfoil (gauge 40, 0·05 mm). This smooths the fitting surface and reduces trauma to the tissues from the rough surface of the denture.

PRESCRIPTION

The prescription to the technician to complete the dentures should include:
1 Materials to be used
2 Any changes in posterior tooth arrangement
3 Any aesthetic improvements to the anterior teeth
4 Reduction of undercuts or thickening of flanges
5 Tinfoiling for relief of hard areas, or to give a smooth fitting surface
6 Gingival contour and colouring required
7 Weight of previous lower denture where necessary.

Chapter 24

Finished Dentures

Despite the rapid growth in the range of available polymers, methyl methacrylate (acrylic resin) with a small degree of copolymerization, still appears to be the most satisfactory denture base material. Polystyrene, epoxy and polycarbonate resins are being used, but whilst their physical properties in the laboratory are good, there is not at present sufficient evidence to show that they are superior to the acrylic resins for oral use. There are occasions, however, when the use of an alternative denture base is to be considered. The three main reasons are: suspected allergy to methyl methacrylate, secondly the desire to create a less traumatic and more hygienic fitting surface, and thirdly, the weakness of an acrylic resin denture base allowing repeated fracture.

ALLERGY

True allergy to methyl methacrylate is a rare occurrence. Polymerized methyl methacrylate causes no tissue reaction but monomer is a tissue irritant. The reaction to monomer may be a primary irritation as occurs with many chemicals placed upon the skin or mucosa. On the other hand, monomer can sensitize tissues so that when this chemical is applied on any subsequent occasion, an allergic reaction occurs. The use of free monomer in the mouth is therefore not advised. With care, a small amount of self-cure base may be added to a denture, but coverage of large areas of tissue with unpolymerized methyl methacrylate dough is to be avoided.

All processed acrylic dentures made from a powder/liquid dough contain some residual monomer. This may be present as single molecules, or as short molecular chains. It is probable that none of the monomer remaining in a correctly processed denture can be leached out in water or saliva. However, if processing is carried out at too low a temperature or for too short a time, more residual monomer is left and this may be washed out into the saliva film between the denture and the tissues. The rate of leaching out depends upon the degree of under-curing and the thickness of the denture itself. It may be assumed that an under-cured, thick, lower denture would continue to release monomer for a longer period of time than a thin upper plate. The monomer released may cause primary irritation or it may produce an allergic reaction in a patient who has previously been sensitized. Skin reaction tests (patch tests) can be performed on patients suspected of having an allergy to methyl methacrylate. However, the interpretation of such tests is not always satisfactory. With a true allergy, all tissues in contact with the polished and the fitting surface of the denture are affected and not only those of the denture bearing area.

Acrylic dentures may be processed at 70 to 75° C for 8 to 10 hours, though it is preferable to always conclude the curing cycle with thirty minutes at 100° C. This reduces the amount of residual monomer to a negligible amount. Processing is just as important when rebasing a denture as it is when making a new one. Frequently, the processing of a rebase is skimped because of lack of time, and on occasions much residual monomer will remain unpolymerized. Self-cure acrylic materials contain more residual monomer after hardening than do heat-cure materials after processing. It is advisable to leave a denture made from self-cure base for as long as possible and so ensure maximum polymerization. If it is then stored in water for at least a day before giving it to the patient, the possibility of monomer irritation will be reduced.

Other possible sources of chemical irritation are the initiator (benzoyl peroxide), the inhibitor (hydroquinone) or the pigment. Whilst these are all possible irritants, it is doubtful whether any of them can be leached out of the denture base. A contact reaction of these constituents with the mucosa is possible, however; but it is probable that the saliva film prevents the actual contact of denture base and tissue necessary to produce such a reaction. In most of the present day acrylic denture bases there is no plasticizer, and therefore irritation from this source can usually be discounted.

Denture cleansers may cause irritation if they are not washed off the denture before it is replaced in the mouth. Those based on perborates may also produce sensitization.

Most cases of burning sensation under dentures are due to trauma from the dentures often associated with a lowered tissue resistance. In a true allergy a denture of another polymer must be made or alternatively a metal based denture provided.

METAL BASED DENTURES

A metal based denture may be advised because of inflammation of the soft tissues of the denture bearing area, or to produce a stronger denture.

The beneficial effect of a metal base is probably due mainly to a reduction in trauma to the tissues and also the achievement of better oral hygiene. The swaged metal base in particular has a smoother contour. As a consequence, its fitting surface does not present sharp abrasive prominences to irritate the tissues and it is also cleaned more easily. Since metal is a good thermal conductor, some additional benefit may arise from an increased blood circulation in the tissues stimulated by warm foodstuffs.

A metal based denture may be recommended for greater strength where

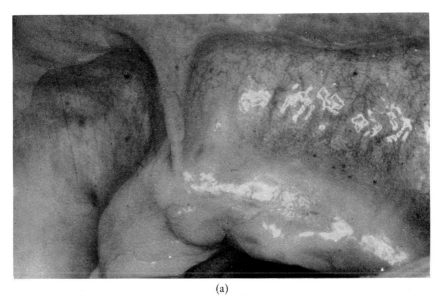

(a)

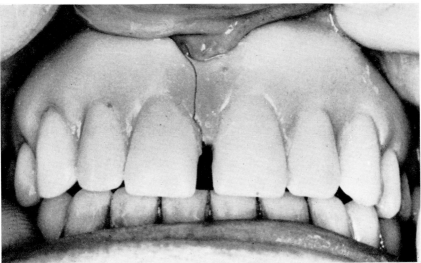

(b)

Fig. 24.1
(a) A large labial frenum;
(b) the resultant midline fracture of the upper denture.

fracture of the denture has recurred. Fracture of a complete upper denture occurs due to:

1 A large frenum attached near to the crest of the ridge, causing a weakening of the denture flange at this point (Fig. 24.1). Acrylic resin is one of the many materials that show notch sensitivity, i.e. small notches in the material are capable of reducing the strength of a part considerably. Midline fracture of an upper denture begins at the base of the incisal notch, gradually spreading along the labial flange and palate. The larger the labial frenum, the greater is the risk of midline fracture.

Whilst a metal denture is stronger than one of acrylic resin, consideration should also be given to resecting a large labial frenum.

2 Large mandibular arch and small maxilla, resulting in the upper teeth being placed outside the ridge.

3 Heavy masticatory force, or tooth clenching and grinding in an anxious patient, particularly with well-developed masseter muscles.

4 Heavy unbalanced forces on the upper denture of a patient who has teeth only in the anterior segment of the lower jaw and who cannot wear a partial lower denture, Naturally, the patient must be encouraged to wear the partial lower denture. At times, however, this is difficult to achieve.

An upper metal based denture may also be advised in cases of nausea where the thinner metal plate is more easily tolerated than the thicker resin palate. It may also be necessary for professional vocalists and speakers to avoid any great effects upon the shape of the oral cavity and therefore on the quality of sound produced. Recurrent fracture of a lower denture occurs if it has to be made very narrow because of a reduction in the width of the neutral zone. The incorporation of a soft lining in a shallow lower denture may weaken it and necessitate the addition, not of a metal base, but of a cast strengthening piece on the lingual aspect of the denture (Fig. 24.2).

The alloys used for metal denture bases are stainless steel, cobalt-chromium and gold. A cast cobalt-chromium denture base is a little heavier than a swaged stainless steel plate, but it is more rigid and better adapted. Therefore it should give slightly better retention and a longer clinical life without fracture. Research on explosive and hydraulic forming of very thin stainless steel plates, however, indicates that the greater detail obtained during this type of swaging produces a light plate with adequate rigidity and good adaptation.

INSERTION OF THE DENTURES

After processing, all dentures should be kept in water until they are inserted into the patient's mouth; otherwise shrinkage of the denture base takes place.

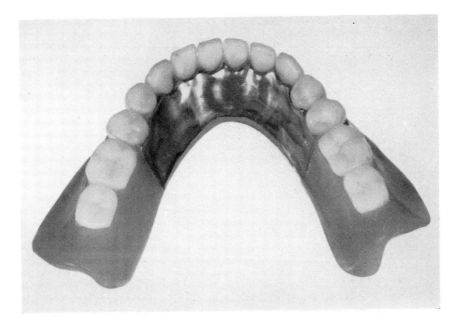

Fig. 24.2 A cast strengthening piece on the lingual aspect of a lower denture based with a soft lining.

Whilst complete sterility of the denture is an ideal to be aimed for, it is difficult to achieve in practice. Immersion of the dentures in a dilute solution of an antiseptic reduces the number of bacteria carried from the laboratory into the dental surgery and the patient's mouth. A simple method of storing dentures in a moist, antiseptic atmosphere, is to place them together with a piece of polyethylene sponge soaked in antiseptic, in a small polythene bag.

Before the patient attends, the fitting surface of the dentures should be examined for pimples and other protuberances due to errors or damage to the casts. Small air bubbles near to the surface of the casts become filled with denture base during processing and if the resultant pimples are left, they produce small ulcers due to high local pressure. Since they are attached to the denture by only a thin stalk, the pimples are readily removed by a blunt scraper. Defects in the cast due to dropping it or cutting it with a knife can be recognized by the shape of surface produced. A raised rosette shape or rough surface indicates damage to the surface of the cast, whilst a tent-shaped ridge shows damage from a knife blade. These areas should be recognized and smoothed with a small carborundum stone. Undue roughness of the palatal surface of a denture detected by moving the finger over it, should also be smoothed either by sandpaper, lightly applied, or with a fine carborundum wheel, followed by lightly smoothing with pumice.

The edges of the dentures are examined to ensure that no angles remain, but that the fitting surface moves in a continuous curve to join the polished surface. Frequently, a sharp edge remains at the sides of frena where the denture periphery has been polished without moving it about sufficiently in relation to the buff.

An assessment is made of the probable difficulty of insertion when marked undercuts are seen to exist. With experience these undercuts may be modified a little at this stage, but generally, it is preferable to await the arrival of the patient and see whether the denture can be inserted. Sometimes a denture with large undercuts may be inserted much more easily than might have been thought when first looking at its fitting surface.

After removing previous dentures, the new upper denture is first inserted. Any resistance to seating the denture due to undercuts is overcome not by force, but by trying different angles of approach. An experienced denture wearer can often place a new denture in position more easily than the operator and it is worthwhile asking the patient to help if the denture almost goes into place. If the denture cannot be inserted, the tissues at the periphery are examined for blanching due to pressure, and the patient is also asked to point out any pressure areas. Reduction of undercuts gradually enables the denture to be inserted. The greatest difficulties occur in persons with large rounded ridges that are only covered by a thin mucoperiosteum. Then, only small undercuts can be tolerated and the denture must be adjusted accordingly.

After insertion, the border of the denture is checked. Overextension is indicated either by displacement of the denture on lip or cheek movement, or by obvious pressure into the sulcus. Due to the vascularity of the sulcus tissues it is not usual to find any blanching except on gross overextension. The posterior border is confirmed by asking the patient to say 'ah', and noting the relation of the denture to the vibration line. The patient is asked to relax the lips and the position and relation of the incisors to the lip together with the amount of support from the denture flange is noted.

Modifications to the denture may be made at the chairside. Alternatively, by drawing on the polished surfaces, instructions of the amount of reduction necessary are given to the technician. Ideally of course, the correct denture extension should have been defined by the impression but on occasions an overextended or bulky denture is seen at the finish stage.

A similar procedure is now followed with the lower denture. In addition, the tongue space is checked and any lingual overextension detected by asking the patient to wet the lips with the tip of the tongue and then to place it in the region of the parotid duct on the inside of each cheek in turn. Movement of the denture on tongue protrusion indicates overextension over the mylohyoid muscle.

OCCLUSION

Next, the patient is asked to occlude the teeth. Even contact of all posterior teeth in the muscular position is the first essential. If a heavy contact can be seen, either of one tooth, or in the posterior segment of the dentures, grinding of the offending teeth of one denture only will usually produce an even occlusion. Smaller uneven occlusal contacts are revealed by the use of articulating paper, carbon paper, wax, or thin cellulose sheets—the patient being asked to occlude the teeth with a light tapping motion. The patient who is experienced in denture wearing can detect small uneven contacts and point out their position. The less experienced patient can usually recognize only larger occlusal defects.

It is not advisable to trim the teeth of both dentures to reduce an occlusal error or much of the cusp formation may be lost.

If a large occlusal error is seen which would be difficult, if not impossible, to rectify by grinding at the chairside, a new intra-oral occlusal record should be made. In such cases the occlusal face height is often too great and a reduction is necessary in addition to achieving balanced occlusal contacts. To make this adjustment the dentures should be mounted in a relation to the hinge-axis on the articulator that is similar to their relation to the patient's condyles. This may be achieved most accurately by using a facebow.

An intra-oral record is obtained using a thin layer of wax. The patient is asked to close *into*, but not *through* the wax. In the laboratory, the dentures are mounted on the articulator, and selective grinding of the offending teeth carried out. Some articulators incorporate a mechanical drive which enables 'grinding in' of an incorrect occlusion to be carried out rapidly.

The incidence of errors of this kind may be reduced by remounting the dentures on the articulator on which they were set up, immediately after processing. Technical errors introduced during processing may then be eliminated. Preparation for remounting the dentures on the articulator in this way is done whilst they are still in the waxed-up state. With care, the cast may be removed from the articulating plaster leaving two intact surfaces which fit accurately together. If similar care is taken to remove the processed denture together with its cast from the flask after processing, it may be replaced in the same position on the articulator. Correction of the error introduced during processing may then be rectified by spot grinding, followed by 'milling' of the occlusal surfaces with a fine abrasive. This reduces the clinical time spent in achieving balanced occlusion and articulation.

When the occlusal error is due to an incorrect recording of the horizontal jaw relation and the teeth have been arranged to occlude in an incorrect protrusive or lateral relation, then the posterior teeth of one or both dentures must be removed and reset in the correct relation.

Only when an even tooth contact is achieved can one assess the occlusal face height and the general effect of the dentures on appearance, and begin to consider balanced articulation. Comparison with the previous dentures enables the operator to assess the amount of increase or decrease in jaw separation which has been achieved, and by comparing old and new dentures he may see whether his prescription for the modifications in the replacement dentures has been accurately carried out.

RETRUSIVE FACETS

If difficulties have been experienced in recording the muscular position, the ligamentous position may have been used. It is then necessary to free the occlusion so that the jaw may slide approximately 1 mm forward in a sagittal plane to the muscular position. This is done by grinding the distal slope of the upper buccal cusps and the mesial slope of the lower lingual cusps. Then the patient has a range of even occlusal contact between the ligamentous and muscular positions but retains retrusive facets preventing any greater backward movement of the mandible beyond the ligamentous position.

It may also be considered necessary to do the reverse of this adjustment, that is to grind the occlusion as seen in the muscular position to allow for use of the retruded position during vigorous mastication. Occlusion is then over a range of horizontal movement of approximately 1 mm between the ligamentous and muscular positions.

BALANCED ARTICULATION

In Chapter 9, the question of whether balanced articulation should be provided with complete dentures was discussed. It was suggested that it was more important to provide for *the possibility* of a smooth interference-free gliding of the posterior teeth than to provide fully balanced articulation in all cases.

Some patients, particularly those receiving dentures for the first time, find difficulty in making lateral and protrusive excursions. It is not advisable to worry the patient unduly at this stage, but to achieve even occlusal contact and then to await the development of some denture experience during the next few days before deciding to what extent balanced contacts in articulation are necessary.

Other patients readily perform jaw movements with new dentures and points of interference can be noted either by direct examination or by recording them with articulating paper, etc. Interference of the anterior teeth is readily seen and is adjusted by grinding the incisal edges of the teeth at an angle until the interference is eliminated.

If it is considered that balanced contacts in articulation are advisable, two colours of articulating paper may be used, one for the left and the other for the right lateral movement. In this way the working and balancing contacts on each side are seen. Heavy contacts are adjusted according to the 'BULL' rule. That is, one should grind the Buccal cusps of the Upper and the Lingual cusps of the Lower teeth. Interference of the posterior teeth in lateral excursions occurs as a result of too great a cusp angle, due to an inadequate curve of Monson. Hence, by grinding the upper buccal cusp, this angle is reduced (Fig 24.3). The lingual cusps of the lower teeth similarly create too steep an angle of movement on the working side. In no circumstances should the lower buccal cusps be ground. Otherwise the even occlusion obtained in the inter-cuspal position will be lost.

After peripheral, bulk, occlusal and articulation adjustments have been completed, the patient is given a hand mirror to examine the dentures in the

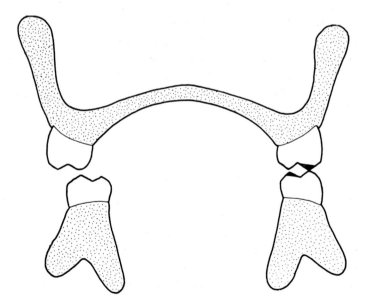

Fig. 24.3 Reduction of the upper buccal cusp angle to obtain balanced contacts on lateral movements.

mouth. Any small aesthetic alterations to incisal edges may then be done before the dentures are dispatched to the laboratory for polishing.

ADVICE TO THE PATIENT

On delivery of new dentures, the patient is advised of the necessity for patience during the period of adaptation. Even though replacement dentures may be very similar to the previous ones, a few days or weeks may pass before the patient has achieved good control over the new denture shape.

The doubting, aggressive, or indifferent patient may not cooperate in overcoming initial discomfort and inconvenience. It is advisable to retain the previous dentures of this type of patient for at least a week. Otherwise they may alternate between old and new dentures and never overcome the difficulties of initial adaptation.

The limitations of dentures will already have deen discussed with the patient when assessing the prognosis at the examination stage. It does little harm, however, to reiterate the amount of improvement to be expected, particularly if only a small improvement has been aimed for. Otherwise, the patient may wonder why the 'new' dentures have not removed all previous difficulties and complaints.

Patients are advised to cut up food at first and not to rely upon incision of large food portions. Until the bulk of the dentures has been accepted, the portions of food placed in the mouth should be small. As a consequence, meals will take a little longer and tough fibrous foods should be avoided for some time. Incision of foodstuffs should not be done in the incisor region, but in the canine region of the dentures, where displacement is resisted by the opposite tuberosity. Instead of breaking the portion of food off by a downward movement, it should be fractured by a slight upward twist which presses the dentures more firmly against the tissues.

Wearing of complete dentures at night is not advised as a routine. Whilst removal every night is ideal, aesthetic reasons and domestic harmony may not allow it. Occasional removal at night, say one night in three, is therefore advised. This reduces the possibility of the development of a denture stomatitis. During the first few nights, however, after delivery of the dentures, the patient is advised to wear them. Stimulation by the denture of nerve endings in the mucosa of the lips, cheeks, tongue and ridges, continues whilst the patient is asleep and awareness of these new sensations fades more quickly than if the dentures are inserted afresh each morning. Naturally, the patient should remove the dentures for cleaning after eating, and before going to bed.

A patient should not experience pain with correctly made dentures. Pain is caused by an error of a half millimetre or more in the dimensions of the fitting surface or 1 to 2 mm of the border. Irritation caused by inaccuracies in the fitting surface should seldom be seen. Inflammation from overextension is more common.

The patient should be seen after 2 days. Then pressure, due to small errors or slight overextension, will have produced inflammation and not ulceration, and the denture can be adjusted before pain is experienced. If the patient does not attend for a week or longer, then ulceration may be produced and the patient may remove the dentures before attending, making it difficult to discover the actual place of irritation.

When a marked change in facial support or tooth appearance has been considered necessary, it is advisable to warn patients of the possible comments of their 'friends'. Only too frequently dentures for a patient with considerable dental difficulty are constructed to their satisfaction and on the basis of advice from the practitioner, yet after a week or so they meet someone who comments upon their changed appearance. The patient should therefore be warned against this type of thoughtless remark.

Chapter 25

Denture Adjustments: Complaints

Unfortunately, many dentists consider the adjustment of dentures after insertion as an unwanted chore. In an effort to dispense with it the dentist may adopt one of two methods of treatment. He may exhort the patient to persevere, notwithstanding discomfort, on the premise that the dentures will 'bed in'. Alternatively, in an over-eagerness to rid the patient of all his troubles at one visit border areas and the occlusal surfaces may be mutilated.

Either course results in future problems. In the case of 'perseverance', severe damage to the oral tissues may ensue. After gross reduction of the denture extension, problems of retention, stability and efficient function increase. Careless trimming of the occlusal surfaces destroys cuspal form and reduces masticatory efficiency. The result is that the patient becomes more and more dissatisfied.

Having entered into a contract to provide the patient with complete dentures, the dentist is under a moral obligation to ensure that the dentures are as satisfactory as can be expected for that particular patient. Apart from obvious injury to the supporting tissues by the dentures and gross errors in denture construction, the patient's complaints and problems must always be assessed in relation to the expectations of both the clinician and the patient regarding the degree of success to be achieved—success in terms of function, aesthetics, retention, stability and comfort.

Before treatment, the dentist discusses with the patient the degree of success to be expected. This is not to say that he should display pessimism in difficult cases, but rather that by discussion and explanation he can gain the patient's confidence and prepare for the degree of compromise that may be necessary— a compromise between the patient's wishes and the dentist's knowledge of what can be done in the particular clinical situation.

During the period of treatment, the dentist has a further opportunity to assess the potentiality of the mouth for denture success and also the attitude of the patient. The clinical examination may have revealed certain inherent dental problems. In some cases, these may have been wholly or partly eliminated during the mouth preparation, but in many others the problems remain.

Unfortunately, many denture patients believe that the onus for success rests solely with the dentist and do not realize the part they must play during the early postinsertion days. They compare the success of their own prostheses with that of their friends and relations who may have better support for dentures or a more equable temperament. The dentist's problems are often considerable if he undertakes treatment for husband and wife or near neighbours. How frequently it seems that one has ideal mouth conditions for denture success whilst the other possesses all the inherent problems that are likely to result in much less than the 100 per cent success the patient inevitably expects.

ASSESSMENT OF THE TREATMENT GIVEN

During the examination and treatment of the patient many decisions have been made with regard to extension of the denture bases, tooth size, shape and position, jaw relations and general denture shape. In cooperation with the technician a prescription has been determined and faithfully carried out.

When seeing the patient at the insertion or first postinsertion visit, an assessment should be made of the accuracy with which these decisions have been interpreted in practice. Human frailty is such that perfection is not possible on every occasion, nor in all cases is it essential to success. Many patients wear dentures successfully though they have many constructional defects. But when the dental condition and the patient's attitude demand near perfection in order to achieve success, then the degree of permissible error is only small. No excuses to the patient at this stage will overcome the effects of an error which has unfortunately been incorporated in the finished dentures. Any attempt to put off the treatment necessary to rectify the error, only reduces the patient's confidence when later, treatment can no longer be avoided and the error is at length rectified. If the dentist is satisfied that no errors in construction have arisen, then the complaints of the patient can be discussed with much greater confidence.

COMPLAINTS

It is advisable to listen carefully to the patient's complaint because the diagnosis and remedy may not be immediately obvious.

Complaints soon after denture insertion fall under one or more of the following headings:

> Discomfort and pain
> Nausea
> Poor retention and stability

Noise
Masticatory inefficiency
Poor aesthetics
Speech difficulties

DISCOMFORT AND PAIN

Patients frequently find difficulty in differentiating between pain and discomfort. By definition, pain is a sensation varying from a prick to an ache aroused by a physical or chemical stimulus. Sherrington's definition of pain is 'the psychical adjunct of an imperative protective reflex'. This is helpful to the organism in that a 'withdrawal' response to the pain prevents further injury. As mucous membrane is richly innervated, the tissues of the denture bearing areas are particularly prone to give pain in response to physical stimulation. Discomfort is less intense and generally less localized than pain and is more a state of physical 'uneasiness'. In attempting to relate the terms discomfort and pain, pain might well be described as *acute discomfort*.

GENERAL DISCOMFORT

This is perhaps the most difficult complaint to assess. Not only do patients often experience difficulty in describing what is troubling them and locating the area involved, but there is also considerable variation in the tolerance of discomfort. This is related to the pain perception threshold. What may be intense and intolerable pain to one person may be only slight discomfort to another. Patients in poor general health, those with nutritional deficiences and those who are psychologically disturbed, are likely to have a low pain threshold. They may well complain of generalized discomfort or pain in the tissues of the whole of the denture bearing areas.

Atrophic changes in the supporting tissues of the older patient contribute to intolerance of dentures, since thinning of the epithelium and atrophy of the mucosa and submucosa, predispose to discomfort under denture pressure. With a thin and often non-resilient mucosa, the nerve endings are compressed between the hard, unyielding denture base and the underlying bone. The painful response will be exaggerated if the crest of the underlying alveolar ridge is irregular and sharp.

One of the commonest causes of general discomfort and a burning sensation is heavy loading of the tissues. This occurs more frequently in the lower jaw since the denture bearing area is smaller. Heavy pressures are caused by dentures with too great an occlusal face height, which encroach on or obliterate the freeway space. Attempts by the patient to 'fit' the dentures better by biting hard, and tooth clenching by a patient under stress, produce similar symptoms.

Treatment is directed at reduction of the stresses applied to the ridges. Confirmation of adequate denture extension, sufficient freeway space and even occlusal contacts are all necessary. A localized alveoloplasty should be considered to reduce bony prominences and smooth an irregular alveolar ridge. A soft lining may be prescribed in cases of atrophy of the tissues of the denture bearing area and low tolerance of denture pressure.

The Particular Problems of the Climacteric

During the climacteric, regressive changes may occur in the oral mucosa and bone in those women in whom there is a sudden and complete deprivation of oestrogen. The oral symptoms that may occur include a burning sensation at the sides, tip and base of the tongue and the soft tissues covered by the dentures, and abnormal taste sensations, together with generalized oral discomfort.

It is not uncommon to find the patient blaming her dentures for the oral discomfort and abnormal taste sensation. Although on examination the dentures may prove to be technically perfect, they do undoubtedly contribute to the patient's unhappiness by directing occlusal forces onto supporting tissues which have a reduced resistance to loading.

The patient requires sympathy and understanding from the dentist. One is likely to be dealing with an alveolar ridge of reduced size covered by an atrophic mucosa. As the pain threshold may also be lowered, dentures must spread the occlusal load widely. When dryness of the mouth is pronounced, a glycerine and lemon mouthwash may be helpful in providing lubrication and reducing the abrasive effect of the denture base on the soft tissues. Where severe atrophic changes have occurred in the surface epithelial layers, a gynaecologist should be consulted with a view to possible local or systemic hormonal treatment in an attempt to increase the thickness of the protective epithelium.

The Particular Problems of Ageing

All the tissues that make up the stomatognathic system are affected by increasing age. In general the tissues lose their adaptability and their tolerance to irritant factors and their potential for repair.

Because nutrition plays a large part in the health of the ageing oral tissues and their ability to respond favourably to denture coverage, the patient should be given advice on diet. The temptation of the old patient to take a diet high in carbohydrate and low in protein should be avoided. He should be advised of the need for adequate protein intake supplemented with vitamins and minerals.

LOCAL PAIN

Compression of nerve endings and pain is likely over prominent parts of the denture bearing area, particularly where there is only a thin covering of soft tissue. Anatomical features particularly prone are the mylohyoid ridges and the genial tubercles.

Normal occlusal loading may result in areas of pain over retained roots or unerupted teeth that are lying just beneath the mucosa. Routine radiographic examination before denture construction would prevent this occurrence.

Where there has been gross alveolar resorption in the lower jaw, the mental foraminae, originally situated on the buccal surface of the mandible, come to lie on its superior surface. Pressure from a denture on the mental nerve fibres emerging from the foramen results in pain. This may be localized, but is more commonly referred as a neuralgic pain to the side of the face and may result in paraesthesia to the lower lip and chin. It can usually be diagnosed by locating the mental foramen and producing the same response by applying pressure either by the finger or with a ball-ended instrument.

Treatment of these causes of pain is directed to local relief of the denture base over the painful areas.

Other common causes of local discomfort and pain beneath a denture are faults in denture design or construction. These may be related to the border, the fitting surface, the occlusal surface or the polished surfaces.

Border Faults

Overextension of the denture borders causes an area of inflammation which may develop into an ulcer unless relieved. Common sites are the labial and buccal frena and the lower buccal and lingual sulci. Careful adjustment of the denture is indicated.

The posterior border of the upper denture will cause trauma if it is positioned incorrectly on the hard palate or is overcompressing the tissues of the soft palate. In the first instance the post dam area must be correctly extended by rebasing the denture but in the second, a reduction of the prominence of the post dam will suffice.

Fitting Surface Faults

Roughness, pimples, sharp ridges may have been missed at the time of insertion of the dentures and the fitting surfaces should be checked again for such defects. The fitting surface may be poorly adapted to the basal tissues because of a faulty impression, processing on a damaged cast, or because dimensional errors have occurred in processing. These will result in local overcompression of the basal tissues. Where the general adaptation is very poor, rebasing or the provision of a new denture is indicated. When there are isolated areas of overcompression, the use of pressure indicating pastes or disclosing waxes will help the operator to accurately locate pressure points and relieve the denture locally. It should be realized that painful irritation and ulceration only arise where an error of $\frac{1}{2}$ mm or more has been made in the shape of the fitting surface of the denture. This is a gross error and, with moderate care in clinical and laboratory work, such pain for the patient can be avoided.

The pressure required to seat a denture over a bony undercut may cause a local laceration of the mucosa as it is pressed into place. The inner aspect of the denture flange should be eased carefully until the denture goes into place under only light pressure.

Occlusal Surface Faults

A common cause of pain beneath dentures, either on the crest of the alveolar ridge or on the inclines, is a lack of balanced contact in occlusion. Failure to record the correct horizontal jaw relation means that the intercuspal and muscular positions do not coincide (Fig. 25.1). It is not uncommon to find that patients, who have given a number of different horizontal relations at registration and trial denture stages, will go into the reproducible muscular position soon after the insertion of the dentures. This may mean that the teeth now assume a cusp to cusp contact, increasing the occlusal face height and overloading the basal tissues.

Even when the correct horizontal jaw relation has been recorded, it is not uncommon to find premature occlusal contacts which cause pain and displacement of the dentures away from the tissues during function. Uneven and premature contacts in articulation cause pain if patients use lateral and incisal contacts in mastication.

Cheek and tongue biting are caused by encroachment by the teeth into the normal areas of action of the cheeks and the tongue, together with the lack of a sufficient buccal overlap of the lower posterior teeth by the uppers. Cheek biting, particularly, is likely to occur in elderly patients where the cheek tissues have lost their earlier elasticity. An addition to the denture base above the upper teeth may help to hold the cheek out of harm's way (Fig. 25.2). Repositioning of the posterior teeth may be necessary but should be delayed to see whether the muscles and soft tissues are able to adapt satisfactorily to the new position of the teeth.

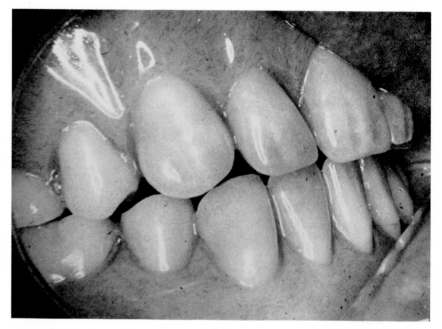

(a)

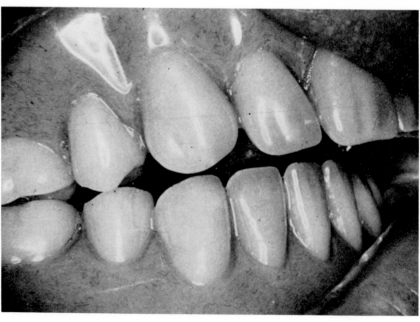

(b)

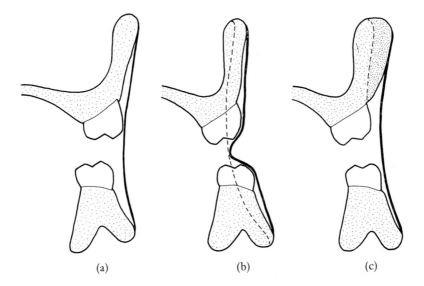

Fig. 25.2 Posterior tooth relation and the possibility of cheek biting:
(a) normal tooth relation—the cheek is held away from the occlusal contact area;
(b) 'crossbite' relation of the teeth—the cheek is likely to get trapped (The dotted line
   indicates the resting position of the cheek without the dentures);
(c) thickening of the upper buccal flange to keep the cheek away from the danger area.

Polished Surface Faults

Over-enthusiastic stippling and contouring of the labial surfaces may result
in irritation of the lip mucosa. A sharp gingival crevice on the lingual or palatal
surface may irritate the tip of the tongue. Improper shaping of the lingual
flanges of the lower denture cramps the tongue which then becomes inflamed
and sore. Discomfort is often felt on the posterolateral tongue surface where
the vertically aligned foliate papillae are to be found.

NAUSEA

There are patients who profess their inability to tolerate dentures because of
the sensation of nausea they provoke. The number of patients who are really
unable to tolerate the presence of dentures in the mouth is fortunately small

Fig. 25.1 Non-coincidence of intercuspal position (a) and muscular position (b) in
finished dentures. The muscular position is distal to the intercuspal position in this
illustration.

and in most cases a period of self discipline by the patient will suffice. This is, of course, assuming that the design of the denture is not a major contributing factor to the feeling of nausea.

The reflex of nausea is triggered off by the stimulation of the posterior third of the tongue and soft palate, conveyed by the glossopharyngeal nerve. The relation of the posterior border of the upper denture to the soft palate is obviously important. On the other hand, it has been suggested that the glossopharyngeal nerve may have, in some patients, a wider distribution than normal.

In patients who are complaining of a feeling of sickness, the sensitive areas of the palate and soft palate should be assessed by firm pressure with a ball-ended plastic instrument. Firm pressure is necessary because light pressure is very likely to induce nausea in patients with supposedly sensitive palates. The acceptable posterior limits of the upper denture should be marked on the tissues. The extent of the denture should then be compared with this line. Common discrepancies are:

OVEREXTENSION

The clinician should not be surprised to find an apparently atypical post dam line in patients susceptible to a feeling of nausea with dentures. It is quite common to locate hypersensitive areas on either side of the midline (Fig. 25.3), and these should be avoided when demarcating the posterior border of the denture.

UNDEREXTENSION

If the denture does not extend as far as the vibrating line of the soft palate, it is usually impossible for adequate compression of the tissues to be achieved in order to make firm and continuous contact. As a result of the inadequate posterior seal, the denture is more likely to move because of loss of retention. The back of the denture falls onto the tongue causing nausea.

Fig. 25.3 The bold line indicates the atypical post dam line sometimes necessary in cases of palatal hypersensitivity. The dotted line illustrates the conventional post dam line.

The treatment in obvious cases of over- or underextension is to correct the extent of the denture base and ensure that adequate compression of soft tissues is achieved.

If the existing post dam of the denture appears to be correctly sited and adapted, there may be other denture errors which are contributing to the patient's difficulties. The palate of the denture may be very thick, and its posterior border prominent. If the degree of jaw separation with the dentures in occlusion is too small, nausea results because of premature and continuous contact of the posterior third of the tongue with the palate of the upper denture. A lack of balance in occlusion or articulation leads to a continuous movement of the dentures away from supporting tissues, resulting in a feeling of nausea.

In cases of severe sensitivity the clinician should consider the possibility of gradually 'conditioning' the tissues to the acceptance of a denture. The mere bulk of a conventional denture may be intolerable, initially, to the patient with very sensitive tissues. Therefore a thin, clear acrylic baseplate is first constructed; this is generally well tolerated and accustoms the patient to stimulation of the palatal tissues and of the dorsum of the tongue. Teeth may then be added to the baseplate in stages, first the incisors and canines and two molars for occlusion and then finally adding all the teeth and rebasing the denture (Fig. 25.4).

In the very rare cases of complete intolerance to palatal coverage, the possible lines of treatment are: (1) the construction of a palateless upper denture,

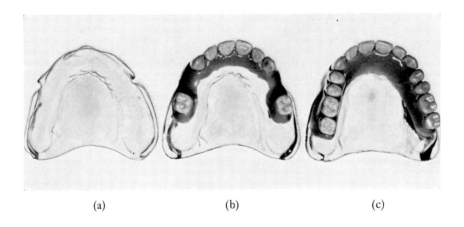

(a)   (b)   (c)

Fig. 25.4 Stages in the provision of a denture for a patient who experiences nausea:
(a) acrylic baseplate;
(b) addition of incisors and two molar teeth;
(c) complete denture.

the prognosis for which can only be considered favourable when the ridge is well formed and covered by a sufficiently resilient mucosa so that some peripheral seal may be achieved; or (2) an implant denture.

POOR RETENTION

Whereas with an upper denture, positive retention can be achieved by virtue of border seal, the lower denture is largely held in place by the retaining pressures of the adjacent musculature. More patients, therefore, have complaints about the retention of the lower denture. This is particularly so during the early postinsertion period before the musculature has adapted to the form of the denture and learnt movement patterns that will maintain it in place. The difficulties of retention will be greatest for patients who either have not had dentures before, or whose previous dentures have proved unsatisfactory and for obvious reasons have not been copied.

There may be certain inherent factors that make the retention of dentures difficult, such as (1) a thin non-resilient mucosa, (2) lack of saliva, (3) saliva of unsuitable viscosity, (4) poor ridge form, and (5) wide variation between the resting and functional depth of the vestibular sulcus. Any incompatibility between the polished, fitting and occlusal surfaces of the dentures and the environmental tissues, when any of these factors are present, is likely to result in diminished retention.

DISPLACEMENT OF THE UPPER DENTURE

With the Teeth out of Contact

The causes are usually (1) overextension of the base, particularly in the areas of the buccal and labial frena, (2) bulky flanges that have been made too thick in an effort to obtain lip and cheek support, (3) interference by the buccal flange with the movement of the coronoid process, (4) anterior teeth positioned too far forward so that the upper lip acts as a displacing force.

Overextension causes rapid displacement with the mouth wide open because the tensed buccal and labial sulcus tissues exert a greater displacing force on the denture border. When the mouth is not so widely opened and when the lips are widely parted as in speech or in laughter, underextension of the denture allows ingress of air and breakdown of seal.

With the Teeth in Contact

Faulty occlusal balance readily brings about denture displacement when the teeth come into contact. If the patient uses lateral and protrusive movements in mastication, lack of balanced articulation also results in denture displacement.

DISPLACEMENT OF THE LOWER DENTURE

This is frequently due to a lack of appreciation on the part of the operator of the extent of the neutral zone. Other common causes of poor retention of the lower denture are (1) under- rather than over-extension of the borders, (2) improper shaping of the polished surface, and (3) anterior teeth that are positioned incorrectly in relation to the lip and tongue (Fig. 25.5).

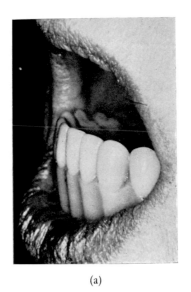
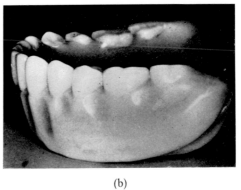

(a)   (b)

Fig. 25.5
(a) Displacement of the lower denture on mouth opening caused by
(b) incorrect positioning of the lower teeth in relation to the ridge.

Excessive thickness of the buccal flange in the premolar region is a common cause of lower denture displacement due to the activity of the modiolus. If the lingual flange is inclined inwards, the tongue gets into this undercut area and lifts the denture. When adjusting a lower denture, all excess buccal, lingual and labial bulk should be eliminated before reducing the extent of the flanges.

Despite suggestions by the patient, the dentist must be very wary about *gradually* reducing the lingual flange so that the border lies on or near the mylohyoid ridge. Extension well below the mylohyoid ridge is preferable.

Such extension provides considerable resistance to lateral movement of the denture. If such extension is not possible, the denture should finish above this ridge.

NOISE

The three main causes of 'noisy dentures' are (1) poor retention, (2) increased occlusal face height, and (3) gross cuspal interferences.

In all cases the upper and lower teeth are brought into contact earlier than expected with consequent noise. The noise will be greater if porcelain teeth have been used.

MASTICATORY INEFFICIENCY

In assessing a complaint of this nature one must be aware that it will always be in evidence if the dentures cause a painful response from the tissues. If this is relieved and greater muscular pressure can be exerted, the patient's masticatory efforts will become more effective.

But there are certain errors in denture construction that prevent adequate mastication of food.

INCORRECT LEVEL OF THE OCCLUSAL PLANE

As the tongue and the buccinator muscles play a major role in the manipulation of the bolus of food, the occlusal level should be in correct relation to these structures. If the level is too high, the buccinator, which apparently has a crest of contraction at one level only, will not be able to return food with ease from the buccal sulcus. Even if this is accomplished the tongue on the inner aspect will have to be elevated unnaturally to help to control the bolus. The correct level of the occlusal plane is just below the level of the dorsum of the tongue when the tongue is in a resting position.

INEFFECTIVE POSTERIOR TEETH

Reduction of cuspal height by gross selective grinding in an attempt to rectify occlusal and articulatory errors, the use of cuspless teeth or a change to acrylic teeth in a patient previously accustomed to porcelain, may all result in a complaint of inefficient mastication.

LACK OF BALANCED CONTACTS

Balanced contacts in articulation are not essential for every patient. The clinician can learn much by examining the patient's masticatory cycle, preferably with a biscuit or some other food in his mouth. If it is obvious that a lateral movement is used, then cuspal interference in lateral movement must be eliminated. Common interferences are found in the canine areas.

INCORRECT OCCLUSAL FACE HEIGHT

It has been said that the most effective muscular loading on the dentures will only occur at the patient's correct occlusal face height. It is fortunate that most patients are able to adapt to various occlusal face heights within a limited range since the accurate assessment of the degree of vertical jaw separation is difficult. The essential need is for an *adequate* freeway space. If this is obliterated, mastication will be difficult, as there will be no room between the occlusal surfaces for the food bolus without a conscious effort to open the mouth further than was previously necessary for mastication.

If the freeway space is too great (an overclosed jaw relation), muscular power is markedly reduced. For old patients, however, a degree of overclosure is acceptable as the reduced masticatory activity is beneficial to the atrophic supporting tissues.

POOR AESTHETICS

Complaints concerning aesthetics occur rarely when the patient has been taken from the natural dentition to the edentulous state by an immediate denture. If a denture copying technique has been adopted when providing replacement dentures, faithful reproduction of the original appearance is possible. If, however, the patient expressed a wish for any modifications in the new dentures these should have been carefully checked and agreed upon at the try-in stage.

With those patients who have never had dentures or whose existing dentures are considered by the dentist or the patient to be aesthetically unsatisfactory, the greatest care should have been taken at the try-in stage to obtain the patient's approval before the dentures are processed. There will always be, however, patients who are dissatisfied with the appearance of the finished dentures even though they accepted them at the try-in stage. Such patients should not necessarily be condemned because the time available for examination and comment at the try-in stage is usually limited.

INADEQUATE LIP AND FACE SUPPORT

This often results from the patient expecting too much from the dentures. Particularly prone are late middle aged females who anticipate that the dentures will obliterate all facial folds. These are more related to atrophy of tissue than to lack of denture support.

APPROXIMATION OF NOSE AND CHIN

This is a normal concomitant of old age and is often caused by age changes in the facial tissues. It may be associated with an insufficient amount of jaw separation; with severe overclosure the chin may become very prominent. As mentioned earlier a measure of overclosure is advised in old patients to reduce the loading on atrophic supporting tissues. It is most important to have explained the reasons for this procedure at the trial denture stage and to have obtained the necessary approval from the patient.

COLOUR, SIZE, SHAPE AND POSITION OF ANTERIOR TEETH

Comments on tooth colour, size and shape are always likely when no pre-extraction records have been available and when there have been no existing dentures to copy.

In instances of complaint about the appearance of the anterior teeth, it should be explained to the patient that an improvement in appearance is likely to occur as tissue adaptation takes place and that the appearance of the teeth immediately on insertion should not necessarily be condemned.

Patients often complain that the anterior teeth are positioned too far forward or too far back. Again the patient should be advised to allow tissue adaptation to occur before passing final comment. Where, because of poor ridge form and low potentiality for retention, the anterior teeth have been placed in close approximation to the ridge crest, the reasons for this should be explained again.

AMOUNT OF TOOTH VISIBLE

This complaint may be because of an inadequate occlusal face height in which case little of the upper or lower anterior teeth will show. Errors in the position-ing of the occlusal plane result in too much of one denture showing and too little of the other.

Where the lower alveolar ridge is grossly resorbed the occlusal plane may have been lowered deliberately to enhance the stability of the denture. If the lower lip is a powerful displacing force it may have been necessary to incline the lower anterior teeth inwards in order to avoid displacement of the denture when the mouth is opened. The patient's complaint will be that no one knows that a lower denture is present.

If the complaints of the patient about appearance are justifiable and due to an error of judgment on the part of the operator, the dentures must either be replaced, or the anterior teeth repositioned on the existing denture base.

Major difficulties exist, however, when the operator is satisfied that the position of the teeth is correct and essential for functional purposes. There will then be a clash between the relative merits of aesthetics and function. Unfortunately, having given some patients comfort and function, they see little reason why appearance cannot now be improved upon. A further discussion is then necessary.

SPEECH DIFFICULTIES

In the production of speech sounds, air from the lungs passes the vocal cords in the larynx, and is then released through the nose or the nose and mouth. The vocal cords may add a vibration to produce a 'voiced' sound such as 'z' or an 'unvoiced' 's'; the latter being simply the passage of air through a small space. During its passage through the mouth the quality of sound is altered and its release controlled by contact of various structures. Lip contact prevents sound escaping except via the nose (m, n, ng) and is also used to create 'plosive' sounds by sudden release of air (p, b). Other contacts are between teeth and lips, teeth and tongue, palate and tongue. The quality of sound released is affected by the resonance of the cavity formed between the palate, teeth and the tongue.

Thus, the removal of natural teeth, or the insertion of a denture of different shape, requires a period of re-education by the patient in order to create suitably shaped spaces and good contacts between lips, teeth, tongue and palate so that clear speech is again possible. This re-education is usually rapid. Obviously speech disturbances are minimal when a previous denture has been copied. For clear speech, the dentures must be well retained and there must be adequate tongue space.

If marked changes in occlusal face height are incorporated in new dentures or if the anterior teeth are positioned further forward of the ridge, difficulties may occur in obtaining lip contact during the sounds 'p, b, m and n'. Attempts to obtain good contact in these circumstances lead to tightening of the circumoral musculature and denture displacement.

Sounds controlled by contact between the lower lip and the upper teeth, (f, v) are affected by a considerable change in the incisal level.

The 'th' sound is affected by an increase in occlusal face height and changes in the incisor relation, particularly horizontal overlap. During speech, one should see a space appear between the teeth, through which, on the pronunciation of certain sounds, the tongue is protruded. After the provision of dentures at too great an occlusal face height, the 'speaking space' is insufficient and the patient talks from behind the teeth and not between them. To produce a clear 'th' sound, the tongue must form a seal against the lower incisors, leaving a small space between its upper surface and the upper teeth. When a large horizontal overlap is present, this type of contact becomes more difficult.

Sounds made by contact of the tongue with the palate behind the upper incisor teeth (j, ch, sh, t, d, l, r) are made difficult by a change in inter-premolar width. Narrowing the arch creates difficulties in applying the tongue firmly to the palate. As a consequence, air leaks often occur, particularly against a smooth polished palate well lubricated with saliva. The tongue 'slips' and the small spaces created are similar to those normally formed to produce an 's' sound. Hence the patient complains of a whistle added to normal speech sounds.

Contact of the dorsum of the tongue with the posterior border of the denture takes place on the formation of sounds 'g, k'. Nausea may occur during speech if the posterior edge of the palate is thick.

As most patients adapt rapidly, no modifications should be made to the dentures unless the speech difficulties persist for more than 2 to 3 weeks. Then, a comparison with any previous dentures will usually indicate that a marked change of incisal position or reduction of tongue space has been made.

The complaints and problems just described are those that commonly occur during the early postinsertion period. After careful diagnosis and correction of the dentures the patient should be able to expect a long period of comfort and efficiency with them. However, there may be occasions during this period when generalized discomfort occurs beneath the dentures and this may be related to a temporary lowering of tissue resistance. In such cases it is inadvisable to modify the dentures as the discomfort will disappear with an increase in tissue resistance. The need for regular inspection of the dentures and their supporting tissues must be emphasized and the patient should be advised to attend for this purpose annually. In this way the dentures may be modified when necessary and remain satisfactory for many years.

Eventually replacement dentures will be necessary: the indications for these were fully discussed in Chapter 17.

Bibliography

BOOKS

ALDRICH C. K. (1955) *Psychiatry for the Family Physician*. McGraw-Hill Book Inc, New York.

ANDERSON W. F. (1967) *Practical Management of the Elderly*. Blackwell Scientific Publications, Oxford.

BATES J. F. & STAFFORD G. D. (1971) *Immediate Complete Dentures. Br dent J*.

BERRY D. C. & WILKIE J. K. (1964) *An Approach to Dental Prosthetics*. Pergamon Press, Oxford.

BLUM R. H. (1960) *The Management of the Doctor-Patient Relationship*. McGraw-Hill Book Inc, New York.

BOURNE G. H. (1961) *Structural Aspects of Ageing*. Pitman, London.

Dental Clinics of North America. April 1971. W. B. Saunders Co.

FENN H. R. B. *et al* (1961) *Clinical Dental Prosthetics*, 2nd ed. Staples, London.

FISH E. W. (1964) *Principles of Full Denture Prosthesis*, 6th ed. Staples, London.

GERSHKOFF A. & GOLDBERG N. I. (1957) *Implant Dentures: Indications and Procedures*. Pitman, London.

HOWE G. L. (1971) *Minor Oral Surgery*, 2nd ed. Wright, Bristol.

HOWELL T. H. (1970) *A Student's Guide to Geriatrics*, 2nd ed. Staples, London.

ISRAEL S. L. (1967) *Menstrual Disorders and Sterility*, 5th ed. Harper-Medical, New York.

JENKINS G. N. (1966) *The Physiology of the Mouth*, 3rd ed. Blackwell Scientific Publications, Oxford.

LEE J. H. (1962) *Dental Aesthetics*. Wright, Bristol.

MACK A. O. (1964) *Complete Dentures. Br dent J*.

McLEAN F. C. & URIST M. R. (1968) *Bone*, 3rd ed. University of Chicago Press, Chicago.

NEILL D. J. & NAIRN R. I. (1968) *Complete Denture Prosthodontics*. Wright, Bristol.

PORTER M. M. (1968) *Dental Problems in Wind Instrument Playing. Br dent J*.

POSSELT U. (1968) *Physiology of Occlusion and Rehabilitation*, 2nd ed. Blackwell Scientific Publications, Oxford.

PREISKEL H. (1973) *Precision Attachments in Dentistry*, 2nd ed. Kimpton, London.

RYCROFT C. (1968) *Anxiety and Neurosis*. Pelican.

SCHLOSSER R. O. (1958) *Complete Denture Prosthesis*, 4th ed. Saunders, Philadelphia.

SHARRY J. J. (1968) *Complete Denture Prosthodontics*, 2nd ed. McGraw-Hill Book Inc, New York.

SWENSON M. G. (1970) *Complete Dentures*, 6th ed. Mosby, St Louis.

WADE A. B. (1965) *Basic Periodontology*, 2nd ed. Wright, Bristol.

WEINMANN J. P. & SICHER H. (1955) *Bone and Bones*, 2nd ed. Mosby, St Louis.

SELECTED PAPERS

AESTHETICS

ASPIN M. E. *et al* (1960) Aesthetics of denture gum work. *Br dent J*, **109**, 271.

CHRISTENSEN L. V. & RUNOW J. (1966) The setting of teeth in cases of an original distoclusion. *Tandlaegebladet*, **70**, 199.

FRUSH J. P. & FISHER R. D. (1959) Dentogenics, its practical application. *J prosth Dent*, **9**, 914.

LIDDELOW K. P. (1967) The edentulous patient who had an Angle's Class II div 2 occlusion on a normal skeletal base. *Dent Mag Oral Top*, **84**, 103.

WILLIAMS J. L. (1911) The esthetic and anatomical basis of dental prosthetics. *Dent Comos*, **53**, 1.

AGEING: THE CLIMACTERIC

ANDERSON W. F. (1972) Modern trends in geriatric medicine. *Dent Practnr*, **22**, 456.

ATKINSON P. J. & WOODHEAD C. (1972) Structural changes in the ageing mandible. *Proc R Soc Med*, **65**, 675.

BJORKSTEN J. (1963) Ageing, primary mechanism. *Gerontologia* (Basel), 8, 179.

COHEN L. (1970) Interpretation of age changes in the oral structures. *J Oral Med*, **25**, 129.

DAVIES M. E. *et al* (1966) Estrogens and the aging process. *J Am med Ass*, **196**, 219.

EXTON-SMITH A. N. & STEWART R. J. C. (1972) Bone resorption in old age. *Proc R Soc Med*, **65**, 674.

FRANKS A. S. T. (1971) Health in old age. *Dent Practnr*, **21**, 349.

GERRISH J. S. *et al* (1972) A dental survey of people living in residential homes for the elderly in Cardiff. *Dent Practnr*, **22**, 433.

HEDEGÅRD B. *et al* (1970) Salivary properties in elderly persons. Svensk Tanklak T. **63**, 997.

HENSCHEN F. (1964) The problem of ageing as seen by the physician. *Int dent J*, **14**, 363.

HERRMANN H. W. (1964) Changes in the oral cavity due to ageing and their effect on prosthetic treatment. *Int dent J*, **14**, 386.

LEVIN B. (1970) Special considerations for the geriatric complete denture patient. *J Am Soc Geriat dent*, **5**, 2.

LIDDELOW K. P. (1964) The prosthetic treatment of the elderly. *Br dent J*, **117**, 307.

MARGULIES R. (1964) Nutritional aspects of ageing. *Int dent J*, **14**, 395.

MASSLER M. (1956) Tissue changes during ageing. *Oral Surg*, **9**, 1185.

RITCHIE G. M. (1973) A report of dental findings in a survey of geriatric patients. *J Dent*, **1**, 106.

SCHWEIGER J. W. (1959) Prosthetic considerations for the ageing. *J prosth Dent*, **9**, 555.

SHELTON E. K. (1954) The use of estrogen after the menopause. *J Am Geriat Soc*, **2**, 627.

SILVERMAN S. jr (1958) Geriatrics and tissue changes—problem of the ageing denture patient. *J prosth Dent*, **8**, 734.

STORER R. (1965) The effect of the climacteric and of ageing on prosthetic diagnosis and treatment planning. *Br dent J*, **119**, 349.

—(1966) Geriatric dentistry. *Br dent J*, **121**, 547.

ARTIFICIAL TOOTH FORM AND MATERIAL

BEARN E. M. (1973) Effect of different occlusal profiles on masticatory forces. *Br dent J*, 134, 7.

CRADDOCK F. W. (1953) The forms of porcelain posterior teeth. *Dent Dig*, 59, 62.

DOCKING A. R. (1952) The relative merits of porcelain and acrylic teeth. *Aust J Dent*, 56, 158.

HARDY I. R. (1951) The developments in the occlusal patterns of artificial teeth. *J prosth Dent*, 1, 14.

KORAN A. *et al* (1972) Coefficient of friction of prosthetic tooth materials. *J prosth Dent*, 27, 269.

MOSES C. H. (1954) Biomechanics and artificial posterior teeth. *J prosth Dent*, 4, 782.

MYERSON R. L. (1957) Use of porcelain and plastic teeth in opposing complete dentures. *J prosth Dent*, 7, 625.

SEARS V. H. (1953) Thirty years of nonanatomic teeth. *J prosth Dent*, 3, 596.

THOMSON J. C. (1971) The load factor in complete denture intolerance. *J prosth Dent*, 25, 4.

DECISION TO RENDER EDENTULOUS

ALLEN E. F. (1944) Statistical study of the primary causes of extractions. *J dent Res*, 23, 453.

BASKER R. M. (1966) Adaptation to dentures. *Br dent J*, 120, 573.

BERRY W. T. C. (1972) Mastication, food and nutrition. *Dent Practnr*, 22, 249.

BOND E. K. & LAWSON W. A. (1968) Speech and its relation to dentistry. *Dent Practnr*, 19, 75 and 113.

CRADDOCK F. W. (1958) Mastication with natural teeth and with full dentures. *N. Z. dent J*, 54, 105.

DAPECI A. & ROD J. (1967) Relationship between dental status and functional gastro-intestinal disturbances. *Zahnaerztl Rundsch*, 76, 243.

ELWOOD P. C. & BATES J. F. (1972) Dentition and nutrition. *Dent Practnr*, 22, 427.

FARRELL J. H. (1956) The effect of mastication on the digestion of food. *Br dent J*, 100, 149.

FISH S. F. (1969) Adaptation and habituation to full dentures. *Br dent J*, 127, 19.

HEATH M. R. (1972) Dietary selection by elderly persons, related to dental state. *Br dent J*, 132, 145.

HOBDELL M. H. *et al* (1970) The prevalence of full and partial dentures in British populations. *Br dent J*, 128, 437.

MÄKILÄ E. (1969) Effects of complete dentures on dietary intake. *Suom Hammasläk Toim*, 65, 299.

MUMMA R. D. & QUINTON K. (1970) Effect of masticatory efficiency on the occurrence of gastric distress. *J dent Res*, 49, 69.

MURPHY W. M. (1971) The effect of complete dentures upon taste perception. *Br dent J*, 130, 201.

NEILL D. J. & PHILLIPS H. I. B. (1970) The masticatory performance, dental state, and dietary intake of a group of elderly army pensioners. *Br dent J*, 128, 581.

PELTON W. J. *et al* (1954) Tooth morbidity experience of adults. *J Am dent Ass*, 49, 439.

SANDLER H. E. & STAHL S. S. (1960) Prevalence of periodontal disease in a hospitalized population. *J dent Res*, 39, 439.

DENTURE BASE MATERIALS

ANDERSON J. N. (1963) Acrylic allergy. *Dent Practnr*, **13**, 480.

— (1963) Metal bases for full upper dentures. *Dent Practnr*, **14**, 17.

— (1963) Acrylic resin as a denture base. *Dent Practnr*, **14**, 110.

AXELSSON B. & NYQUIST G. (1962) The leaching and biological effect of the residual monomer of methyl methacrylate. *Odont Revy*, **13**, 370.

BAHRANI A. S. *et al* (1965) Slow-rate hydraulic forming of stainless steel dentures. *Br dent J*, **118**, 425.

BLAIR G. A. S. & CROSSLAND B. (1963) Explosive forming of stainless steel upper dentures. *Dent Practnr*, **13**, 413.

BRADEN M. & CLARKE R. L. (1972) Viscoelastic properties of soft lining materials. *J dent Res*, **51**, 1525.

CRAIG R. G. & GIBBONS P. (1961) Properties of resilient denture liners. *J Am dent Ass*, **63**, 382.

DAVENPORT J. C. (1972) The denture surface. *Br dent J*, **133**, 101.

SMITH D. C. (1961) The acrylic denture: mechanical evaluation of mid-line fracture. *Br dent J*, **110**, 257.

STORER R. (1962) Resilient denture base materials. *Br dent J*, **113**, 195 and 231.

TURRELL A. J. W. (1966) Allergy to denture-base materials—fallacy or reality. *Br dent J*, **120**, 415.

DENTURE COPYING

ADAM C. E. (1958) Technique for duplicating an acrylic resin denture. *J prosth Dent*, **8**, 406.

BASKER R. M. & CHAMBERLAIN J. D. (1971) A method for duplicating dentures. *Br dent J*, **131**, 549.

CHICK A. O. (1962) The copying of full dentures. *Dent Practnr*, **13**, 96.

SCHER E. A. (1964) A replacement denture technique. *Dent Practnr*, **14**, 464.

EXAMINATION OF THE MOUTH; EXAMINATION OF DENTURES

BERGMAN B. *et al* (1964) A longitudinal two-year study of a number of full denture cases. *Acta odont scand*, **22**, 3.

BODINE R. L. (1969) Oral lesions caused by ill-fitting dentures. *J prosth Dent*, **21**, 580.

BREMNER V. A. & GRANT A. A. (1971) A radiographic survey of edentulous mouths. *Aust dent J*, **16**, 17.

BUDTZ-JØRGENSEN E. & BERTRAM U. (1970) Denture stomatitis. *Acta odont scand*, **28**, 71, 283 and 551.

CAWSON R. A. (1963) Denture sore mouth and angular cheilitis. *Br dent J*, **115**, 441.

CHERASKIN E. (1959) The arithmetic of disease. *J dent Med*, **14**, 71.

COHEN L. (1972) Oral candidiasis—its diagnosis and treatment. *J oral Med*, **27**, 7.

CRADDOCK F. W. (1953) Retromolar region of the mandible. *J Am dent Ass*, **47**, 453.

DAVIES G. N. & WALSH J. P. (1953) Survey of denture-wearers in New Zealand. *N Z dent J*, **49**, 124.

DEELEY R. A. (1965) The effect of protein versus placebo supplementation upon denture tolerance. *J prosth Dent*, **15**, 65.

DESJARDINS R. P. *et al* (1971) Comparison of nerve endings in normal gingiva with those in mucosa covering edentulous ridges. *J dent Res*, **50**, 867.

FROST H. M. (1962) A model of endocrine control of bone remodelling. *Henry Ford Hosp med Bull*, **10**, 119.

GOULD A. W. (1964) An investigation of the inheritance of *torus palatinus* and *torus mandibularis*. *J dent Res*, **43**, 159.

GRATY T. C. *et al* (1964) The mylohyoid ridge problem. *Br dent J*, **116**, 203.

KAPUR K. K. & SHKLAR G. (1963) Effect of complete dentures on alveolar mucosa. *J prosth Dent*, **13**, 1030.

KIMBALL H. D. (1954) Factors to be considered in the control and elimination of soreness beneath dentures. *J prosth Dent*, **4**, 298.

KING D. R. & MOORE G. E. (1971) The prevalence of *torus palatinus*. *J oral Med*, **26**, 113.

LITTLE K. (1963) Bone resorption and osteoporosis. *Lancet*, **2**, 752.

LYON D. G. & CHICK A. O. (1957) Denture sore mouth and angular cheilitis. *Dent Practnr*, **7**, 212.

MCCRORIE J. W. (1963) The origin of the pear-shaped pad. *Dent Practnr*, **13**, 517.

— (1971) An orthopantomogram survey of edentulous mouths. *Dent Practnr*, **22**, 83.

MCMILLAN D. R. (1972) The cytological response of the palatal mucosa to dentures. *Dent Practnr*, **22**, 302.

MARSLAND E. A. & FOX E. C. (1958) Some abnormalities in the nerve supply of the oral mucosa. *Proc R Soc Med*, **51**, 951 (Section of Odontology, 31).

MATTHEWS E. *et al* (1961) The full denture problem. *Br dent J*, **111**, 401.

MOLLER P. & CHERASKIN E. (1961) The relationship of three-hour blood glucose to oral signs (dental findings). *J dent Med*, **16**, 124.

NEWTON A. V. (1962) Denture sore mouth: a possible aetiology. *Br dent J*, **112**, 357.

NYQUIST G. (1953) The influence of denture hygiene and bacterial flora on the condition of the oral mucosa in full denture cases. *Acta odont scand*, **11**, 24.

OSBORN J. W. (1964) Mucosal reactions to dentures. *Int dent J*, **14**, 373.

OSBORNE J. (1960) The full lower denture. *Br dent J*, **109**, 481.

ÖSTLUND S. G. (1958) The effect of complete dentures on the gum tissues. *Acta odont scand*, **16**, 1.

PLIESS G. & BORNEMANN G. (1957) Oral lesions and atypical growth of epithelial tissue in patients wearing dentures. *Fortschr, Kiefer- u. Gesichts-Chir*, **3**, 41.

RALPH J. P. & STENHOUSE D. (1972) Denture-induced hyperplasia of the oral soft tissues. *Br dent J*, **132**, 68.

REGLI C. P. & GASKILL H. L. (1954) Denture base deformation during function. *J prosth Dent*, **4**, 548.

REITHER W. (1959) Denture stomatitis—a dental as well as a medical problem. *Munch med Wschr*, **101**, 606.

ROBINSON J. E. (1964) Dental management of the oral effects of radiotherapy. *J prosth Dent*, **14**, 582.

ROSE J. A. (1968) Etiology of angular cheilosis. *Br dent J*, **125**, 67.

SEWERIN I. (1971) Prevalence of variations and anomalies at the upper labial frenum. *Acta odont scand*, **29**, 487.

SHARP G. S. (1960) Treatment for low tolerance to dentures. *J prosth Dent*, **10**, 47.

SHEPPARD I. M. *et al* (1972) Survey of the oral status of complete denture patients. *J prosth Dent*, **28**, 121.

STORER R. (1957) A radiographic survey of edentulous mouths. *Br dent J*, **103**, 344.
— (1972) Oral cancer. *Lancet*, **1**, 430.
TAYLOR P. F. *et al* (1964) Nerve endings in the anterior part of the human hard palate. *J dent Res*, **43**, 447.
WALLENUS K. & HEYDEN G. (1972) Histochemical studies of flabby ridges. *Odont Revy*, **23**, 169.
WOELFEL J. B. & PAFFENBARGER G. C. (1959) Method of evaluating the clinical effect of warping a denture: report of a case. *J Am dent Ass*, **59**, 250.
YUDKIN J. (1967) Evolutionary and historical changes in dietary carbohydrates. *Am J clin Nutr*, **20**, 108.

IMMEDIATE DENTURES

ATKINSON H. F. (1960) Some aspects of immediate denture treatment. *Aust dent J*, **5**, 221.
CARLSSON G. E. *et al* (1967) Changes in contour of the maxillary alveolar process under immediate dentures. *Acta odont scand*, **25**, 21 and 45.
DEMER W. J. (1972) Minimizing problems in placement of immediate dentures. *J prosth Dent*, **27**, 275.
GIMSON A. P. (1955) Immediate dentures: alveolar ridge trauma from socketed anteriors. *Br dent J*, **98**, 387.
HEDEGÅRD B. (1962) Some observations on tissue changes with immediate maxillary dentures. *Dent Practnr*, **13**, 70.
HEARTWELL C. M. & SALISBURY F. W. (1965) Immediate complete dentures: an evaluation. *J prosth Dent*, **15**, 615.
JERBI F. C. (1966) Trimming the cast in the construction of immediate dentures. *J prosth Dent*, **16**, 1047.
JOHNSON K. (1969) A study of the dimensional changes occurring in the maxilla following closed-face immediate denture treatment. *Aust dent J*, **14**, 370.
NAIRN R. I. & CUTRESS T. W. (1967) Changes in mandibular position following removal of the remaining teeth and insertion of immediate complete dentures. *Br dent J*, **122**, 303.
WICTORIN L. (1969) Evaluation of bone surgery in patients with immediate dentures. *J prosth Dent*, **21**, 6.

IMPLANTS

BJORLIN G. *et al* (1971) Silicone implants for reconstruction of flabby alveolar ridges. *Svensk Tandlak T*, **64**, 789.
BODINE R. L. (1963) Implant dentures. *J Am dent Ass*, **67**, 352.
BOYNE P. J. (1971) Transplantation, implantation and grafts. *Dent clin N Amer*, **15**, 433.
DOMASCHK W. & LHOTSKY B. (1971) Problems in subperiosteal implantation in the jaws. *Deutsch zahnaerztl Z*, **26**, 961.
L'ESTRANGE P. R. (1971) Aids to the insertion of endosseous implants. *Dent Practnr*, **21**, 389.
FITZPATRICK B. (1968) A comparative study of some implant materials. *Aust Dent J*, **13**, 360 and 422.
LINKOW L. I. (1970) Endosseous oral implantology. *Dent clin N Amer*, **14**, 185.
MACK A. O. (1968) Reactions of the oral tissues to subperiosteal appliances. *Int dent J*, **18**, 779.

MANDERSON R. D. (1972) Experimental intra-osseous implantation in the jaws of pigs. *Dent Practnr*, **22**, 225.

TIDEMAN H. (1971) Preprosthetic surgery. *Nederl T Tand*, **78**, 224 and 264.

IMPRESSION MATERIALS AND TECHNIQUES

ANDERSON J. N. (1960) Flow and elastic properties of alginate impression materials. *Dent Prog*, **1**, 63.

BOUCHER C. O. (1951) A critical analysis of mid-century impression techniques for full dentures. *J prosth Dent*, **1**, 472.

BRILL N. *et al* (1965) The dynamic nature of the lower denture space. *J prosth Dent*, **15**, 401.

DOUGLAS W. H. *et al* (1965) Pressures involved in taking impressions. *Dent Practnr*, **15**, 248.

FAIGENBLUM M. J. (1968) Retching, its causes and management in prosthetic practice. *Br dent J*, **125**, 485.

FOURNET S. C. & TULLER C. S. (1936) A revolutionary mechanical principle utilized to produce full lower dentures surpassing in stability the best modern upper dentures. *J Am dent Ass*, **23**, 1028.

HEATH R. (1971) A study of the morphology of the denture space. *Dent Practnr*, **21**, 109.

MOSES C. W. (1953) Physical considerations in impression making. *J prosth Dent*, **3**, 449.

MURPHY W. M. (1966) The neutral zone and the polished surfaces of full dentures. *Dent Practnr*, **16**, 244.

OHASHI M. *et al* (1966) Pressures exerted on complete dentures during swallowing. *J Am dent Ass*, **73**, 625.

SCHWARZKOPF H. (1969) A new method for edentulous jaw impressions. *Deutsch zahnaerztl Z*, **23**, 30.

WOELFEL J. B. (1962) Contour variation in impressions of one edentulous patient. *J prosth Dent*, **12**, 229.

MANDIBULAR POSITIONS AND MOVEMENTS

AGERBERG G. (1971) The distances between different occlusal positions and their reproducibility of registration. *Svensk Tandlak T*, **64**, 185.

AHLGREN J. (1966) Mechanisms of mastication. *Acta odont scand*, **24**, Suppl 44.

BAIKIE M. W. (1970) The Gothic arch tracing and its relation to mandibular dimensions. *J dent Ass S Afr*, **25**, 357.

BERRY D. C. (1960) The constancy of the rest position of the mandible. *Dent Practnr*, **10**, 129.

BERRY D. C. & WILKIE J. K. (1964) Muscle activity in the edentulous mouth. *Br dent J*, **116**, 441.

BONAGURO J. G. *et al* (1969) Ability of human subjects to discriminate forces applied to certain teeth. *J dent Res*, **48**, 236.

BRILL N. *et al* (1962) Aspects of occlusal sense in natural and artificial teeth. *J prosth Dent*, **12**, 123.

FISH S. F. (1961) Functional anatomy of the rest position of the mandible. *Dent Practnr*, **11**, 178.

GRASSO J. E. & SHARRY J. (1968) The duplicability of arrow-point tracings in dentulous subjects. *J prosth Dent*, **20**, 106.

HEDEGÅRD B. *et al* (1970) Masticatory function—a cineradiographic study. *Acta odont scand*, **28**, 859.

JERGE C. R. (1964) The neurologic mechanism underlying cyclic jaw movements. *J prosth Dent*, **14**, 667.

KAWAMURA Y. & NISHIYAMA T. (1966) Projection of dental afferent impulses to the trigeminal nuclei of the cat. *Jap J Physiol*, **16**, 584.

KLINEBERG I. J. *et al* (1971) Contributions to the reflex control of mastication from mechanoreceptors in the temporomandibular joint capsule. *Dent Practnr*, **21**, 73.

LAURITZEN A. G. & BODNER G. H. (1961) Variations in location of arbitrary and true hinge axis points. *J prosth Dent*, **11**, 224.

McMILLAN D. R. & IMBER S. (1968) The accuracy of facial measurements using the Willis bite gauge. *Dent Practnr*, **18**, 213.

MIROSHNICHENCO I. T. (1971) Bioelectric activity of masticatory muscles during adaptation to removable complete dentures. *Stomatologiya Mosk*, **50**, 47.

MUNRO R. R. (1972) Coordination of activity of the two bellies of the digastric muscle in basic jaw movements. *J dent Res*, **51**, 1663.

MURPHY T. R. (1967) Rest position of the mandible. *J prosth Dent*, **17**, 329.

NAGLE R. J. (1956) Temporomandibular function. *J prosth Dent*, **6**, 350.

NAVAKARI K. (1956) An analysis of the mandibular movement from rest to occlusal position. *Acta odont scand*, **14**, suppl 19.

NEILL D. J. (1967) Studies of tooth contact in complete dentures. *Br dent J*, **123**, 369.

NISWONGER M. E. (1934) The rest position of the mandible and the centric relation. *J Am dent Ass*, **21**, 1572.

NYFFENEGGAR J. W. (1971) Opening movements of the mandible. *Schweiz Mschr Zahnheilk*, **81**, 961.

OSBORNE J. (1949) Recording centric occlusion for edentulous cases. *Dent Rec*, **69**, 6.

OWALL B. (1970) Oral tactility during chewing. *Scand J dent Res*, **78**, 431.

PAYNE A. G. L. (1969) Gothic arch tracing in the edentulous. *Br dent J*, **126**, 220.

PERRY H. T. (1957) Muscular changes associated with temporomandibular joint dysfunction. *J Am dent Ass*, **54**, 644.

POSSELT U. (1957) Movement areas of the mandible. *J prosth Dent*, **7**, 375.

POSSELT U. & NEVSTEDT P. (1961) Registration of the condyle path inclination by intraoral wax records—its practical value. *J prosth Dent*, **11**, 43.

PREISKEL H. (1970) Bennett's movement. *Br dent J*, **129**, 372.

RAMFJORD S. P. (1961) Dysfunctional temporomandibular joint and muscle pain. *J prosth Dent*, **11**, 353.

ROTHMAN R. (1961) Phonetic considerations in denture prosthesis. *J prosth Dent*, **11**, 214.

SCHWEIZER H. (1971) The myomonitor. *Schweiz Mschr Zahnheilk*, **81**, 1187.

SHEPPARD S. & SHEPPARD I. (1971) Incidence of lateral excursions during function with complete dentures. *J prosth Dent*, **26**, 258.

SIIRILA H. S. & LAINE P. (1968) Occlusal tactile threshold in denture wearers. *Acta odont scand*, **27**, 193.

SILVERMAN M. M. (1956) Determination of vertical dimension by phonetics. *J prosth Dent*, **6**, 465.

TALLGREN A. (1957) Changes in adult face height. *Acta odont scand*, **15**, suppl 24.

THOMSON J. C. & McDONALD N. S. (1969) Monitoring mandibular posture. *J Biomechanics*, **2**, 319.

THOMPSON J. R. (1946) Rest position of the mandible and its significance to dental science. *J Am dent Ass*, **33**, 151.

TIMMER L. H. (1970) An objective method for the determination of vertical dimension. *Deutsch zahnaerztl Z*, **25**, 596.

TUELLER V. M. (1969) The relationship between the vertical dimension of occlusion and forces generated by closing muscles of mastication. *J prosth Dent*, **22**, 284.

TURRELL A. J. W. (1972) Clinical assessment of vertical dimension. *J prosth Dent*, **28**, 238.

YEMM R. (1972) Stress-induced muscle activity. *J prosth Dent*, **28**, 133.

YURKSTAS A. A. (1951) Compensation for inadequate mastication. *Br dent J*, **91**, 261.

YURKSTAS A. A. & KAPUR K. K. (1964) Factors influencing centric relation records in edentulous mouths. *J prosth Dent*, **14**, 1054.

OCCLUSION, ARTICULATION AND ARTICULATORS

ADAMS S. H. & ZANDER H. A. (1964) Functional tooth contacts in lateral and centric occlusion. *J Am dent Ass*, **69**, 495.

ANDERSON D. J. (1956) Measurement of stress in mastication. *J dent Res*, **35**, 664 and 671.

ANDERSON D. J. & PICTON D. C. A. (1957) Tooth contact during chewing. *J dent Res*, **36**, 21.

BERGSTRÖM G. (1950) On the reproduction of dental articulation by means of articulators. *Acta odont scand*, **9**, suppl 4.

BERRY D. C. (1957) Denture fractures resulting from occlusal wear of acrylic teeth. *Dent Practnr*, **7**, 292.

BLOMBERG S. *et al* (1961) Articulators. *Odont Revy*, **12**, 180.

BORGH O. & POSSELT U. (1958) Hinge-axis registration: experiments on the articulator. *J prosth Dent*, **8**, 35.

GERBER A. (1970) Aspects of the theory, diagnosis and treatment of occlusions. *Schweiz Mschr Zahnheilk*, **80**, 447.

HANAU R. L. (1926) Articulation defined, analysed and formulated. *J Am dent Ass*, **13**, 1694.

KAPUR K. K. & SOMAN S. (1965) The effect of denture factors on masticatory performance. *J prosth Dent*, **15**, 54, 231, 451 and 662.

LAMMIE G. A. *et al* (1958) Certain observations on a complete denture patient. *J prosth Dent*, **8**, 786.

LINDBLOM G. (1949) Term 'balanced articulation', its origin, development and present significance in modern odontology. *Dent Rec*, **69**, 304.

MANLY R. S. & VINTON P. (1951) A survey of the chewing ability of denture wearers. *J dent Res*, **30**, 314.

POSSELT U. (1952) Studies in the mobility of the human mandible. *Acta odont scand*, **10**, suppl 10.

SCHWEITZER J. M. (1962) Masticatory function in man. *J prosth Dent*, **12**, 262.

SHARRY J. J. *et al* (1956) A study of the influence of occlusal planes on strains in the edentulous maxillae and mandible. *J prosth Dent*, **6**, 768.

SINGER F. (1969) Porcelain or plastic artificial teeth, anatomical cusps or flat masticatory surfaces in complete dentures? *Oest Z Stomat*, **66**, 206.

VINTON P. & MANLY R. S. (1955) Masticatory efficiency during the period of adjustment to dentures. *J prosth Dent*, **5**, 477.

WATT D. M. (1969) Recording the sounds of tooth contact. *Int dent J*, **19**, 221.

WEINBERG L. A. (1963) An evaluation of basic articulators and their concepts. *J prosth Dent*, **13**, 622, 645, 873 and 1038.

WOELFEL J. B. *et al* (1962) Effect of posterior tooth form on jaw and denture movement. *J prosth Dent*, **12**, 922.

WOELFEL J. B. & PAFFENBARGER G. C. (1963) Change in occlusion of complete dentures caused by a pipe habit: a case report. *J Am dent Ass*, **66**, 478.

YURKSTAS A. A. (1965) The masticatory act. *J prosth Dent*, **15**, 248.

OVERLAY DENTURES

BIAGGI A (1952) Die anker-bifra-prothese. *Schweiz Mschr Zahnheilk*, **62**, 463.

BRILL N. (1955) Adaptation and the hybrid prosthesis. *J prosth Dent*, **5**, 811.

CRUM R. J. & LOISELLE R. J. (1972) Oral perception and proprioception. *J prosth Dent*, **28**, 215.

DOLDER E. J. (1968) A complete denture supported by a bar type frame. *Praxis*, **57**, 264.

LÖFBERG P. G. (1966) Post-examination of patients treated with alveolar bar construction dentures in the mandible. *Svensk Tandlak T*, **59**, 81.

MORROW R. M. *et al* (1969) Tooth supported complete dentures. *J prosth Dent*, **22**, 414.

PLISCHKA G. (1968) The preservation of the last remaining tooth in prosthetic care. *Oest Z Stomat*, **64**, 145.

PREISKEL H. (1967) Prefabricated attachments for complete overlay dentures. *Br dent J*, **123**, 161.

— (1968) An impression technique for complete overlay dentures. *Br dent J*, **124**, 9.

VON ROSSBACH A. (1971) The crown edge and the marginal periodontium with telescopic crowns. *Deutsch zahnaerztl Z*, **26**, 730.

WIRZ J. (1970) Endodontic implant posts (Dolder) in root-supported complete denture patients. *Z W R*, **79**, 721.

POSTEXTRACTION CHANGES IN ALVEOLAR BONE

ATWOOD A. D. (1971) Reduction of residual ridges. *J prosth Dent*, **26**, 266.

COOLBAUGH C. C. (1952) Effects of reduced blood supply on bone. *Am J Physiol*, **169**, 26.

HARRISON A (1972) Alveolar bone resorption in two edentulous populations. *J Dent*, **1**, 77.

JOHANSEN J. R. & GILHUUS-MOE O. (1969) Repair of the post extraction alveolus in the guinea pig. *Acta odont scand*, **27**, 249.

KOIVUMAA K. K. & MÄKILÄ E. (1970) Formation of residual alveolar ridges in edentulous persons after extraction of teeth for periodontal reasons. *Suom Hammaslaak Toim*, **66**, 372.

LAVELLE C. L. B. (1970) Age changes in dental arch shape. *J dent Res*, **49**, 1517.

ORTMAN H. R. (1962) Factors of bone resorption of the residual ridge. *J prosth Dent*, **12**, 429.

RADDEN H. G. (1959) Local factors in healing of the alveolar tissues. *Ann R Coll Surg*, **24**, 366.

SHARRY J. J. *et al* (1960) Influence of artificial tooth forms on bone deformation beneath complete dentures. *J dent Res*, **39**, 253.

SIMPSON H. E. (1960) Experimental investigation into the healing of extraction wounds in macacus rhesus monkeys. *J oral Surg Anesth Hosp dent Serv*, **18**, 391.

SOBOLIK C. F. (1960) Alveolar bone resorption. *J prosth Dent*, **10**, 612.

STAHL S. S. *et al* (1952) The influence of systemic diseases on alveolar bone. *J Am dent Ass*, **45**, 277.

TALLGREN A. (1972) The continuing reduction of the residual alveolar ridges in complete denture wearers. *J prosth Dent*, **27**, 120.

WATT D. M. (1960) Morphological changes in the denture bearing area following the extraction of maxillary teeth. PhD Thesis, University of Edinburgh.

PREPARATION OF THE MOUTH

BEHRMAN S. J. (1961) Surgical preparation of edentulous ridges for complete dentures. *J prosth Dent*, **11**, 404.

BOUCHER L. J. (1965) Injected Silastic for tissue protection. *J prosth Dent*, **15**, 73.

BRADEN M. & CAUSTON B. E. (1971) Tissue conditioners. *J dent Res*, **49**, 145 and 496; **50**, 1544.

COOLEY DE ORR (1952) A method for deepening the mandibular and maxillary sulci to correct deficient edentulous ridges. *J oral Surg*, **10**, 279.

CRADDOCK F. W. & WALSH J. P. (1946) Surgical preparation of the mouth for dentures. *N Z dent J*, **42**, 165.

DOWNTON D. (1954) Mylohyoid ridge resection. *Dent Rec*, **74**, 212.

GUERNSEY L. H. (1971) Preprosthetic surgery. *Dent clin N Amer*, **15**, 455.

HOWE G. L. (1965) Preprosthetic surgery in the lower labial sulcus. *Dent Practnr*, **16**, 119.

KELLY E. (1970) Tissue preparation for the complete denture patient—a simplified approach. *Dent clin N Amer*, **14**, 441.

KENNEDY D. R. & WELLINGTON J. S. (1963) Use of despeciated calf bone in freshly prepared tooth sockets and mandibular defects in dogs. *J dent Res*, **42**, 599.

LEE J. H. & DOWNTON D. (1958) Frenoplasty. *J prosth Dent*, **8**, 19.

LEWIS E. T. (1958) Repositioning of the sublingual fold for complete dentures. *J prosth Dent*, **8**, 22.

MEYER I. (1966) Alveoloplasty—the oral surgeon's point of view. *Oral Surg*, **22**, 441.

SINCLAIR-HALL A. H. (1964) Repair of bony and dentinal defects following implantation of polyvinyl alcohol sponge. *J dent Res*, **43**, 476.

TASSAROTTI B. (1972) A clinical and histologic evaluation of a conditioning material. *J prosth Dent*, **28**, 13.

REBASING

OSBORNE J. (1952) Relining and rebasing. *Br dent J*, **92**, 149.

WOELFEL J. B. *et al* (1962) Deformed lower ridge caused by the relining of a denture by a patient. *J Am dent Ass*, **64**, 763.

RETENTION AND STABILITY

BARBENEL J. C. (1971) Physical retention of complete dentures. *J prosth Dent*, **26**, 592.

BRILL N. *et al* (1960) The role of learning in denture retention. *J prosth Dent*, **10**, 468.

CRAIG R. G. *et al* (1960) Physical factors related to denture retention. *J prosth Dent*, **10**, 459.

LAWSON W. A. (1961) Influence of the sublingual fold on retention of complete lower dentures. *J prosth Dent*, **11**, 1038.

LEDLEY R. S. (1954) The relation of occlusal surfaces to the stability of artificial dentures. *J Am dent Ass*, **48**, 508.

ÖSTLUND S. G. (1960) Saliva and denture retention. *J prosth Dent*, **10**, 658.

RYGE G. & FAIRHURST C. W. (1959) An evaluation of denture adaptation on the basis of contour meter recordings. *J prosth Dent*, **9**, 755.

SMITH D. E. *et al* (1963) The mobility of artificial dentures during comminution. *J prosth Dent*, **13**, 839.

SNYDER F. C. *et al* (1945) Effect of reduced atmospheric pressure upon retention of dentures. *J Am dent Ass*, **32**, 445.

STAFFORD G. D. & RUSSELL C. (1971) Efficiency of denture adhesives. *J dent Res*, **50**, 832.

TAYLOR R. L. (1962) The stability of complete dentures. *Aust dent J*, **7**, 145.

TYSON K. W. (1967) Physical factors in retention of complete upper dentures. *J prosth Dent*, **18**, 90.

VAN WILLIGEN J. D. & MOOK W. G. (1967) An analysis of the physical properties which might play a part in the retention of complete dentures. *Nederl T Tand*, **74**, 478.

Index